The Health of the
First Ladies

ALSO BY LUDWIG M. DEPPISCH, M.D.

*The White House Physician: A History from
Washington to George W. Bush* (McFarland, 2007)

The Health of the First Ladies

Medical Histories from Martha Washington to Michelle Obama

LUDWIG M. DEPPISCH, M.D.

Foreword by Dr. Connie Mariano

McFarland & Company, Inc., Publishers
Jefferson, North Carolina

Library of Congress Cataloguing-in-Publication Data

Deppisch, Ludwig M., 1938–
The health of the first ladies : medical histories from
Martha Washington to Michelle Obama /
Ludwig M. Deppisch, M.D. ; foreword by Dr. Connie Mariano.
p.   cm.
Includes bibliographical references and index.

ISBN 978-0-7864-7436-3 (softcover : acid free paper) ∞
ISBN 978-1-4766-1766-4 (ebook)

1. Presidents' spouses—Health and hygiene—United States.
2. Presidents' spouses—United States—History.
3. Presidents' spouses—United States—Biography.
I. Title.

E176.2.D47 2015   973.09'9—dc23   [B]   2014043494

British Library cataloguing data are available

On the cover: top to bottom First Ladies Martha Washington,
Louisa Catherine Adams, Eleanor Roosevelt, Jackie Kennedy
and Nancy Reagan (all photographs Library of Congress);
background the White House (iStock/Thinkstock)

Manufactured in the United States of America

McFarland & Company, Inc., Publishers
Box 611, Jefferson, North Carolina 28640
www.mcfarlandpub.com

To Barbara and Carl
with pride and love

Table of Contents

Part III: Modern Times and
Into the Twenty-First Century

Acknowledgments

Once again I have discovered that the writing of a book of history is a long, arduous, and complex undertaking. For an author to complete this task, the assistance of many is a necessity. To those people, the following acknowledgments in print are but a modest and inadequate expression of my appreciation.

I owe special thanks to Dr. Jeanne Clarke for her unselfish commentary and copyediting of the manuscript; to Dr. Connie Mariano for her generosity in sharing her unique perspective on the workings of the White House Medical Unit; to Dr. Katherine Morrissey, teacher extraordinaire, for her encouragement and insights; to Andre Sobocinski, a splendid public servant, for his knowledge and assistance in innumerable ways.

Hannah Fisher, research librarian of the University of Arizona Health Sciences Library, was never presented with the name of an obscure physician whose biography she failed to locate. Carl Sferrazza Anthony, historian to the National First Ladies' Library, graciously answered my many requests for information. Mike Shaw's computer skills were of great assistance in the final organization of the manuscript.

Special thanks are owed to the National First Ladies' Library, Canton, Ohio. This unique institution has become a comprehensive repository of information related to America's first ladies. Its extensive bibliography became for me an indispensible source of first ladies information.

I am grateful to the many librarians and archivists who responded to my requests with generosity and patience: Kevin Bailey, Ellen Brightly, Jennifer Capps, Tiffany Cole, Peggy Dillard, Judith Graham, David Haugard, Nancy Johnson, Laura Karas, Patrick Kerwin, Pat Krider, Nancy Miller, Nancy Hord Patterson, Arlene Shaner, Heidi Stello, Cynthia Van Ness. My sincere apologies to anyone whose assistance I may have neglected to acknowledge.

Thank you to my medical colleagues whose insights and counsel have been most helpful in the writing of this book: Doctors Rob Darling, Jonathan Davidson, Emanuel Husu, Howard Lein, Alan Levenson, Hugh Smith and Dick Tubb.

And finally, and most important, thank you to my wonderful family: my children, Barbara, Carl and Rich, my grandchildren Nick, Joey and Jake, and, above all, my dear wife, Rosemarie. The book is done. I am back in your lives.

Foreword
Dr. Connie Mariano

When I first arrived at the White House in 1992 as the new White House physician, I received a detailed orientation covering my responsibilities. I was to take care of the president but was also responsible for the care of the first lady. I was instructed early in my nine-year White House tour that any statements regarding the president's health were to be issued though the White House press secretary with the approval of the president. On the other hand, there were to be no statements issued about the health of the first lady. Since the wife of the president was not an elected official, her health and medical history were considered private issues and not for discussion in the press.

In his *The Health of the First Ladies,* Dr. Lud Deppisch breaks taboo and tradition. He explores the health history of each of the first ladies in a scholarly and comprehensive manner. He demonstrates that each first lady is representative of the women of her ea. He divulges through his meticulous research their medical issues, access to care, and the way they were each treated in sickness and in health.

Why is the health of the first lady significant? When you look at the inner circle of the president of the United States, no one has greater access to, and intimacy with, the president than the first lady. She is the first voice he hears every morning and the last voice he hears every night. If the first lady suffers from an illness, her condition most likely would impact the president's attention, concern, and, ultimately, his ability to function in office. Dr. Deppisch offers an illuminating and fascinating look at the importance of the health of the presidential spouse.

Dr. Connie Mariano was the White House physician from 1992 to 2001 and is the author of *The White House Doctor: My Patients Were Presidents*

Preface

Rising Interest in the Lady in the White House

Eleanor Roosevelt shattered the mold that traditionally confined presidential spouses to the background, if not to obscurity.[1] Mrs. Roosevelt stepped far beyond the shadow cast by the formidable figure of her quadruple-elected husband to become a public political figure in her own right. Later, in a different fashion, Jacqueline Kennedy illuminated the visual and print media with her stylish success in fulfilling the social and ceremonial responsibilities of a first lady. Pat Nixon, Hillary Clinton, Laura Bush and Michelle Obama increasingly traveled abroad without their presidential husbands and attracted significant attention while doing so. At the onset of the twenty-first century, the president's wife has become a celebrity, not a subsidiary. A simple expression by first lady Michelle Obama that Americans should drink more water received disproportionate and substantial wide publication and commentary.[2] Consequently, it is timely to examine in detail a significant aspect of their lives: their health and medical histories. To my knowledge this subject has not been addressed in either a systematic or comprehensive manner.

Dispositive proof of increased interest was the establishment of the National First Ladies' Library. This institution was founded in 1998 in Canton, Ohio, the hometown of President and Mrs. William McKinley. Mary Regula, social science teacher and wife of Ohio state legislator Ralph Regula who later became congressman was the force behind its establishment. She was both frustrated and dismayed by the dearth of published information about presidential spouses. Consequently Regula focused her leadership, drive and political savvy to combine the renovation of a historic house in downtown Canton with the establishment of a first ladies bibliography of 40,000 entries. The result was the National First Ladies' Library located within the renovated Saxton-McKinley House, in which president-to-be William McKinley and his wife, Ida Saxton McKinley, resided for fourteen years while he was a congressman. The library also serves as the museum of the Saxton-McKinley homestead. It presents frequent exhibits and events and has become an important and invaluable resource for education and research about America's first ladies.[3]

Biographies and autobiographies of individual presidential spouses have long filled the shelves of university libraries. Occasionally these books have reached prominence either by placement on best-seller lists or by the published accolades of prestigious academic panels.[4] Several writers have broadened the scholarship on this topic; these historians have either authored or edited biographical synopses inclusive of all first ladies at the time of this publication. Perhaps the first to attempt this task was the prolific Laura C. Holloway. Her *The Ladies of the White House: Or, In the Home of the Presidents; Being a Complete History of the Social and Domestic Lives of the Presidents from Washington to the Present Time, 1789–1881* was published in 1881 by the Bradley publishing house in Philadelphia.[5]

Historian Betty Boyd Caroli has updated her compendium, *First Ladies*, at least three times since 1987. In the introduction to her initial edition, she wrote the following: "In the beginning, I considered writing a history of the institution of first lady, a book that would have documented the decision making process, the level of staff performance, and the rise in power of the distaff side of the White House. I abandoned the project when I realized that most readers would want more biographical information than that volume would have involved…. Whatever the future, the bicentennial of the Constitution approaches, and it seems appropriate to look at presidents' wives and see how the role of First Lady was transformed from ceremonial backup to substantive world figure."[6]

Carl Sferrazza Anthony is the consultant historian to the National First Ladies' Library. In his two-volume 1990 biography, *First Ladies: The Saga of the Presidents' Wives and Their Power, 1789–1961*, he wrote: "What intrigued me most was their varying degrees of power…. How much power did she exercise? How much influence did she seek to wield, and how successful was she? … Another consideration was how well they embodied their eras…. So I have placed great emphasis on the times, and one woman is used to represent each of

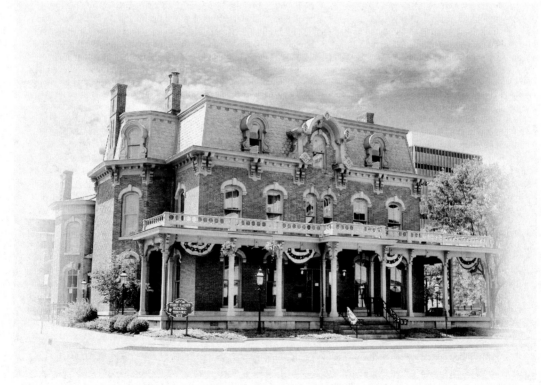

The First Ladies' National Library, Canton, Ohio, the Saxton McKinley House, the family home of first lady Ida Saxton McKinley and longtime residence of President and Mrs. McKinley (courtesy National First Ladies' Library).

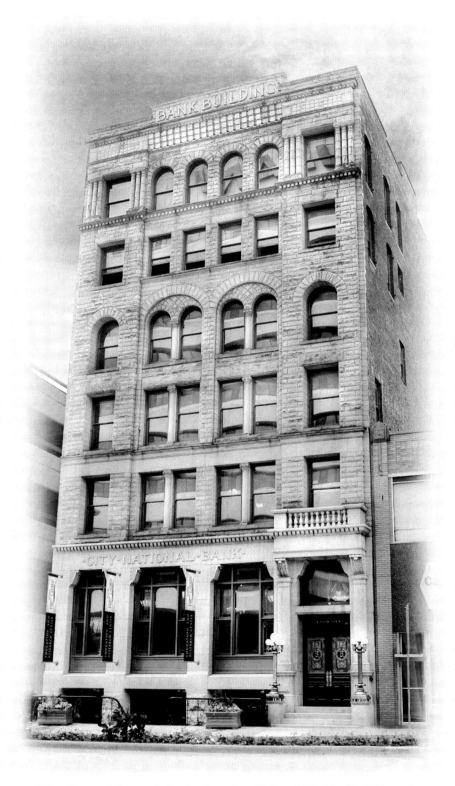

Education and Research Center (courtesy National First Ladies' Library).

the periods. Particular to each, like civil rights, women's issues, the press and public, technology, and how the women responded to or were affected by them—are woven through the two hundred year story." In the end, he said, "almost every one of them missed the power."[7]

Margaret Truman, the daughter of President Harry and first lady Bess Wallace Truman, scrutinized the lives of these women from an insider's perspective. Her biographical work, *First Ladies*, was released by Random House in 1995.[8] Professor Robert P. Watson in his 2000 book, *The Presidents' Wives: Reassessing the Office of First Lady*, analyzed the evolving social, ceremonial and political responsibilities of this unofficial position and has measured the success of each in fulfilling these responsibilities.[9]

In 2001 Louis L. Gould edited and contributed to *America's First Ladies: Their Lives and Their Legacy*. The book was a compendium of short biographies of all of the first ladies up to the publication date. Gould's purpose for the work was stated in the introduction: "By the early 1990s the outlines of a distinct research area devoted to First Ladies had emerged where history, political science, and women's studies intersected.... Despite these constructive achievements the new field lacked a reliable up to date reference work that included the essential facts about each First Lady in a brief biographical essay." Therefore, he produced his book as an "effort to assess ... place in the development of the institution of the First Lady."[10]

Both professors Robert Watson and Louis Gould have edited an ongoing series of concise biographies of individual first ladies. *The Presidential Wives* series is edited by Watson and published by Nova History of New York. *Modern First Ladies* is edited by Gould and published by the University of Kansas Press. Watson's purpose is public enlightenment regarding the important office of first lady and the power and influence of its occupants.[11] Gould's foreword to his series' biography of Grace Coolidge is more personal and specific: "[It] will leave readers ... with the real sense of Grace Coolidge as a human being and a contributor to the historical legacy of presidential wives."[12]

The Genesis of This Book

My previous book, *The White House Physician: A History from George Washington to George W. Bush*, focused on the complex nexus of the health of American presidents, their medical care, their medical practitioners, and the evolution of medical practice in the United States. During my research, I discovered that presidential wives lived compelling and interesting histories. They were frequently ill; their health often suffered because of their husbands' ambitions; some were crushed by the responsibilities of a first lady, while others thrived. The influence of their health on their spouses' executive performance was both complicated and at times ambiguous. The subject of the health of the first ladies of the United States became too intriguing and enticing to abandon. Hence this book. The chapters that follow explore various aspects of the first ladies' health. The histories are presented in a broadly chronological sequence. However, in a few instances, exceptions will occur when individual stories from different times will be conflated for purposes of interest and explanation.

The medical histories of the first ladies will be examined. Focus will be upon, but not restricted to, their years in the White House. Their medical care will be analyzed, with respect to both diagnostic and therapeutic standards of the times and the qualifications and competence of their physicians. With the passage of time, public and preventative health measures, refined medical skills and major scientific advances have influenced the types and severity of illness. Over two and a quarter centuries, America's first ladies have battled in rough sequence: infections (yellow fever, malaria, tuberculosis); pregnancy-related disorders; mental problems; kidney ailments; vascular disease, including stroke; cancer; and, lastly, autoimmune disorders such as Barbara Bush's bout with Graves' disease.

Particular attention will be given to this question: Did health influence performance as first lady? The role of the first lady encompasses social, ceremonial, familial and political responsibilities in variable degrees. Did illness affect any first lady's success in accomplishing her duties? Conversely, did these responsibilities affect the health of the first lady? Also, does marriage to a very ambitious man take a toll on the health of his wife? Admittedly this is a question that in many cases has no definitive answer.

Illness may plausibly affect the performance of a president who is confronted with the sickness of a loved one. However, any generalization is a Herculean task far beyond the scope of this book. The specific responses of two presidents, Franklin Pierce and William McKinley, when faced with this situation will be described.

The position of first lady accrues medical advantages that may be unavailable to other citizens, which gives rise to the following questions: What sort of medical attention did the first ladies receive and from whom? Was their care equivalent to that received by other women of that era? Therefore, the selection, training, and success or failure of the treatments by their physicians will be discussed. Moreover, it was possible that presidents were given different, and possibly better, medical care and attention than their wives. Over the years physicians to the first ladies were burdened with additional conflicts: patient confidentiality versus the public's right to know; homeopathic care versus orthodox medicine; and when and whom to employ as medical consultants.

Lastly, consideration will be given to the use by the first lady of the "bully pulpit," or, more appropriately, the "velvet voice," to raise public awareness through a personal experience with a disease. This has occurred with increasing frequency since the mid-twentieth century and has become a significant point of political discourse.

Introduction

"First Lady" Usage and Acceptance

The Constitution does not mention the title "First Lady." Moreover there is neither a law nor a job description that authorizes the use of a specific title for the president's spouse.[1] Martha Washington was hailed with shouts of "Long live Lady Washington" as she was rowed across the Hudson River on the presidential barge after her husband's 1789 inauguration in New York City. These shouts were accompanied by a thirteen-gun cannonade.[2]

Inconsistent titles were applied to early and mid-nineteenth century presidential wives. Abigail Adams was called "Mrs. President" and "Her Majesty," mainly by her husband's political opponents. Dolley Madison, the wife of James Madison, the fourth chief executive of the United States, was called respectfully "Lady Presidentress." Additionally, at her death in 1849, President Zachary in his eulogy referred to Dolley as "our First Lady for half a century."[3]

Historians and biographers generally agree that the title "First Lady" achieved acceptance and general usage during the presidency of Rutherford B. Hayes (1877–1881). Hayes' wife, Lucy, was the first presidential wife to secure a college degree (from Cincinnati Wesleyan). Lucy Hayes was a prominent personage during the Hayes administration; additionally she accompanied her spouse on a transcontinental train trip. In 1877 reporter Mary Clemmer Ames, writing in the *Independent*, referred to Lucy Hayes as "First Lady of the Land." Historian Stanley Pillsbury, writing in the *Dictionary of American History*, applied the title "First Lady" to Lucy Hayes in his narration describing her husband's inauguration in 1877.[4]

Caroli noticed that dictionaries gradually began to use "First Lady," but only after the country's political attention had been drawn to Washington, D.C., in the twentieth century. Beginning with Webster's *New International Dictionary* in 1934, other dictionaries began adopting the title. Two plays solidified its usage by the general public: the 1911 production by Charles F. Nirdlinger about Dolley Madison, *The First Lady of the Land*, and a 1935 play by Katherine Dayton and George S. Kaufman, titled *First Lady*.[5]

For clarification, "First Lady" as used in this book refers only to the wives of sitting presidents of the United States. The deceased wives of the four presidents who were widowers (Thomas Jefferson, Andrew Jackson, Martin Van Buren and Chester Arthur) are not included. Moreover, surrogates, either family members or others, who assisted disabled first ladies with their ceremonial and social responsibilities are neither considered nor analyzed.

The National First Ladies' Library lists Harriet Lane as a first lady. Miss Lane was the orphaned niece of President James Buchanan (1857–1861). When his sister's daughter was orphaned Buchanan adopted her, directed her schooling, and provided for her welfare. Over time Harriet Lane became not only her uncle's political consort, but also his personal confidante. When Buchanan became president, his niece acted as his "First Lady." Harriet was twenty-seven years of age at his inauguration and married only after her uncle's death. She is not included in the profiles that follow.[6]

Caroline Fillmore and Mary Harrison married presidents after the chief executive left the White House; neither were first ladies. Conversely, two sitting presidents, John Tyler and Woodrow Wilson, remarried shortly after the death of their wives. Both second wives, Julia Gardiner Tyler and Edith Bolling Gault Wilson, deservedly are listed as first ladies. Benjamin Harrison, a third president who was widowered in the executive mansion, married his deceased wife's niece, but only after leaving the presidency. Three wives of presidents died in the White House, while a disproportionate eight presidents died or were killed in office.

Chapter One

Martha Washington and Dolley Madison

The First First Lady and the First Mistress in the White House

It was my wish to have continued in Philadelphia longer, [George Washington wrote to his personal secretary, Tobias Lear] but Mrs. Washington was unwilling to leave me surrounded by the malignant fever wch. prevailed, I could not think of hazarding her ... any longer by my continuing in the City the house in which we lived being, in a manner, blockaded by the disorder and was becoming every day more and more fatal.[1]

Martha Washington never lived in the White House; its construction was not completed until after George Washington's death. Abigail Adams, the spouse of the second United States president, John Adams, occupied the still unfinished building for four brief months during the winter of 1800–1801.[2] The third American president, Thomas Jefferson, was a widower. Mrs. Dolley Madison, the wife of his secretary of state and successor as president, officiated as White House hostess for both Jefferson and James Madison, and thus may correctly be identified as its first mistress.

Both Mrs. Washington and Mrs. Madison were confronted by infectious diseases (yellow fever, smallpox), scourges of a bygone era, and both suffered from chronic maladies (gall bladder disease [Washington] and arthritis [Madison]), still prevalent in modern times. A physician was not officially assigned to either president during their husbands' tenures, although both George Washington and James Madison were seriously ill while president. Neither Martha nor Dolley was significantly sick or the recipient of medical attention during her tenure as first lady. As a result, both were able to successfully fulfill the responsibilities of wife and first lady.

Martha Washington and Dolley Madison were Virginia born. Both experienced early widowhood upon the deaths of their first husbands. Both bore children during their first marriages but were unable to become pregnant during long second marriages. Children with both first husbands died at an early age. Both ladies outlived their presidential husbands, Dolley by many years. Martha and Dolley had auditioned for their roles as first lady. Washington was the wife of the Revolutionary War American commander in chief; Madison served as hostess for the widower Thomas Jefferson while her husband James was Jefferson's secretary of state.

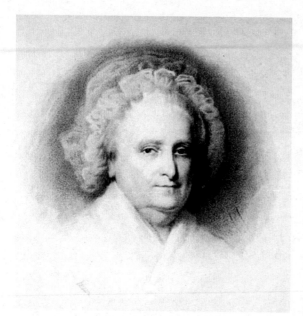

Martha Washington, the first first lady (Library of Congress).

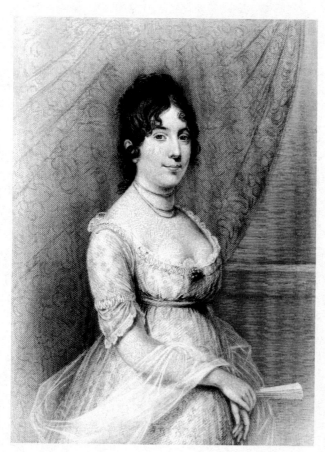

Dolley Madison, the first mistress of the White House. Yellow fever killed her first husband and her infant son (Library of Congress).

Martha Washington was often addressed as Lady Washington.[3] While serving as Jefferson's hostess, Dolley Madison acquired the unofficial title of Presidentress. During her husband's administration she received the nicknames of "Lady Presidentress" and "Queen Dolley."[4]

Yellow Fever

In 1793, Philadelphia, Pennsylvania, was the largest city in North America, with a population of nearly 51,000.[5] It was also the capital of the infant American republic, the United States of America. The seat of national government officially moved from New York City to Philadelphia on December 6, 1790. The city would remain the nation's capital until 1800, when the next and permanent center of government would be established in Washington, D.C.[6]

In mid–August a familiar yet mysterious pestilence affected the city. Yellow fever disrupted not only the personal lives of its inhabitants but also the institutions of federal and state governments. Yellow fever killed five thousand, or 10 percent, of Philadelphia's population, sickened thousands, impelled twenty thousand into exile, and cast two of the city's residents, Martha Washington and the future Dolley Madison, into decisive roles. Lady Washington was the country's first first lady when the epidemic struck. Her principal goal was to assure the medical safety of her husband by removing him from Philadelphia's pestilence. The future Queen Dolley was the young wife of John Todd, a local attorney, with a newborn child and fearful of any ill consequences for her family.

On Sunday, August 3, 1793, "a young French sailor rooming at Richard Denny's boarding house, over on North Water Street, was desperately ill with a fever.... All we know is that his fever worsened and was accompanied by violent seizures, and that a few days later he died."[7] Thereafter the numbers of deaths increased by geometric progression. The usual course of the disease began with chills and a high fever, headache, and generalized muscle aches. This state would persist for approximately three days until the fever broke, with an apparent recovery. However, fever returned almost immediately accompanied by jaundice of the eyes and skin. Hence the diagnosis "yellow fever." Subsequently the nose, gums and intestines would experience spontaneous bleeding, with the vomitus of black blood. Neurological symptoms of depression, confusion and delirium climaxed in death.[8]

The leading practitioner of medicine in Philadelphia at the time was Dr. Benjamin Rush. On August 19, Rush, recalling the signs and symptoms of a 1762 epidemic that ravaged the city, was quick to make the diagnosis of yellow fever. He worked tirelessly to serve the victims of the "American plague" while many of his professional colleagues fled and others sickened and died. Rush was twice infected, on September 12 and on October 20, 1793.[9] An August 28 newspaper article authored by a committee of the Philadelphia College of Physicians panicked the city's population rather than reassuring it. Its inhabitants fled and private business was abandoned. The term of the U.S. Supreme Court was interrupted, and the Pennsylvania General Assembly adjourned on September 5 after only eight days in session.[10]

Yellow fever brushed close to, but did not infect, Martha Washington. Her close companion was Polly Lear, the wife of the president's secretary, Tobias Lear. The Lears lived in the presidential mansion with the Washingtons. Polly Lear was one of the first fatalities of the epidemic.[11] Then, Alexander Hamilton, the country's treasury secretary and Washington's closest friend in the cabinet, came down with the illness. Other members of the cabinet were absent: attorney general Edmund Randolph was away negotiating an Indian treaty and secretary of state Thomas Jefferson had resigned and remained at Monticello, his country retreat. Almost all the clerks in the Treasury Department and the Post Office became ill, leaving the people's business at a standstill. Washington was very reluctant to depart from the city. He worried about Hamilton's well-being. He was also dismayed by the floundering functioning of the government, complaining that nearly everyone had "matters of private concernment which required them to be absent."[12]

There was great anxiety among Washington's friends for his physical well-being as the epidemic raged through August into September. Deaths from the epidemic reached one hundred per day. The president had great anxiety for Martha; he urged her to retreat to the safety of their Mount Vernon, Virginia, home. Martha refused to leave her husband and insisted that she would remain with him in Philadelphia. Finally, Washington acquiesced and left the nation's capital for his Virginia home.[13]

First lady-to-be Dolley Madison, then Dolley Todd, had lived in Philadelphia for some years. Dolley married attorney John Todd in January 1790, and bore him a son, John Payne, in February 1792, and a second son, William Temple, in the summer of 1793.[14] Dolley Todd, her husband, her two sons, her mother, her two sisters and a brother, were among the thousands who fled the epidemic. They reached Gray's Ferry, a resort fourteen miles away. Dolley, still weak after her recent pregnancy, required a litter to reach their hoped-for refuge. John Todd returned to Philadelphia to be with his parents and to tend to his infected law student. After the deaths of all three from yellow fever, he departed for Gray's Ferry, where he became chilled and succumbed to the disease on October 14.[15] Their infant son, William, died the same day, despite departing Philadelphia with his mother and older brother two months earlier. "Mr. Todd on his return bore with him the dread disease. At the threshold, he said to Dolley's mother: 'I feel the fever in my veins, but I must see her once more.' In a few hours he was dead—'a martyr to professional duty.' In the embrace was contamination. The younger child died and Dolley recovered. Mr. Todd died October 24, 1793."[16]

Katherine Anthony suggests that Dolley had contracted yellow fever, which in her case was prolonged and severe. In late autumn Dolley returned to the city, recovered from her own illness: "[W]hether she contracted yellow fever is unclear; certainly a woman weakened from childbirth must have been susceptible."[17] "And even though she had removed herself and her two-year-old son to a farm at Gray's Ferry, they had both become infected and been close to death themselves." She returned to the city in November 1793 to set up a boardinghouse.[18] It is intriguing to speculate whether the future first lady developed yellow fever. However, she probably did not. Yellow fever is infectious from a mosquito bite, not contagious from another infected individual. Dolley had been absent from the epidemic's epicenter for two months prior to her farewell embrace with her husband. His return to Philadelphia from the haven at Gray's Ferry, although heroic, was deadly.

When yellow fever returned to Philadelphia in the summer of 1794, George Washington wasted no time in removing Martha, himself, and the rest of his household along with his official papers to Germantown, Pennsylvania, over seven miles from the seat of government.

President and Mrs. John Adams' arrival in Philadelphia from their summer residence in Quincy, Massachusetts, was delayed in 1797: "Yellow fever raged again in Philadelphia, as they learned en route, and so it was necessary to stop and wait in East Chester.... Adams was kept apprised by daily reports. Two thirds of the population of Philadelphia had fled the city." During the summer of 1799 John Adams' administration evacuated to Trenton, New Jersey, to avoid another outbreak of the disease.[19]

In 1793 both the medical community and the lay population were ignorant of the cause and the treatment of yellow fever. The miasma of summer was widely considered to be the culprit. It was only in 1900 that Dr. Jesse Lazear of the U.S. Army Yellow Fever Commission conclusively demonstrated that a mosquito was the vector of yellow fever.[20] That same year, Lazear's superior, Dr. Walter Reed, publicly announced that mosquitoes transmitted the disease and identified the female Aedes aegypti mosquito as the carrier.[21] Since many French refugees fled Haiti's revolution in 1793 to reach Philadelphia, it is possible that some previously infected with the yellow fever virus might have provided the necessary viral reservoir for summer-abundant mosquitoes to transmit the infection to Philadelphia's unsuspecting denizens.[22]

The aforementioned Benjamin Rush claimed that only heroic, aggressive measures could cure the disease. These included toxic doses of mercury and jalap to purge the gastrointestinal system through vomiting and explosive diarrhea. Copious bloodletting completed his heroic regimen.[23] The Philadelphia epidemic waned and then disappeared with the onset of cold weather, which destroyed the adult mosquito population. Today yellow fever is controlled by isolation, destruction of a breeding mosquito population by swamp clearage and insecticides, and vaccination against the yellow fever virus.[24] Fortunately for the widow Todd, geographic distance spared her from Rush's heroic ministrations.

Smallpox

Smallpox was widespread in America during the 1700s. Vaccination using cowpox virus did not become accepted until later. During Revolutionary times, protection against the smallpox virus was by inoculation with fluid from a skin pustule of a patient with active smallpox. The inoculant would often develop significant but nonfatal smallpox symptoms.

Martha Washington was well aware of the ravages of active smallpox; her husband was stricken in Barbados as a young man, and his face was permanently marked with scars of the disease.[25] Martha underwent inoculation in May 1776. The procedure was performed by Dr. John Morgan, a graduate of the Medical College of Edinburgh and a professor and founder of the first American medical school in Philadelphia.[26] The procedure went well. Martha received a June 9, 1776, letter from her son John Parke Custis: "My dear Momma … [I] hear You were in so fair a Way of getting favorably through the Smalpox … which I doubt less should have felt on the inoculation of so dear a Mother."[27]

Martha Washington's Medical History

During her first marriage, to Daniel Parke Custis, Martha gave birth to four children, two of whom died in childhood.[28] Her second marriage, to George Washington, was childless, but it was generally blessed with good health.[29]

Although Washington during his two-term presidency (1789–1797) was beset by serious medical afflictions for which he was cared for by the elite of the New York and Philadelphia medical establishments, there is no record that the first lady sought any doctor's care during her husband's presidential tenure.[30] Her singular complaint was gallbladder disease. In May 1781, she came down with abdominal pain, "biliousness" and jaundice that lasted five weeks.[31] In an April 1792 letter to Fanny Bassett Washington she complained: "I have been unwell for some weeks with chollick complaints."[32] Elizabeth Willing Powel wrote to the first lady on December 7, 1796: "[Y]ou mentioned that you had taken Noyan as a Medicine to cure the Colick, but that you did not think it was as pure as that you then tasted, knowing that the true Martinique Noyan is not to be purchased as this time, I have taken the liberty to send you a Bottle, tho I hope you will not have occasion to use it as a Remedy for any complaint half so distressing as the Colick."[33] Martha's physique was that of a gallstone victim: "At 5 feet tall, Martha put on weight easily. She no longer rode horseback and frequently indulged her fondness for candy and desserts. The pleasing plumpness of her middle age had become grandmotherly stoutness, complete with double chin. She often suffered from colic and severe stomach pains."[34]

Reports of the physicians who assisted Martha during her life are few. In June and July 1757, Dr. James Carter of Williamsburg treated the Custis family, first by dispatching drugs.

When there was no improvement, he traveled the twenty-five miles to the Custis farm with a vast array of medicines. Not only did he unsuccessfully treat Martha's husband, Daniel Custis, who died at age 45, he also stayed for five days and in August returned to treat Martha for an undisclosed illness.[35] The Custis estate received the following bills from Dr. Carter for services rendered: 132 British pounds (November 28, 1757), 27 pounds, eight shillings, nine pence (December 1, 1758, to November 16, 1759). Carter set up an apothecary shop and practiced medicine and surgery at the Unicorn's Horn in Williamsburg as early as 1751. He served in the Virginia militia during the Revolutionary War and continued practice until his death about 1800.[36] In January 1760, Martha's second husband, George Washington, used the services of the Rev. Charles Green, a local clergyman with medical training, when Martha contacted measles. In April 1760, Martha was ill once more and Washington contacted another physician, who showed up drunk. Nevertheless the doctor spent the night at Mount Vernon and bled Martha in the morning.[37]

The only credentialed physician, by modern standards, who treated Martha was James Craik of Alexandria, Virginia. Craik had been the first president's personal doctor for many years before Washington's presidency and was unwilling to forego his lucrative Virginia medical practice in order to become the first presidential physician—in either New York or Philadelphia.[38] However, when the Washingtons returned to Mount Vernon after leaving office in 1797, Craik reassumed his role as George's personal physician and eventually attended his death. On several occasions in 1799 the doctor was requested to treat Martha for probable malaria. He used the usual remedy, "the bark" (quinine).[39] In 1802 he was present during Martha Washington's final illness and death at 70 years. At the end of her life Martha Washington suffered from some sort of mental distress or possibly dementia.[40]

Dolley Madison's Medical History

Dolley Madison, a robust and attractive woman, was notable not only for her extravagant sociability but also for her physical appearance. She stood five feet, six and one half inches tall and had blue eyes and black hair. The latter was usually adorned by her signature turban. Born Dorothea Payne, she was early on familiarly addressed as Dolley and the name stuck.

While providing sturdy physical and emotional support props for her second husband, James Madison, during his secretary of state, presidential and retirement years, Dolley had several illnesses. A major problem occurred midway during her service as President Jefferson's social hostess. While at the Madison home in Virginia—Montpelier—"In the fourth year at Washington, Mrs. Madison succumbed to a physical ailment. She had an attack of rheumatism, the inflammatory kind. From Montpellier [sic], June 3, 1804, she tells her sister, Anna, of the painfulness of it; of the bleeding by Dr. Willis and the nursing by Mother Madison, and of her intended return to Washington the week later." "Then Mrs. Madison was at Montpellier, held by rheumatism." The lesion of her right knee was variously described as a "sore," an "ulcer," and a "tumor." Its true nature remains unsettled; Ketcham described the lesion as "a complaint near her knee, which from a very slight tumor had ulcerated into a very obstinate sore."[41] Washington doctors were consulted: "Two doctors have applied caustic with the hope of getting me well, but heaven knows! I feel as if I should never walk again." It is unsurprising that the fierceness of these remedies was directly proportional to the distress of the patient, since she was confined to her room in Washington with no clinical relief.[42]

After a month of unsuccessful treatment, James Madison accompanied his wife to Philadelphia for treatment by the famous and respected physician with the memorable last name—Dr. Philip Synge Physick. A benefit, then and now, generally reserved for the prominent, especially America's first ladies, is access to the most famous and skilled practitioners of the day. Philadelphia native Physick had received his medical degree in 1792 from the prestigious University of Edinburgh.[43] Returning home, he was shortly appointed surgeon to the Pennsylvania Hospital. Ten years later he became the first chair of surgery at the University of Pennsylvania School of Medicine.[44] Physick returned to Philadelphia just in time to assist during the 1793 yellow fever epidemic which "afforded ... his first opportunity for proving to his fellow citizens his entire devotion to his

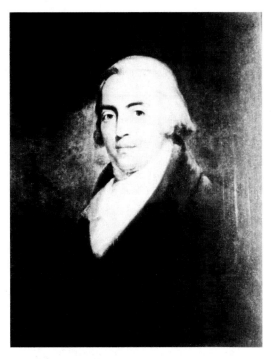

Dr. Philip Syng Physick, prominent Philadelphia surgeon. He treated future first ladies Dolley Madison and Louisa Catherine Adams (courtesy National Library of Medicine).

professional disputes, his utter disregard of his personal considerations ... and the fearless intrepidity with which he exposed himself to danger, in order to contribute to the safety of others."[45] Physick autopsied yellow fever deaths, but, like all his contemporaries, erroneously ascribed its cause. He attributed its pathogenesis to gastritis.[46] Physick was sickened with yellow fever during the 1798 Philadelphia epidemic but survived.[47] (Dolley may have had a previous connection with Physick. As a student, Physick boarded in Philadelphia "with the family of the late Mr. John Todd, the father in law of the present venerable Mrs. Madison.")[48]

The eminent Physick confined Dolley to a bed and treated her with splints that bound her knee. Although a noted surgeon, he did not operate. She wrote her sister: "I am on my bed." At first she was afraid that she would never walk again. She remained under his care for four months. Then, cured, she returned to Washington in November 1805. A November 1, 1805, letter from Dolley in Philadelphia to James Madison in Washington states the following: "I have great pleasure, my beloved, in repeating to you what the doctor has just told me—that I may reasonably hope to leave this place in a fortnight."[49]

Physick's fame was such that he treated President Andrew Jackson and Louisa Johnson Adams in later years. On August 19, 1811, Mrs. Madison wrote Anna Custis advising her to consult Physick for her daughter's foot problem: "...but your precious daughter—What shall we do? when you are able, come on, & stop with Dr. Physick—many, many, have been made perfect by [his] care, & why may we not hope that her dr. foot will be streighten'd with care—Yes, I am sure it will."[50]

Dolley suffered one other illness before her husband's inauguration that occurred after an arduous journey from Washington to the Madisons' Montpelier estate. Her June 3, 1808, letter stated: "I have been quite ill since I wrote you last, with the Infamitory Rumatism [*sic*]—never had I more extreme sickness and pain—Doct Willis bled me and gave me medcin [*sic*]." (Dr. John Willis had married Nelly, Dolley's niece, in 1804.)[51]

Wife of the President

"Queen Dolley" was nothing less than regal during James Madison's eight-year, two-term presidential reign. Catherine Allgor characterized the tenure of this first lady: "Despite an eye ailment. rheumatism, ear trouble with temporary deafness, and several other bouts of ill health, Dolley Madison presented a healthy, energetic, robust appearance to the political world: "A confident, easy Dolley, cheeks ablaze, dominating the room, not only balanced James's [Madison] lack of vigor, it allowed him to be himself."[52] "[U]nder Dolley's presiding genius ... the years of Madison's presidency were a social triumph." "The Madisons set entertaining standards that dominated Washington social life until the Civil War."[53] The first wedding in the White House was that of Dolley's widowed sister Lucy to associate Supreme Court justice Thomas Todd.[54]

Her correspondence, however, disclosed several episodes of significant illness. Her June 1811 letters refer to "a dangerous and severe illness" and being "extremely ill," an illness that confined her to her room for three weeks. A July 29, 1812, letter explained: "For the past 10 days I have been sick, so much so, that I could not write or do anything but nurse myself." A February 1, 1816, letter by a Mrs. Crowninshield recounts the following: "Mrs. Madison has been sick since Sunday—bilious colic." The nature of her sicknesses remains undetermined. In neither instance did she seek medical advice. At this time there was no official physician in attendance at the White House.[55] However, one chronic medical problem was identified—an eye ailment. For this she was treated with brandy and water by Scottish physician Robert Honyman. She refused to take "physick" other than a cream of tartar, and magnesia now and then. Honyman practiced in Hanover County, Virginia, and was a friend of Dolley's aunt and uncle and acquainted with the Madisons.[56]

After the presidency, the Madisons returned to their plantation at Montpelier, where James Madison died in 1836. The former president was chronically unhealthy; Dolley was in far better condition but continued to suffer from rheumatism, stress, and the recurrent eye ailment. Her "ophthalmia, so draining of her reading pleasure grew worse. With weakening painful eyes, she could be less useful in rearranging Madison's papers."[57] In letters she wrote that "my eyes are troubling me," "the continuing and very severe affection of my eyes, not permitting, but with much difficulty, even the signature of my name, has deferred ... the acknowledgements due to your very kind and very acceptable letter."[58] In 1837 she journeyed to White Sulphur Springs for her eyes. Despite episodic improvements, there was a negative net loss.[59]

After her husband's death, Dolley Madison eventually returned to Washington, where she led an active social life and was revered both by presidents and by the social-political elite. She died from a stroke on July 12, 1849, at age seventy-seven.[60]

Chapter Two

Malaria in the White House

Abigail Adams, Sarah Polk and Lucretia Garfield

> Abigail's malaria and rheumatism had both acted up in Philadelphia, and she had been especially miserable the previous spring. The malaria "still hangs about me & prevents my intire recovery," she reported to her sister Mary ... in April, 1792.[1]

Malaria was a significant illness in colonial and nineteenth-century America. It affected at least three presidential wives: Abigail Adams (1797–1801), Sarah Polk (1845–1849) and Lucretia Garfield (1881). (Malaria still infects 225 million people worldwide each year and almost 800,000, mostly in Africa, die annually from this disease.)[2]

Prior to the discovery of its infectious agent and its mode of transmission during the late nineteenth and early twentieth centuries, malaria in North America was commonly known as the "ague," "fever and ague," "intermittent fever," and, less frequently, "remittent fever" or "bilious fever." Its symptoms—the cyclic occurrence every two days of sudden coolness followed by rigor, and then fever and sweating lasting four to six hours—were familiar to both the medical and lay population. Malaria's intermittent character is related to the cyclic multiplication of its causative agent within the patient's red blood cells. There was an early recognition that proximity to swamps or still water was a requirement for infection. Seasonality was connected to the appearance of the disease; symptoms would arise in the summer and disappear in the cold of winter. For centuries there was an erroneous association with the miasma, i.e., noxious air, arising from decomposing waste. Hence arises the derivation of its name: foul or bad (mal) air (aria).

It was not until 1880 that the Frenchman Charles Laveran discovered the protozoan parasite (plasmodium) in human blood as the agent that caused the disease. Furthermore, it was only at the dawn of the twentieth century that Ronald Ross proved that this protozoan was transmitted by mosquitoes.[3]

Abigail Adams

Malaria

The formidable wife of John Adams, much admired and a frequent subject of biographers, suffered from many physical ills, one of which was malaria. Readers may inquire

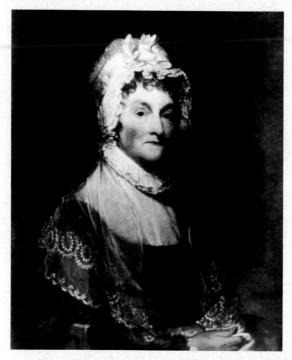

Abigail Adams, wife of John Adams. She was the second first lady (Library of Congress).

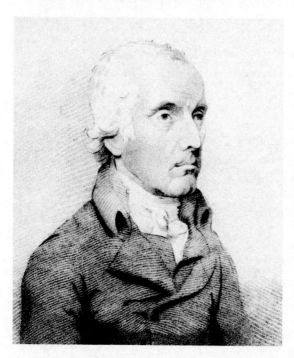

Dr. Benjamin Rush, physician to Abigail Adams in Philadelphia (courtesy National Library of Medicine).

how this hardy New Englander, who rarely spent the months of summer south of New England, was able to contract malaria, considered at present to be a neotropical disease. Her husband, John Adams, was inaugurated as the first vice president of the United States in 1789. He importuned Abigail to join him in New York City, the first capital; she acquiesced and joined him in June 1789.[4] The Adamses remained in the city until the nation's seat of government transferred to Philadelphia in late 1790. Mrs. Adams left for the new capital during mid-autumn of 1790.[5] A biographer described New York City at the time as "steamy and unsanitary." In the 1700s, the city neighborhood known as Five Points (now near city hall) was the site of a swampish lake, called the Collect, which was rimmed by slaughterhouses: "Due to the conditions, malaria was not uncommon."[6]

The prospect of moving the household back to Massachusetts and back again to New York City and then to Philadelphia proved too daunting, and consequently Abigail remained eighteen months, including the summers of 1789 and 1790, in New York. This episode was one of the few times she spent these months south of New England.[7]

On the evening of October 10, 1790, "she contracted an illness she called 'intermitting Fever' ... Abigail 'was taken with a shaking fit which held me 2 hours and was succeeded by a fever which lasted till near morning.'" Historians believe she had contracted malaria. It would periodically flare up throughout the rest of her life. The usually sturdy Mrs. Adams was diminished by her illness, becoming so weakened that any effort made her ill: "Despite her illness she managed to finish the packing, and in late October they moved to Philadelphia.... Her ill health had made the trip slow and tedious, she could stand to travel only about 20 miles a day, so it took them five days to go from New York to Philadelphia."[8] Her symptoms, the early autumn onset, her summer residence in a "steamy and unsanitary" port city, and her own description of the fever as "intermitting" convince one that the disease was malaria, a conclusion shared by her biographers. A feature of the type of malaria endemic to America is its chronic periodicity, with several annual flare-ups that produce morbidity but rarely mortality.[9]

After an uninterrupted year and a half in New York and Philadelphia (1790–1791), the Adamses decided never again to spend a summer in the nation's capital. The restorative effects of a few months at home far outweighed the inconvenience of moving their household twice a year. The Adamses journeyed to their Massachusetts home to spend the 1791 summer and subsequently returned to Philadelphia for the congressional session that commenced in October. "For the remainder of his term as Vice President, the Adamses settled into a comfortable if hectic routine. From late fall when Congress convened until sometime in the spring when it adjourned, they lived in Philadelphia; the moment Congress completed its session they went home."[10] Abigail was miserable during her 1791–1792 stay in Philadelphia. Physical complaints from rheumatism and malaria increased to the point that she worried how she could manage the journey home when Congress adjourned. In a March 20, 1792, letter to her sister, Abigail explained: "It was necessary to quell the inflamtory disease first, & Bark could not be administered for that. I am now reduced low enough to drive away the Rhumatism but the old Enemy yet keeps possession. The Dr. promises me the Bark in a few days."[11]

The physician referred to in the letter was the famous Dr. Benjamin Rush; the bark was the material wherein quinine was administered at the time. Benjamin Rush was well known to both Adamses; he was a friend of John and both were signers of the Declaration of Independence. The doctor had previously treated their youngest son, Thomas, in Philadelphia in 1790. At that time, Abigail "found him a kind friend as well as Physician." During her miserable 1791–2 interlude in Philadelphia, Rush visited several times to draw blood from her. She also consulted Rush regarding her niece's tuberculosis. "The (future) first lady's reliance upon Dr. Rush stemmed in part from her agreement … on the value of bleeding as an almost universal remedy. Emetics, bleeding, and the bark, in Abigail's catechism of health, the holy trinity of treatment." Abigail's faith in Rush was enduring. In 1811 she wrote him in Philadelphia from her home in Massachusetts about the breast tumor that afflicted Nabby, the Adamses' daughter. From afar, Rush diagnosed cancer. He urged a mastectomy—an exceedingly rare surgery at that time—upon the Adamses' reluctant Boston doctors. The operation was performed and Nabby lived for three more years.[12]

John Adams' political activity was the nexus connecting the most renowned Philadelphia physician of the period to Abigail and the Adams children. The courageous doctoring of Benjamin Rush during Philadelphia's yellow fever plague of 1793 has already been noted. Rush, with fellow American graduates of the University of Edinburgh Medical School, founded the first medical college in North America. He was a charter member of the faculty of the Medical School of the College of Philadelphia. His long tenure there allowed him to become the most influential teacher of future American physicians during the late eighteenth and early nineteenth centuries. His "heroic" approach to a patient, which encompassed significant blood-letting and both adventuresome emetics and purgatives, may have endeared him to the future first lady but also corrupted medical therapeutics for decades to come.[13]

In the early 1600s, Jesuit missionaries noted that the bark of the cinchona tree was used by the northern Peru Indians as a cure for "shivering diseases." Assuming that "Jesuit's bark" or the "bark," would be equally effective for treating the shaking chills associated with "marsh fever," as malaria was commonly called in Rome, the bark was exported to Italy. Later, quinine was identified as the active ingredient of the bark. It was introduced to colonial America by English physicians. Its use would temper the symptoms but not cure the disease.[14]

During the summer of 1792, "Abigail was sick through most of the summer with malaria, or 'intermittent fever,' as she called it…. Abigail was debilitated for several weeks with the disease. When it came time to return to Philadelphia in the fall, she had neither the strength nor enthusiasm for the journey." She did not leave her Massachusetts home for the capital for five years, even missing her husband's second vice presidential inaugural in 1793.[15]

Malaria sickened Abigail Adams periodically through 1798. It occurred annually, sometimes attacking her twice a year. Its symptoms seldom kept her bedridden for more than a few days. There is no record of medical attendance or type of treatment for these chronic attacks during the Massachusetts interval. Perhaps her uncle, Cotton Tufts, provided for her care. He was a Harvard undergraduate, studied medicine as an apprentice to his brother, and later received an honorary degree in medicine from Harvard. Tufts was a well-known physician and was an incorporator and later president of the Massachusetts Medical Society.[16]

Abigail's sense of civic responsibility overcame her reluctance to serve as her husband's first lady in Philadelphia. But the late summer journey home in 1798 was the most unpleasant of her several journeys. She was seriously ill when the Adamses reached their Quincy, Massachusetts, home. She "felt so close to death that she directed her relatives to assemble so she might take care of them properly." This attack was the most serious she had ever experienced. Her physicians were perplexed by the disease but finally made the diagnosis of "bilious fever." Her symptoms subsided and she revived to the extent that John Adams, in early November, returned by himself to the nation's capital city. Abigail's physicians during this episode are not identified.[17]

Rheumatoid Arthritis

Even more debilitating than malaria was near-crippling rheumatism, probably rheumatoid arthritis. In 1775, "the middle of Abigail's right hand was so sore that she could not hold her pen for three weeks." A significant handicap for this inveterate scribe! Her age (30 years) and the location (middle finger joint) are characteristic of rheumatoid arthritis. Her rheumatism prohibited her journeying to Philadelphia that year for the smallpox inoculation urged by her husband. The sea journey to England in August 1784, as John Adams became the first ambassador to Great Britain, aggravated her symptoms and produced headaches.[18]

Her rheumatism—and it was always called this by Abigail—continued to affect her in Philadelphia. In autumn 1791, the rheumatism combined to lay her low. After six weeks in bed, she was still too feeble to go downstairs without being carried. It was during this episode that Dr. Rush came several times to bleed her.[19] This visit would be Mrs. Adams' last visit to the nation's capital for five years: "Her body was worn with rheumatic pains and fevers that, at times, left her wrists lame and her eyes so sensitive that she could not read, write, or sew by candlelight, let alone leave her bed."[20] In a March 20, 1792, letter to her sister, she wrote: "Tis now the sixth week since I have been out of the door of this chamber…. I was taken six weeks ago very ill with an Inflammatory Rheumatism and tho it did not totally deprive me of the use of my limbs, it swelld and inflamed them to a high degree, and the distress I sufferd in my head was almost intolerable."[21]

The arthritis, like malaria, was a chronic problem. On a return to Philadelphia in 1798 she wrote her sister, referring to it: "I have it floting about, sometimes in my head, Breast, Stomack etc, but if I can keep of fever I can Parry it so not to be confined." In an aside about her favorite physician, she continued: "Dr. Rush is for calling it gout, but I will not believe a word of all that, for Rheumatism I have had ever since I was a child." Apparently her physician continued to be Dr. Rush and bleeding remained his primary treatment.[22] Arthritis continued to oppress the first lady when she took up residence in the unfinished White House in the District of Columbia in November 1800: "When she arrived, she 'suffered from feverish chills, rheumatism and depression.'"[23] In retirement in Quincy, Massachusetts, she continued to suffer from rheumatism.[24]

Smallpox Inoculation

After the British army quit Boston in the spring of 1776, the mingling of colonists, both those exiting the city after being sequestered by the British and those returning to their Boston homes after having been expelled, led to a major smallpox epidemic by June. Abigail determined that smallpox inoculation was required for her, her sisters, and her four children. The process had changed little since John Adams' inoculation more than a decade before. In preparation the Adams family isolated themselves for several weeks. Seven thousand people received the smallpox virus through inoculation in Boston during this period, many, like the Adams contingent, in smallpox hospitals. Their inoculation doctor, Thomas Bullfinch (a 1756 graduate of the University of Edinburgh), had modified the usual ten-day preparation period of self-induced vomiting and a strict debilitating diet. Instead he prescribed medicines that caused the children to "puke every morning." "The practice in colonial Boston … was to insert into the patient's bloodstream a small quantity of the smallpox virus itself. The only way to obtain immunity to the disease was to deliberately contract a minor case of it. About one in every one hundred cases of self-inflicted infection proved fatal. It was widely believed that inoculation patients could improve their odds by preparing themselves with a week of isolation, purgatives, and abstention from meat and dairy products. After a patient had been infected, he or she became a highly contagious carrier of the virus and therefore had to be quarantined for at least three weeks." Boston was a reservoir of the disease, and since John Adams practiced law in the city he was previously inoculated, in 1764.[25] After Dr. Bullfinch inoculated the Adams family, Abigail and two of her children broke out with smallpox pustules, a sign that the infection took and immunity was conferred. However, the inoculation did not take for daughter Nabby and son Charles. Both required a second inoculation that rendered Nabby very sick.

Charles required a third inoculation. When he finally broke out with pustules, it was not the mild form usually associated with inoculation but in the "Natural way," a contagion from a sickened individual. The whole experience lasted more than two months. Fortunately, this inconvenience did not deter Abigail from participating in Boston's celebration of the Declaration of Independence.[26]

Both Martha Washington and Abigail Adams, the future first and second first ladies, had the foresight and the courage to suffer the rigors of smallpox inoculation, not only to protect themselves and their families from an often fatal disease but also to fortify themselves in advance for the rigors of future national prominence.

In 1796 English physician Edward Jenner inoculated an eight-year-old boy with the pus of a patient with active cowpox. He subsequently inoculated the lad with smallpox discharge with no reaction. In this fashion Jenner determined that injection with cowpox (vaccinia) virus would render a person immune to the smallpox virus. Vaccination rapidly replaced inoculation; by 1801, over a hundred thousand people had been vaccinated in Great Britain. Thomas Jefferson, then the third U.S. president, became a strong proponent of vaccination in the United States.[27]

The Adamses: Separation and Influence

Mrs. Adams was an absentee "Second Lady." The vice president's wife resided in Philadelphia for only fourteen of the seventy-seven months John served there as vice president. Her reasons were several, the most significant being her health[28]: "Given Abigail's anxieties about the hazards of office, age, and her poor health, which was only accentuated by Philadelphia's seasonal heat and disease, retirement to Braintree seemed more 'eligible' to her on the eve of the presidency."[29] Additionally, Abigail did not like Philadelphia, basing her judgment on her first visit as wife of the vice president. She observed that the city was filled with Jacobins, not perceiving any difference between urban Republicans and French revolutionaries. Also, despite Philadelphia's reputation for religious diversity and tolerance, there was no church that fit her spiritual tastes.[30] Perhaps a further reason for her absence was the unimportance of the vice presidency. In Adams' own words, "My country in its wisdom contrived for me the most insignificant office that ever the invention of man contrived or his imagination conceived."[31]

Abigail Adams was also for the most part an absentee first lady, remaining in the capital cities of Philadelphia and Washington for less than half the time Adams was president (only 21 out of 48 months). On New Year's Day 1797, John urged Abigail to join him in Philadelphia for his March 4 inauguration. She demurred and the new president was forced to plead for her presence once again. This time Mrs. Adams acquiesced and departed from Massachusetts at the end of April.[32]

After fewer than three months in the capital, she accompanied John Adams home in July. In early October of 1797, both left Massachusetts for Philadelphia. Since yellow fever still raged in that city, as a precaution the Adamses tarried in New York until the end of month.[33] Their return journey to Massachusetts at the end of July 1798 was a very arduous one for Mrs. Adams, and she became very ill, as detailed previously. Her illness determined that the president return to Philadelphia alone. Therefore, he was without his most trusted advisor, alone in the nation's capital for five months. Moreover, upon his return home in late March 1799, he remained for seven months, a far longer absence than his predecessor, George Washington, spent at Mount Vernon, and never during a political crisis.[34]

John Adams left his home the last day of September 1799. However, he was unable to reach Philadelphia because the capital was again in the midst of a yellow fever epidemic. The cabinet had to meet in Trenton, New Jersey. It was December 1799 when Abigail departed for Philadelphia; she remained there only until spring 1800.[35] Her final trip south as first lady was to the unfinished White House in the desolate and sparsely populated new capital city of Washington, D.C. She thus became the first first lady to reside in the White House. She remained only briefly from November 16, 1800, to February 15, 1801.[36]

A salient question, in light of this historical examination, is whether Abigail's illnesses deprived the president of her advice, analysis, and encouragement. Did his months of lonely isolation in Philadelphia lead to policies that might have been altered or thwarted by her presence? Her absence excluded her from "political disquisitions" regarding the initiation of an American peace mission to France's Talleyrand. On February 19, 1799, Adams informed Congress that he had just authorized William Vans Murray, then American minister to The Netherlands, to reopen peace negotiations with France.[37] Conflict between the two countries had approached open warfare. To counter a feared French invasion, Congress previously had authorized the formation of a Provisional Army, to be led by George Washington and Alexander Hamilton. In this context, Adams' peace initiative shocked the country, especially the members of his own Federalist party. Many Federalists concluded that John Adams had gone soft and "they wisht the old woman had been there," "she surely would have shot it down"; "Oh how they lament Mrs. Adams absence…. If she had been there, Murray would never have been named nor his Mission instituted." In Massachusetts the first lady was amused by these laments. Although Abigail was more warlike than her husband regarding France, this time she agreed with John's " master stroke of policy."[38]

The Responsibilities, Problems and Rewards of a First Lady

Abigail Adams' service to the young American republic as its first "Second Lady" and as its second first lady came with a significant price. Her physical well-being was assailed by malarial infection and by debilitating rheumatoid arthritis. Previously in her American travels she had rarely left New England, but the responsibilities of a vice president's wife placed her in New York City, where she became a target of the Anopheles mosquito. Late eighteenth-century carriage travel over America's roads was slow, arduous and physically harmful. Her trips between Boston, Philadelphia, and Washington, D.C., exacerbated the injuries to her joints and muscles, already under the grip of chronic rheumatoid arthritis.

With her prominence as a member of the new government's elite came the availability of the best physicians. Whether the attention of Dr. Benjamin Rush was a benefit to her is subject to conjecture. Rush provided Mrs. Adams with quinine, the standard remedy at the time for malaria. However, his standard treatment for rheumatism—bleeding—was both therapeutically ineffective and pernicious to her well-being.

Abigail Adams was her husband's political soulmate. Their separations were lengthy during John Adams' tenures as vice president and as president. The distance between them probably did not affect his decision making, but this issue remains unresolved.

Sarah Polk

Overview

Robert Watson described Mrs. Polk's role as first lady (1845–1849): "Sarah Polk was a full political and presidential partner.... She was his political partner and leading political advisor ... edited her husband's speeches, discussed politics with him, campaigned with him, was his constant traveling partner, and ... even briefed him on current events. The Polk partnership was well known. Samuel L. Laughlin, a newspaper editor from Nashville, even referred to Sarah as 'Membress of Congress.'"[39]

Sarah Polk was described as having large brown eyes, long dark hair, and a rich olive complexion. She was vivacious and outgoing, and her formal education was far above the norm for women of her generation. There is a possibly apocryphal story that James Polk asked his mentor and fellow Tennessean Andrew Jackson what Polk should do to further his political career. After Jackson had advised the younger man to find a wife and settle down, Polk asked his mentor who Jackson had in mind. He responded, "The one who will never give you any trouble. Her wealthy family, education, health, and appearance are all superior. You know her well."[40] Sarah Childress, born September 4, 1803, married aspiring politician James Knox Polk, nearly eight years her senior, in 1824. Together they formed a successful and intimate social and political union that dissolved only with James's death from cholera in 1849, twenty-five years later.[41] The Polks' political partnership was continuous and successful, he emerging from Tennessee state legislative office to the United States House of Representatives, 1825–1839, where he held the position of Speaker, then rising to the governorship of Tennessee in 1839, and culminating in his election as the eleventh president of the United States in 1840.[42]

However, the Polks' bond was an infertile one, speculatively the consequence of a ghastly surgical procedure performed upon young Polk just shy of his seventeenth birthday. James was frail and in chronic poor health as a teenager. Urinary bladder stones were deemed to be the cause of his physical problems. Sam Polk, his father, decided that a surgical cure was required to ensure a robust manhood for his son. The Polks commenced an eight-hundred-mile journey from Tennessee to Philadelphia where the eminent surgeon Philip Syng Physick would operate. This will not be this good doctor's final appearance in this narrative. However, violent spasms of pain interrupted the Polks' odyssey and James was urgently placed into the surgical hands of Dr. Ephraim McDowell of Danville, Kentucky. Using brandy as an anesthetic, the surgeon "made an incision behind the young man's scrotum and forced a sharp, pointed instrument called a gorget through his prostate and into the bladder. The stone was removed with forceps." It is no surprise, then, that the Polk union was without progeny.[43]

Malaria

Sarah Polk's life prior to the White House was a healthy one. The single exception was a severe case of measles she suffered in the fall of 1828.[44]

Bumgarner, in his biography of Sarah Polk, described the capital's summer political hiatus when James Polk was a congressman: "In Polk's time Washington was deserted by the politicians and the affluent during the warm season, when they fled to the mountains and the seashore to escape the heat. The south side of the president's mansion overlooked the Potomac and a canal laden with malaria-carrying mosquitoes. Quinine was available, but there was a high incidence of malaria among those who stayed in the capital in the hot season and exposed themselves to infection." Sarah and James Polk always took advantage of this interlude to return home to Tennessee.[45] However, when they were president and first lady, the Polks never traveled far from the capital and spent their 1845–1848 summers vulnerable to the pestilence of the District of Columbia. Their dedication to their civic responsibilities was rewarded with episodes of malaria: In May and again in September–October 1847 in the case of Sarah, and in late September 1847 and June 1848 in the case of James.

The diary of President Polk from April 30 to May 8, 1847, recorded a classical textbook description of an attack of tertian malaria (plasmodium vivax), the species endemic to the Washington swamp. His entry for April 30 read: "She [Sarah] had slight symptoms of a chill Friday last, which had not attracted much attention as she had casually mentioned it, but had not complained of much indisposition of it." However, two days later, on May 2, his entry was more alarming: "When Mrs. Polk returned from Church she complained of being very cold, and it was manifest she had a chill, and a short time later a reaction took place and she had a fever." Both she and the president remained in bed for the rest of the day. Predictably the symptoms of periodic chills and fever resumed two days later on Tuesday, May 4. Polk recorded it in his diary: "I soon discovered she had a chill and threw more covering on the bed. Her chill continued for more than three hours. I have never seen her suffer or complain more than she did for several hours. After the chill subsided, the fever rose." Again, characteristically, Sarah was much better the next day. However, on the succeeding day, Thursday, May 6, the chills and fever diagnostic of "intermittent fever," which are now recognized as tertian malaria, returned. A violent chill shook her, leaving her sick all day. Two days later the anticipated symptoms did not appear. Sarah commented, "Well, I guess I am getting better because I did not have my usual chill this morning. This has certainly been a severe attack of intermittent fever."[46] Mrs. Polk underwent a second bout of malaria during late September to mid October 1847. Polk's diary recounted "she had another chill and suffered much and rested badly during the night and day." During this period one of the president's malarial episodes coincided with his wife's.[47]

Sarah Polk's position as first lady attracted the best medical care then available. Two of the most prestigious physicians in practice in Washington attended her during her illnesses. Doctors James Crowdhill Hall and Thomas Miller also treated her husband. Hall and Miller were "Pillars of the Profession," two of an elite group of Washington physicians whose patients included presidents of the United States, among other notables. In Hall's case, he cared for five presidents; Miller was the physician to three. Dr. Hall holds the ghoulish distinction of attending at the deathbed of three presidents: Harrison, Taylor and Lincoln. Although James Polk was successful in escaping becoming president number four on Hall's mortality list, the former president died from cholera in Nashville three months after the conclusion of his presidency.[48]

Both physicians were well trained, unlike the vast majority of "doctors" at the time. Both had an apprenticeship before attending and completing medical school. In the mid-nineteenth century most physicians' training ceased with the completion of an apprenticeship. Formal medical school education was obtained only by a minority. Miller and Hall were graduates of the University of Pennsylvania School of Medicine and both had previously graduated from college before medical school. Both served as presidents of the District of Columbia Medical Society. Miller was the president of the District's board of health and established the practice of recording Washington births during his tenure. Moreover, he was active in the establishment of St. Elizabeth's Asylum and was the physician to the District's jail.[49]

Drs. Hall and Miller prescribed medicine for Mrs. Polk's malaria, undoubtedly quinine.[50] One might ask why a congressman's wife, whose husband had spent seven terms over fourteen years in Washington as a congressman, was not stricken earlier by malaria. At the time, congressional sessions commenced in late autumn or December and adjourned before summer's heat enveloped the capital. A review of the Polks' travels during his congressional tenure indicates that they escaped D.C. and spent their summers in Tennessee.[51] There is no evidence that either episode of malaria affected Sarah's partnership with, and her support of, the president.

Mrs. Polk was one of the widows who long outlived their ex-president husbands. She never remarried. She died in her Nashville, Tennessee, home in her eighty-ninth year in late summer 1891, forty-two years after the death of James.[52]

Lucretia Garfield

Overview

Lucretia Garfield was 48 years old when her husband, James, was inaugurated as the United States' twentieth chief executive on March 4, 1881. Their twenty-two-year marriage resulted in ten pregnancies. Five children—only one a girl—survived into adulthood.[53]

James Garfield served as a U.S. Representative from Ohio between 1863 and 1880. At that time it was still the practice for congressional families to flee Washington in the summer for cooler and healthier locations: "The Garfield family ... was now settling into a yearly routine of life in Washington during the Congressional season and summer vacations in Ohio, or occasionally on the Jersey coast."[54]

Malaria

Lucretia Garfield's May 1881 episode with malaria distinguishes her illness in the following ways: The first huddling of doctors in the practice on "VIP Medicine"; the first female physician to treat a first lady; the first doctor of the homeopathic school to render care; and widespread newspaper coverage of a president's wife's illness.

In early May 1881, Mrs. Garfield was seen huddled before "a rather unseasonable wood fire" and appeared "pale but animated." Garfield's diary entry for May 4, 1881, recorded: "Crete has been quite ill all day with something like chill fever. She has been too hard worked during the past two months."[55] The morning after huddling before the wood fire, the chill of the previous night "turned into malaria." Her fever spiked to 104 degrees and her pulse raced to 100 beats per minute. "Her hair fell out in patches," and ominously "for a time it seemed as if she could not possibly live."[56]

James Garfield, as president, had the capacity to summon as many physicians as he thought necessary to cure the first lady, in this instance at least four. Included in the professional huddle were prominent Washington physician Col. Jedediah Baxter, who was also James Garfield's doctor; Dr. Gustavus Polk, who was trained as an allopathic doctor but who treated homeopathically; and two true homeopathic doctors, Susan Edson and Silas Boynton. Fortunately for Lucretia, Thomas Jefferson's famous maxim about group medicine did not apply in her case: "That whenever he saw three physicians together, he looked upward to discover whether there was not a turkey buzzard in the neighborhood."[57]

Homeopath doctor Susan Edson was the first female physician to practice in Washington, D.C., and the first female doctor to tend to a first lady. Edson at some undetermined time had assumed the medical care of Lucretia Garfield. Edson was a favorite of the entire Garfield family, and son Abe Garfield addressed her as "Dr. Edson, full of Med'cin." Edson made the diagnoses of malaria and nervous exhaustion and proclaimed her prognosis that the patient would recover. But President Garfield was dissatisfied with the slow pace of his wife's improvement and summoned his cousin, prominent homeopath Silas Boynton, from his ranch near Wichita, Kansas. Eventually all the medical consultants agreed with Edson's original diagnosis.[58] Lucretia Garfield had a predilection for homeopathic doctors. These physicians, in contrast to the doctors of the predominant orthodox or allopathic school, were considered to be more patient-friendly and to employ gentler remedies, not the bleeding and purging in vogue among orthodox practitioners. Other first ladies in the future would also seek the assistance of homeopaths for their physical ills.

Mrs. Garfield's illness inserted itself into the public's awareness. On May 11, one week after the onset of the illness, Washington's newspapers began commenting on it: "Early reports stated ... [she] had fallen victim to typhoid fever; later the diagnosis was changed to typhoid-malaria. Finally it was said she suffered from malaria and nervous exhaustion." Later, "her illness was followed across the country in headlines and editorials."[59] By mid–May her condition had improved somewhat, and on June 12, Silas Boynton declared that she was past her illness. There was a long convalescence. On June 12, still weak and thin, Lucretia was carried downstairs to attend dinner with the family for the first time since she had become ill. On June 18, she left Washington by train for the Atlantic seaside cottage at Long Branch, New Jersey. At the time, future assassin Charles Guiteau, then stalking President Garfield, was at the Washington train depot with his pistol. Later he recalled that Mrs. Garfield "looked so thin and clung so tenderly to the president's arm, my heart failed me to part them." The first lady wrote her husband on June 30 that her recovery was complete.

On July 2, 1881, she was well enough to plan to travel to New York City to meet her husband. Meanwhile the president arrived at Washington's Baltimore and Potomac depot for his train to New York. This time Charles Guiteau did not hesitate and shot Garfield twice. Mrs. Garfield hastened to Washington to care for her husband. The president lingered in pain for many weeks. Despite the ministrations of multiple physicians he died on the eightieth day after the attack. Jefferson's foreboding epigram proved correct in the case of President Garfield's condition.[60]

The Garfields and the Effects of Lucretia's Malaria

Lucretia's illness and convalescence lasted six weeks, during which Garfield refused to see anyone, not even senators. The gates of the White House were closed to visitors.[61]

Instead, Garfield spent much of his time beside his wife's bed or sleeping on a nearby daybed. "I sat up with Crete until 4 hours past midnight."[62] It is questionable whether the president's distraction significantly interfered with the performance of his responsibilities. A principal function of many 19th-century presidencies was completing patronage appointments. In the opinion of one biographer, "the president could pay only fitful attention to the last critical stages of the struggle with Conkling. Instead he devoted all his energies to nursing his wife back to health."[63] Sen. Roscoe Conkling was the political boss of New York State and a leader of the Republican faction opposed to Garfield. During May 1881, Garfield all but recused himself from participating in the intra-party feud. On the month's last day, Lucretia's doctors pronounced her recovered; coincidentally this was same day that Conkling resigned from the Senate and doomed his political career.[64]

The District of Columbia: No Place for the Squeamish

It was recognized early that a proximity to stagnant water or swamps was a prerequisite for the existence of malaria. Only later was it understood that these venues provided the breeding grounds for the mosquitoes that functioned as the vectors for human transmission. Draining the swamps improved the health of those in their proximity.[65] Malaria flourished for centuries in the American South and in port cities like Boston and New York. Swamp drainage and residential spread gradually removed malaria from the North, but Walter Reed's 1895 study of two army posts on the Virginia side of the Potomac River showed that "intermittent and remittent" fevers were constantly present from 1871 to 1895.[66] Packard described late nineteenth-century Washington: "But more than just the weather gave the city its notable unpleasantness. Washington's water supply was not only the dirty and the polluted but represented in all its permutations a mortal threat to the health of the capital's inhabitants. The lowest parts of the city, which unfortunately included the White House and its precincts, rose mere inches above the sluggishly tidal Potomac River, some stretches of which were lined with swamps. As the stream coursed past the District, its most troubling habit was overflowing onto lower Pennsylvania Avenue."[67]

The city's reputation was so negative that a committee of its medical society was formed to combat the widely held belief that Washington was a very unhealthy place. The committee reported that "there has been a gradual but decided diminution in the extent and intensity of diseases of a malarial nature, owing, no doubt, to improved drainage, better paved streets, the filling of low lands, and other improvements.... Malarial diseases are almost entirely confined to those portions of the city immediately bordering on the Potomac river and its tributaries, the Eastern Branch and Rock Creek." The timing of the society's attempt at marketing was unfortunate, since its 1881 report was issued the same year that the country's first lady contracted malaria in the same city.[68]

Two years earlier the *New York Times* had reported that President Hayes arranged to be absent from the District "in order to escape the malarial atmosphere which will necessarily arise and be carried by the southerly winds across the parking to the mansion [White House] as soon as the vegetation begins decaying." He was determined to submit legislation to Congress to have the decaying and dangerous vegetation removed.[69]

As was the case of first lady Sarah Polk, Lucretia Garfield's commitment to the White

House during Washington's malarial season made her vulnerable to its disease-carrying mosquitoes. Both received the care of the best available physicians and both recovered to lead long lives. Lucretia Garfield died March 13, 1918, in her California home after a brief bout with pneumonia. She did not remarry; her widowhood lasted almost thirty-seven years.[70]

Presidents Who Contracted Malaria

At least nine presidents contracted malaria, most of them prior to their tenure in the White House but several during their presidency. George Washington was treated for malaria with quinine in August and September 1786. His physician, Dr. James Craik, gave him eight doses of "red bark" at a time.[71] Presidents James Monroe[72] and James Polk were infected in the executive mansion. James Garfield's malaria preceded that of his wife's by many years. The young Garfield drove horses that pulled barges along Ohio's many canals. At age sixteen, he fell many times into the canals' miasmic waters and caught the disease.[73]

Andrew Jackson was no stranger to diseases, one of which was malaria,[74] and in the summer of 1835 Abraham Lincoln had chills and fever on alternate days for over a month, for which he took "heroic doses of Peruvian bark."[75] John Kennedy contracted malaria during his navy service in the South Pacific, a fact that was prominently stated in his 1960 campaign literature.[76]

In 1858 Ulysses Grant gave up his attempt at farming as his "health was not good. He had what he believed to be the ague."[77] Finally, Theodore Roosevelt, during his post-presidential African safari, developed malaria's well-recognized symptoms: "He knows this is not African malaria, but the Cuban variety that has plagued him since Rough Rider days. Always the sudden convulsions, the cracking headache, then zero at the bone."[78]

Chapter Three

Letitia Tyler

A First Lady Dies in the White House

[In September 1839, Robert Tyler, son of John and Letitia Tyler, married Priscilla Cooper:] Yet the happy occasion was marred by the absence of Mrs. Tyler, who shortly before the wedding had suffered a stroke that left her partially paralyzed.[1]

Letitia Tyler

Letitia Christian Tyler, a daughter of the antebellum plantation South, fulfilled all expectations assigned her as wife, as mother, and as mistress of the Tyler homestead. Unfortunately, her exemplary success in satisfying these roles, wearying and debilitating as they were, undoubtedly diminished her ability to perform the social role as first lady of the United States. Mrs. Tyler died in the White House on September 10, 1842, at age fifty-one years and ten months and after more than twenty-one years of marriage. Her husband, John Tyler, had become president seventeen months earlier upon the death of William Henry Harrison. Mrs. Tyler was the first of three first ladies whose deathbeds were located in the presidential mansion.

In the previous two chapters, the focus was on infectious diseases prevalent in eighteenth- and nineteenth-century America. This chapter introduces consideration of a physical state unique to women that often led to severe consequences, especially in the nineteenth century. Pregnancy was a significant maternal health risk during a period when obstetrical care was primitive by twentieth- and twenty-first-century standards. First ladies were not spared, as exemplified by Letitia Tyler (probable pregnancy-related hypertension); Louisa Johnson Adams (postpartum depression); Ida McKinley (eclampsia with cerebrovascular accident); and Ellen Wilson (probable post-eclamptic chronic renal failure).

A "paralytic stroke" in 1839 incapacitated Letitia Tyler, and she was significantly disabled during her husband's presidency. To what extent did her illness affect her functioning as first lady? Conversely, did her position as first lady affect the course of her disease? Moreover, was her medical care as the president's wife comparable to that received by her husband? Did her position privilege her in the care she received in contrast to the care expected by the average male and female American in the early 1840s. Finally, did her illness affect Tyler's functioning as president? The following discussion attempts to answer these questions.

Medical History

Letitia Christian married John Tyler in 1813. By 1830 she had given birth to eight children.[2] John Tyler was an absentee father, his political career being nearly continuous. He was gone much of the time during his service in the Virginia house of delegates (1811–1816), the United States House of Representatives (1816–1821), as a returnee to the Virginia house (1823–1825), as governor of Virginia (1825–1827), in the United States Senate (1827–1836), and back again to the Virginia house of delegates (1838–1840) before his selection as William H. Harrison's vice president.[3]

Unlike the growing number of wives who traveled to Washington with their husbands to participate in the congressional social season, Letitia chose to accompany her husband to the District only once. She rarely traveled to Richmond when Tyler served in the Virginia legislature. (Williamsburg, Virginia, was the Tylers' home.)[4] However, when John was Virginia governor, she "presided over the governor's mansion with charm and set a high standard for social life" in Richmond. An interview with a Richmond woman of the time appeared in the *Washington Globe*, and the woman recalled she was "then in perfect health and adorned with beauty."[5]

Yet Letitia was plagued by ill health for most of her marriage to John. Tyler was very concerned about his wife's physical condition but not to the extent that he abandoned his political career. Instead the husband relied on their oldest child, Mary, to look after her sickly mother. As time passed, Mary became her mother's caretaker: "Letitia's health worsened with each passing year; she was ever more prone to excruciating headaches and debilitating illness as she got older. After her husband's election to the [United States] Senate in 1827, she never seemed well."[6]

Her symptoms, other than severe headaches and a nonspecific debility, were undefined. One biographer ascribed her condition to "difficult pregnancies and the demands of a large family." Mrs. Tyler's condition continued to cause Tyler a great deal of unease, and he worried about her delicate health constantly. However, he hewed to his climb up the political ladder. "He relied on Mary to look after her mother when she suffered from headaches and to keep him apprised of her condition." Tyler purchased a large bathtub for his wife and converted their farm's dairy to a room where she could soak in salt water for some relief: "Mary enjoined a slave to fill the tub with salt water once or twice a week, whenever her mother appeared to need treatment."[7]

In a June 16, 1832, letter to his daughter, Tyler, then a United States senator wrote to her, somewhat condescendingly: "[I am] concerned to learn from your mother that she had suffered from a severe headache the day after.... This proceeds from over anxiety on her part, aided by a predisposition to disease. Tell her that Doctor Gaither says a free use of the pills I gave her would serve to keep off those attacks, and that she would derive great benefit by using the bath."[8] The Tylers employed another tactic to fortify Letitia's declining health. On several occasions when her health required it, Mrs. Tyler sought a respite at the Greenbrier in the (then) Virginia mountains.[9] Ironically Greenbrier became the site of President Tyler's honeymoon with his second wife, less than two years after his first wife's demise. (The Greenbrier resort in White Sulphur Springs, West Virginia, continues as a famous vacation destination today.[10])

Stroke (Cerebrovascular Accident, CVA)

In 1839, shortly before the wedding of the Tylers' oldest son, Letitia suffered a stroke in Williamsburg, Virginia. Its extent was "extremely severe." She was partially paralyzed and lost her powers of speech: "She could not express her joy in words when she heard the news of the happy outcome of her son's courtship." It is unclear whether she regained her ability to speak, either partially or completely. Despite medical care, "her system remained greatly shattered and her health continued evermore precarious." It is also unclear whether she overcame the partial paralysis, but it is unambiguous that Letitia Tyler was even more physically dependent after this medical emergency.[11] The identities of the treating physicians are unrecorded, as was the nature of their treatments. John Tyler, at the time a delegate to the Virginia house, should have understood the gravity of his wife's condition, since in April 1797, when Tyler was seven, his mother died of a paralytic stroke.[12]

The new Tyler daughter-in-law, Priscilla Cooper Tyler, wrote about her mother-in-law's partial recovery in a letter to her sisters: "[She reads] her bible and her prayer-book—with her knitting usually in her hands.... Notwithstanding her very delicate health, mother attends to and regulates all household duties.... All the clothes for the children, and for the servants, are cut out under her immediate eye, and all the sewing is personally super-intended by her." "She must have been very beautiful in her youth, for she is still beautiful in her declining years and wretched health." Unfortunately Mrs. Tyler remained in her bed-chamber after this illness.[13]

Motherhood in the Old South was both difficult and demanding. Women approached their due date in fear of pain and death for either themselves or their infants. Southern mothers emerged from their repeated pregnancies with physical ailments, infections, and debilitating illnesses. Southern families, as in the case of the Tylers, were large, thereby increasing a woman's physical risks. "Malaria was another danger for Southern women during and after childbirth. For the most part it did its harm by causing debilitation and a susceptibility to other diseases."[14]

Letitia Tyler's debility was no doubt in part a result of physical exhaustion from her repeated pregnancies. However, hypertension may be linked to grand multiparity; additionally a salient symptom in this patient was recurrent, frequently severe, headaches, another linkage with hypertension. The rudimentary medicine of the era could not document her blood pressure or laboratory values. However, one may speculate strongly that an elevated blood pressure would explain her medical problems, at least in part.[15]

First Lady

John Tyler, after his election (November 1840) as William Henry Harrison's vice pres-ident, planned to continue living in his Williamsburg home. He decided that the ailing Letitia would be more comfortable there than in Washington. Such an arrangement was possible since the vice presidency continued to remain a nonessential office.[16] This plan dramatically changed with President Harrison's death one month after his inauguration. Tyler became the first vice president to succeed to the presidency upon the death of a pres-ident. Daniel Webster's son, Fletcher, chief clerk in the State Department, and Mr. Beall, an officer of the Senate, interrupted the Tylers' rustic peaceful existence with the shocking news. It was then decided that Letitia would move to the White House, but it was apparent that she was unequal to the role of first lady. Her daughter-in-law Priscilla, a former actress, became the social mistress of the executive mansion, the second of the surrogate first ladies. Fortunately, an old and successful hand was available for guidance, as we shall see.[17]

As President Tyler had the social intuition to select as his official White House hostess one who could match his easy informality, he accordingly asked his daughter-in-law Priscilla to perform this responsibility and took her consent for granted as his wife was an invalid; his two older daughters were married; and his two younger daughters were either inexperienced or too young. Priscilla's responsibilities included presiding at biweekly receptions, triweekly dinners, monthly public levees, and the entertainment of callers who every night crowded the White House Green Room. Occasionally one or several of the Tyler daughters would assist, but from April 1841 to March 1844 the responsibility was chiefly that of Priscilla Cooper Tyler.[18]

When in doubt, she had that most experienced of White House hostesses available for advice. Dolley Madison had returned to Washington and subsequently assisted Priscilla in her social duties. The widow Madison, "turbaned, painted, powdered, and dipping snuff was in and out of the White House like a good neighbor." Mrs. Madison, who had frequently served as the hostess for the widower Thomas Jefferson, was the first surrogate first lady[19]: "After a short time she became more accustomed to her stellar role and pleased the President and amazed herself by performing her duties with what seemed easy grace."[20]

Priscilla continued in this role until her husband accepted a government job in Philadelphia. The Tylers' second daughter, Letitia Semple, briefly acted as hostess until the president's young wife, Julia Gardiner, took on the role after her wedding in June 1844. John Tyler's new bride was thirty-one years his junior. The ex-president went on to sire seven more children with his much younger wife.[21]

Elizabeth Tyler, the third Tyler daughter, married William Waller in a White House ceremony on January 31, 1842. The wedding and the reception afterwards were the only public occasions at which Letitia Tyler appeared. She generally remained in her room, an invalid who avoided excitement of any kind. However, on the night of the wedding, she emerged, beautifully dressed, to celebrate with the bride and groom.[22]

Mrs. Tyler's death was both unexpected and sudden. Daughter Letitia wrote her brother: "From the time she had been first stricken with paralysis, her health had been frail, but none of us anticipated an immediate, or even an early renewal of an attack, and far less, a sudden dissolution of her system."[23]

On the morning of Friday, September 9, 1842, Dr. Thomas, the family physician, noted a significant change in the first lady and became alarmed that a recurrent stroke was imminent. He immediately called for the consultation of Dr. Sewall. The methods used by these practitioners to prevent a cerebrovascular accident are unrecorded. Whatever treatments that were employed were unsuccessful. Mrs. Tyler declined rapidly and expired at 8:00 p.m. on Saturday, September 10, 1842.[24]

Medical Care in the Tyler White House

President John Tyler, by all accounts, was healthy during his White House tenure (1841–1845). There is no record either of illness or of professional medical care during his presidency. However, his term in office was not tranquil. Tyler was confronted by contentious foreign issues, domestic policy disputes, political disappointments, and the illness and demise of his wife. After he departed from the White House, he devoted himself to his much younger second wife, a growing family, and his Virginia farm. He occasionally involved himself in politics, the most notable example his election to the Confederate House of Representatives in 1862. He died in Richmond, the capital city of the confederacy, seventeen years after leaving the presidency.[25]

John Moylan Thomas and Thomas Sewall were the two District physicians who attended the first lady at the end of her life. Moreover Dr. Thomas had made "almost daily visits" to the failing first lady for many months prior to her demise. Thomas was also the doctor to President Tyler, although any medical care for the president is undocumented.[26] Thomas was well trained, receiving his medical degree from the University of Maryland. He started a medical practice in Washington, D.C., and also became involved in the profession's organizational and academic activities. He was active in the District of Columbia Medical Society and represented the society at the 1848 inaugural meeting of the American Medical Association in Baltimore. He later became a professor at Washington's Columbian Medical College.[27]

However, Dr. Samuel Busey, a contemporaneous practitioner in the District, was very critical of Thomas' personal character. He recollected that Tyler "came leisurely, after time, to his lectures on physiology (at the Columbian College), which were brief, polished, and unsatisfactory. He was always neatly dressed in the latest style, dignified, polite, but very reserved. At that time he had a very large business among the better class of citizens, and lived sumptuously." A later citation by Busey even suggested an addiction to alcohol: "Some years later I parted with him in front of John Foy's saloon about one hour before he wrote a prescription, it was alleged, killed a porter at Fuller's Hotel, and the last time I saw him he was struggling, with assistance, to respond to a summons to see Mrs. Adams."[28]

Dr. Busey was more complimentary of Dr. Thomas Sewall, the second physician present at Mrs. Tyler's deathbed: "In 1825 Thomas Sewall, a native of Massachusetts and a graduate of Harvard University, delivered the first lecture in the Medical Department of Columbian University. From that date until his death in 1845, at the age of fifty-nine years, Sewall was one of the most conspicuous and popular physicians of the city." Sewall's professional career in Washington was both prominent and successful: Charter professor of Anatomy and Physiology at Columbian University, the predecessor of the George Washington School of Medicine; astute promoter of William Beaumont's groundbreaking experiments on gastric physiology; and assistant surgeon in the 1839 removal of a seven-and-a-half pound tumor of the jaw of a prisoner at the Washington almshouse.[29] Sewall's civic accomplishments were also numerous. He had been known to President Tyler since the chief executive appointed him as one of the three medical inspectors of the federal penitentiary in the District and reappointed him in 1844.[30]

During his career, Sewall was involved with some of the more colorful aspects of nineteenth-century medicine in America: grave robbing (body snatching), phrenology, and temperance. The unavailability of bodies for medical teaching purposes was decidedly an impediment to eighteenth- and nineteenth-century physicians in England and the United States. The number of legally available cadavers was greatly inadequate for the development of anatomical familiarity and surgical skill. The only lawful sources of bodies were executed criminals and bodies bequeathed to medical schools for study. As a consequence there was an enormous imbalance between what numbers were available and the numbers required. It was estimated that in 1878 in the United States, at least half of the cadavers studied in medical schools were illegally acquired: "A body will sell for five dollars anywhere, and in Ohio and other states thirty dollars is the usual price."[31]

Sewall had commenced his medical practice in Massachusetts, but in 1818 he was convicted of digging up a corpse for the purpose of dissection. *The History of the Medical Society of the District of Columbia* elaborated: "Sewall … came to Washington under a cloud, having robbed the grave of a near relative in his devotion to the study of medicine. Hingham's loss was Washington's gain."[32] Fortunately for the physician, his attorney was Daniel Webster, then a Massachusetts congressman, a future U.S. senator and later the secretary of state for president John Tyler. Webster invited Dr. Sewall, his client, to the more forgiving milieu of Washington. Sewall accepted this invitation and his career prospered.[33]

Phrenology was the study of the relationship between a person's character and the morphology of the skull. Its practitioners were convinced that an examination of the skull's shape predicted the size and development of the brain beneath. Its popularity in England in the early 1800s led to its spread and use in the United States between 1830 and 1850.[34] Sewall, in two lectures delivered to the students of the Columbian College in February 1837, debunked the "science" of phrenology, concluding, "Is it strange, then, when we are told that a science that has been discovered, by which the character and capabilities of the human mind can be ascertained; the secrets of the heart disclosed, and this, too, by a momentary examination of the exterior of the head, that we should find men who will study and advocate its doctrines?" The following year Sewall loaned former first lady Dolley Madison a book on phrenology for reasons unknown.[35]

Sewall was very active in the national and international temperance movement. His lecture to the Maryland State Temperance Society, "On the Pathology of Drunkenness," was widely reported. The lecture used as props transparent paintings of the stomach in a state of health, the stomach of a confirmed alcoholic, and the stomach of an alcoholic who died from delirium tremens.[36]

As a famous physician in the still small city of Washington, his professional connection with other inhabitants of the White House in addition to Mrs. Tyler should not surprise one. Sewall was called in consultation to the deathbed of William Henry Harrison, Tyler's predecessor. It has been a frequent practice of doctors, when confronted with an unhappy or complex outcome for a prominent patient, to spread the blame for any treatment failure among as many physicians as possible. Sewall was prestigious enough to have his name included with other doctors in the medical statement issued to the public and press upon Harrison's demise.[37]

In early 1835, Richard Lawrence attempted to assassinate President Andrew Jackson. The attempt failed when Lawrence's pistols failed to discharge. Sewall and a second physician were charged to determine "the state of mind" of the assailant. Their widely disseminated report was comprehensive and factual but devoid of conclusions. A clarification was asked of the examiners, who replied, "[W]e therefore do not hesitate to state, as our opinion, that this unfortunate man is laboring under extensive mental hallucination upon some subjects."[38]

A third connection was with the flamboyant congressman Franklin Pierce in late February 1836, seventeen years before Pierce was inaugurated as the fourteenth president. The congressman, inebriated, was embroiled in a fight with two other representatives at a Washington theater. Subsequently Pierce was awakened at night with a fever and pleuritic pain: "Dr. Sewall visited Pierce and removed 16 oz. of blood from him. On the next visit, 24 hours later, the doctor removed 10–12 more ounces of blood by cupping. To this treatment was attributed his recovery.... During the second week of March, he was well enough to resume his work in Congress." Whether Sewall repeated this treatment on the dying Letitia Tyler remains unknown.[39]

Diagnosis and Treatment of Stroke in the Nineteenth Century

In the nineteenth century, medical understanding of "paralytic stroke" was limited. Physicians were able to recognize it as an abrupt change in cerebral function and in muscle motor control. By the 1840s, it was accepted that its cause was an obstruction of the blood vessels to the brain. The accepted treatment for paralysis could be calamitous. Mushet wrote that "much evidence might be collected in favor of bleeding in cases of sudden hemiplegia." According to Taylor, remedial treatment included rapid venesection, which "should be early and extensively employed, a frequent repetition of the bleedings being indispensable in most instances." He further proposed that the bleeding be initiated in the jugular vein of the neck to the point that the radial pulse weakened.[40] Adjunctive treatment also could be deleterious and included hot brandy. cayenne pepper, the cathartic calomel, emetics and blistering. There is no record of the treatment received by Letitia Tyler either for the stroke in 1839 or for her terminal cerebrovascular accident.[41]

Outcome

The burdens of being first lady did not affect Letitia Tyler's health, since she was already disabled when she first took up residence in her White House quarters. She was unable to perform any of the required tasks, and as a consequence the question is moot. She was incapable of accomplishing any of a first lady's requisite social and ceremonial tasks. Her prominent position gave her access to the best D.C. physicians available. Dr. Thomas may not have merited such prestigious consideration, but Dr. Sewall certainly did. Letitia died at an earlier age—just shy of fifty-two years—then the life expectancy of that of white American females in 1850. The very first mortality statistics for the United States appeared as part of the seventh census of the United States in 1850. In 1850, a white female at age 10 would be expected to live for 47.2 more years, i.e., until age 57.2.[42]

John Tyler was well during his presidency and his medical care in the White House was minimal or absent. Letitia's illness drove him to work harder: "He buried himself in work. Rising with the sun, he stayed at his desk without a break until three-thirty in the afternoon, at which time the family dined together. After candlelight he interviewed visitors and performed miscellaneous social chores until bedtime at ten o'clock. Tyler worked arduous hours to avoid dealing with the approaching death of his wife."[43] His wife's illness apparently did not effect the performance of his presidential duties.

Chapter Four

Retiring and Sickly First Ladies in Antebellum Washington

Elizabeth Monroe, Anna Harrison, Margaret Taylor and Abigail Fillmore

Elizabeth Monroe, the Sickly First Lady

> [Elizabeth Monroe suffered from] an unidentified ailment that forced her to curtail her activities as First Lady.[1]

Social Challenges

Elizabeth Monroe, the wife of James Monroe, the fifth United States president (1817–1825), succeeded the effervescent and extremely popular Dolley Madison as first lady. Mrs. Monroe suffered greatly in comparison to Mrs. Madison. During the eight years of the Monroe presidency Dolley's tradition of returning courtesy calls was abandoned and the previous sparkle of White House ceremonial dinners, drawing room mixers, and social teas was dimmed. Mrs. Monroe was accused of snobbery for her French manners, and the grande dames of the capital initially boycotted her parties.[2] The criticism of the capital's social elite assailed the first lady's plans for her daughter Maria's White House wedding, and the invitation list was limited to forty-four guests. Maria's March 1820 wedding was the first for a daughter of a sitting president in the White House.[3]

First lady Monroe frequently missed social events where her presence was either anticipated or expected, and there were periods when she was absent from public view. Additionally she had the hauteur of an aristocrat and projected the image of a grande dame. Carl Anthony may have surmised the thoughts of her contemporaries: "But though the words were unspoken, it was understood that America now had its first Queen Elizabeth."[4]

Someone needed to stand in for the often absent president's wife. The surrogate was the Monroe's older daughter, Eliza Hay. Almost immediately after her husband's inauguration, Elizabeth began to rely upon her daughter to fulfill social commitments. This dependency increased during Monroe's second term, since the first lady was said to be increasingly troubled by illness. Eliza Hay's personality complicated rather than alleviated

39

the sensitive social situation. Eliza was both abrasive and snobbish. Her schooling in France contributed to her aloofness and condescending behavior. Louisa Adams, the wife of Monroe's secretary of state, was also schooled in France. The opinionated but perceptive Louisa described Eliza as so "full of agreeables and disagreeables, so accomplished and ill bred, so proud and mean," with such a "love of scandal that no reputation is safe in her hands."[5]

Elizabeth Monroe eventually overcame the early criticisms of her management of White House's social and ceremonial affairs. Her charm, beauty and sincerity won the admiration and esteem of all, including her most severe critics. "In spite of her poor health, Mrs. Monroe still looked younger than her years and her beauty was much admired." Although she had been ill during much of the winter, the first lady presided at the White House dinner that honored the Marquis de Lafayette upon the fiftieth anniversary of his initial visit to America. She impressed all with her remarkable beauty in spite of her sixty years.[6] Ammon summarized the role of the nation's fourth first lady: "In public, her formal manners left an impression of coldness and reserve, but in private she was a devoted wife and a doting mother, possessing to the full the domestic virtues then so highly prized—a complete absorption in the affairs of her family and household and a total detachment from the world of politics and business."[7]

The only public political action undertaken by Elizabeth Monroe during her husband's forty plus years in government service was her role in the release from a Paris prison of Madame de Lafayette, the wife of the French hero of the American Revolution. James Monroe was twice the American ambassador to France, the first time being 1793 to 1796 during the French Revolution. The aristocratic Madame de Lafayette was imprisoned under the sentence of death; her mother and her sister had already been executed. Ambassador Monroe was diplomatically constrained from any personal action to free the prisoner. However, the ambassador's wife, Elizabeth, not shackled by similar restraints, became a willing coconspirator in the plan to free this prisoner. Mrs. Monroe boldly drove to the prison in a very elegant and conspicuous carriage to meet with Madame de Lafayette. The meeting between the two women became public knowledge almost immediately. Consequently the French government, made aware of the significance of Madame Lafayette to its American ally, freed her shortly thereafter.[8]

The Monroe presidency concluded in March 1825. Monroe welcomed the release from the responsibilities of office. His principal concern was that Elizabeth would regain her health in the quiet of their Virginia home. She was in such poor health that she and her husband were compelled to remain in the White House for three weeks after the inauguration of his successor, John Quincy Adams.[9]

Illnesses

Chronic illness or illnesses, rather than social maladroitness or a pretentious personality, prevented Elizabeth Monroe from performing successfully as a first lady. Without doubt she was sick in the White House both before and after Monroe's presidency. Illness was chronic and persistent, and more than a single disease likely was present. Primary sources are largely silent regarding her symptoms, diagnoses, treatments, and even the identity of her physicians. Almost everything written on this subject in biographies is either inference or speculation.

James Monroe, age twenty-seven, married Elizabeth Kortright, only seventeen, in New York City's historic Trinity Episcopal Church on February 16, 1786. Their devoted marriage produced three children: Eliza, born December 5, 1787; James Spence, born 1799 (died from pertussis on September 28, 1800); and Maria Hester, born in Paris in 1803.[10] During the Monroes' early married life, Elizabeth was healthy. James Monroe's letters, mainly to fellow Virginians Thomas Jefferson and James Madison between 1786 and 1794, contain few references to Elizabeth's health. There is no reference to a chronic illness. His epistolary references to Elizabeth were then, and would be later, habitually succinct.[11]

Rheumatoid Arthritis

Elizabeth Monroe likely was afflicted by three diseases: rheumatoid arthritis, epilepsy, and a gastrointestinal malady. The first of these is the most documented. Her health problems began during Monroe's terms as governor of Virginia (1799–1803) when she developed "rheumatism." Her symptoms intensified during a March 1803 transatlantic voyage to France, where her husband negotiated the Louisiana Purchase. Elizabeth was thirty-five when this journey commenced.[12]

The age of onset of her illness and her generalized symptoms, including fatigue, convict rheumatoid arthritis as the offender. Unfortunately the specific joints affected and a clinical description of their appearance are missing. Therefore one should conclude that all references to "rheumatism" in this patient's medical history would in today's parlance be rheumatoid arthritis. The first description of rheumatoid arthritis appeared in the dissertation of Augustin Jacob Landre Beauvais in 1800. However, it was not until 1890 that the diagnostic term "rheumatoid arthritis" was coined by the French physician Archibald Garrod.[13]

Immediately upon the conclusion of his mission to France, James Monroe was dispatched to London as American ambassador to the Court of St. James. London's cold damp weather worsened Mrs. Monroe's symptoms, as such weather characteristically affects patients with arthritis. The ambassador was forced to move his family to the English countryside to escape both the dampness and the city's deleterious air quality.[14]

A legendary palliative for arthritic sufferers is bathing in hot springs and mineral waters. The ambassador took his wife and daughters to the fabled therapeutic waters of Bath, England in early 1806.[15] A second visit to therapeutic waters is mentioned in an 1806 letter from Ambassador Monroe to his boss, secretary of state James Madison. The letter also reveals the chronicity and severity of Elizabeth's arthritis:

> The delicate state of my family's health especially Mrs. Monroe's who has been much affected by rheumatism, more than 13 months past … makes it necessary that she should be as little exposed as possible to moisture. It is owing to her indisposition and that of my daughter just before we left London (but who is now recovered) that we passed some time at Cheltenham, whose waters are composed of salts and steel…. These waters are a compound of sulphur and steel, and are said to be excellent in the rheumatic complaints.[16]

"Rheumatism" continued to vex the future first lady after the Monroes returned to America. James wrote to his Albemarle neighbor, Dr. Charles Everett, that Elizabeth Monroe is ill with rheumatism. Later, that March, the husband complained to his Albemarle County neighbor, Elizabeth Trist, that his wife was suffering from rheumatism.[17]

James Monroe served as a very successful secretary of state (1811–1817) during the

Madison administration. Elizabeth, still in her forties, suffered constantly from rheumatoid arthritis. She often ignored the pain and was a good hostess. The wife of a secretary of state had the significant social responsibility of entertaining many of the foreign dignitaries who either resided in or visited Washington in an official capacity. Louisa Adams, Elizabeth's successor as both the wife of secretary of state and president, was also a very good hostess. However, Louisa's talents were similarly eclipsed as first lady, but for a different reason. When Mrs. Monroe's pain was too great, their daughter Eliza would come from Richmond to substitute for her mother at dinners and receptions. A prominent newspaper editor of the time wrote that when Elizabeth was well, she had "an appearance of youth which would induce a stranger to suppose her age to be thirty." In 1815, both Monroes visited the therapeutic mineral springs of Sweet Springs, White Sulfur Springs, and Warm Springs, all then in Virginia. They spent ten days at each spa and the prolonged rest proved beneficial.[18]

When Elizabeth was first lady, rheumatism is cited as a major factor in limiting the size of the 1818 New Year's reception and her absence at her husband's formal dinners during his second term.[19] Controversy continues whether Elizabeth's semiretirement as first lady was due to an illness other than rheumatoid arthritis. However, there is no disputing the fact that her disability worsened during Monroe's second term. Her health deteriorated, leaving her infirm when Monroe began his last year in office.[20]

In late August 1824, an auditor in the treasury confirmed her dire condition: "Mrs. Monroe is very ill. I fear she will die. If she does, the President will not survive her long."[21]

Epilepsy

Many biographers have speculated that epilepsy was a major reason for Elizabeth's disability and inability to function as a first lady.[22] However, a strong inference and later a documentation of epilepsy are found in two letters, written by James Monroe, the first while still president, and the second in retirement. A letter dated September 1, 1824, to physician Charles Everett declared: "Since we have been in London, Mrs. Monroe has had a very serious attack of the kind to which she has been subject of late, in the head, but was recover'd from it, in a great measure, when I left her Saturday."[23]

A December 29, 1826, letter to son-in-law Samuel Gourveneur is more diagnostic. It refers to a "fit," a "convulsion" and implies that the episode was a recurrent event: "[She fell ill] shortly after I left home, of a fit, a convulsion, which was attended with the painful consequences. Occurred unattended in her room and burned herself severely by falling into the fireplace … and found her senseless, at some distance from the fire, incapable of motion. Burned herself very severely in many places. Three days before she could be restored to her senses. 250 drops of laudanum and some glasses of pure brandy, rubbed with spirit, and her feet immersed in hot spirit and water, with a portion of salt in it. She has since been rapidly recovering—her wounds are healing. She still takes fifty drops of laudanum every night." Monroe elaborated that no physician was called but daughter Eliza, the aforementioned surrogate to the first lady, "is altogether ignorant of the disease of convulsive fits, and would wish to know how she is to act, before they come on … before, by great irritability of temper, or deep melancholy, and unhappiness of mind. Mrs. Hay thinks these fits occur once in three months."[24]

Further evidence for epilepsy is theoretical and conjectural. Epilepsy is offered as an explanation as to why first lady Monroe was "alternatively in good, and then bad, condition, and sometimes unavailable for weeks at a time."[25] Biographies that suggest this diagnosis reference no other primary sources than the two letters cited above.[26]

A parallel conjecture argues that rheumatoid arthritis (rheumatism) by itself is insufficient to explain the secretive nature of Elizabeth's disappearances and absences in the White House. Epilepsy, then called the "falling disease," had emotional and mental connotations, and its diagnosis would bring both shame and embarrassment to the affected parties, especially if they were prominent. Therefore "it was natural that it was kept very private, particularly in a first Lady."[27]

Medical Care of the First Lady

A third medical ailment, characterized by a congeries of digestive symptoms, was treated by Dr. Charles Everett. Dr. Charles Everett was James Monroe's Virginia neighbor, friend, political confidante, and occasional physician. His medical care of the first couple during his two-term presidency seems to have been episodic. He was a 1795 graduate of the University of Pennsylvania School of Medicine,[28] and his medical practice was based in and around Charlottesville (Albemarle County), Virginia. Proximity to Monticello and Ash Lawn-Highland exposed both Thomas Jefferson and James Monroe to Everett's professional care. However, the doctor preferred to maintain his Virginia practice rather than move to the nation's capital to tend to the medical needs of his famous patients.

The president and his first lady vacationed at their Albemarle County home during the summer of 1820, and on July 1 Monroe urgently requested the medical assistance of Doctor Everett, who was nearby. Elizabeth Monroe became seriously indisposed with "digestive disorders, particularly her problem with her bile.... So strong are the evidences of a disorder'd bilious affection, that we are induced if you do not forbid it, or we do not hear from you this evening, to give her 10 grains of calomel." On July 9, Monroe wrote the doctor to thank him for bringing medicine. The identity of the medicinals and the nature of Everett's treatment are undocumented.[29]

Curiously, Everett frequented the White House not in the role of a physician but as a political appointee. On December 2, 1822, the president invited Everett, then practicing in Richmond, to move to Washington to become his presidential secretary "in the station lately held by my brother, & after him, by Mr. Governeur."[30] The position paid six hundred dollars a year, and Monroe attempted to make his offer more appealing by offering a good room and other allowances. The president wished that the position were more attractive and concluded the invitation by mentioning their friendship. When Everett accepted his friend's overture is unclear, but a letter to Everett dated November 13, 1823, encouraged the physician to return to the White House since Elizabeth "has been much indisposed." At the time, there was no government payment for a civilian physician to serve as "White House Physician." Perhaps the offered monies as a government employee might have eased this assignment.[31]

The same letter narrated the course of Mrs. Monroe's illness, calling it a "debility of the stomach," then "bile" and finally "erysipelas fixing on her stomach." Weakness, frequent fevers and loss of appetite accompanied her illness. Dr. Henry Huntt, a prominent physician of the District, treated the first lady with stimulants, calomel in strong doses, quinine, tartar emetic plasters, Jennings steam bath and port wine. Most of Huntt's prescriptions exacerbated Elizabeth's illness and only later did the gentler remedies calm her symptoms. Monroe's dispatch to his trusted friend can be interpreted as a plea to preserve his wife from the aggressive practices of an elite Washington doctor.[32] Mrs. Monroe's digestive complaints were chronic and episodic, but remain without a definitive diagnosis. In the nineteenth century, "bilious fever," a bile disease with an elevated temperature, referred to intestinal disorders of any cause, malaria and typhus. What ailed this patient is highly speculative.[33]

After his presidency ended, Monroe's letters frequently mentioned his wife's illnesses, which seemed to be episodic but frequent. The only specificities, other than his 1826 letter to his son-in-law, were mentions of "influenza" and having a "fever."[34] Elizabeth Monroe died six years after leaving the White House, on September 23, 1830, likely from a pulmonary infection. She was sixty-two years old. James Monroe died in New York City less than a year later.[35]

Anna Harrison: The Absent First Lady

Anna Harrison, the wife of General William Henry Harrison, America's ninth President (1841), was one of the antebellum first ladies whose tenure was inconsequential and unmemorable. In her case it was with good reason. She was an absent first lady who never visited Washington, D.C., or entered the White House. Anna Harrison was a first lady only in the literal sense, as the wife of a sitting president, but not in the geographic sense as she never resided in the executive mansion of the United States.

William Henry Harrison was elected president as the top half of the famous 1840 "Tippecanoe and Tyler Too" national ticket. At sixty-eight years of age, Harrison was the oldest incoming American president until Ronald Reagan in 1980. Harrison traveled from his North Bend, Ohio, home to Washington, and as a hardy and sturdy former military commander, proceeded to deliver a lengthy inauguration address in the outdoors and in the rain. Hatless and without an overcoat, he spoke before fifty thousand for one and a half hours. He relied on his physical well-being to shield him. It didn't. He developed a respiratory infection that evolved into pneumonia. He died exactly one month after his inauguration, thus becoming the first president to die in office and the one with the shortest tenure.[36]

Anna Harrison previously had decided not to accompany her husband to Washington. She planned to travel there in May when the road conditions from North Bend to the East would be better. There is a single reference that she was too ill to accompany William's coterie to the nation's capital. This report may be erroneous, because she was in good health and was prepared to travel by stagecoach to Washington when news of her husband's demise reached her. She remained at home to prepare for the president's burial.

Anna Harrison was not enthusiastic over the prospect that William would be president and she first lady. She had opposed his running for the presidency both in 1836 and in 1840. In this she was persistent, saying, "I wish that my husband's friends had left him where he is, happy and contented in retirement."[37] However, disinterested as she was, Mrs. Harrison did contemplate her Washington future. She dispatched her daughter-in-law with her husband to serve as the official White House hostess until Anna's later arrival. The daughter-in-law, Jane Irwin Harrison, was thirty-six years old and a widow.[38]

Anna Harrison was sixty-six in March 1841. She bore ten children, nine of whom survived to adulthood. This number of adult surviving children is a record for a first lady. (Louisa Johnson Adams was pregnant twelve times, but only four children were born alive.) It is unknown whether Mrs. Harrison suffered any miscarriages. She viewed her responsibilities as lying in—and achieved her satisfaction from—the traditional role of mother and wife and as a devoted member of her church. She lived with her children in North Bend, Ohio, when her husband was campaigning during the War of 1812; while he was In Washington serving as a United States representative and senator; and when he resided in Bogotá, Columbia, as U.S. minister.[39]

When Harrison was territorial governor of Indiana, Anna was a successful hostess at the territorial capital. Moreover, her health was robust enough to rear her many children

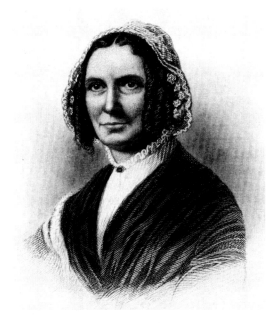

Anna Harrison, wife of William Henry Harrison and also the absent first lady (Library of Congress).

and to manage her household. There is no documentation of any medical illness or any treating physician during her life. She lived until she was eighty-eight and died at North Bend. She outlived all but one of her children.

Margaret Taylor: The Reluctant First Lady

"Betty Bliss agreed to serve as the official hostess in her mother's stead."[40]

Margaret Taylor was another presidential wife during the antebellum period who delegated the performance of her social and ceremonial roles to a family member. Other first ladies of the first half of the nineteenth century were hobbled by physical or mental disability: Elizabeth Monroe was disabled by rheumatoid arthritis and a mystery illness, possibly epilepsy; Letitia Tyler by a stroke; Mildred Fillmore by a leg injury; and Jane Pierce by a crippling depression. None of the members of this quiescent quintet is ranked high in polls of the most successful first ladies.[41]

Twenty-one-year-old Margaret Mackall Smith married Lieutenant Zachary Taylor in Louisville, Kentucky, on June 21, 1810. The Taylors raised a family of five daughters and one son in a series of frontier army posts that stretched from Minnesota to the Deep South. Although the Taylors were determined to remain together, several extended periods of separation were inevitable. One such period was during the Mexican War. General Taylor commanded the United States forces that successfully battled the enemy in northern Mexico. The public fame that resulted from his victories made him a candidate for the 1848 Whig nomination for president. However, Margaret was ready for retirement and so strongly opposed her husband's nomination that she prayed that Henry Clay would get the nod.[42]

Margaret Smith Taylor, this wife of thirty-eight years of an itinerant United States army officer, decided that a public role in the political glare of the nation's capital was not what she fancied as the capstone to a successful and devoted marriage. She designated her twenty-four-year-old daughter, Mary Elizabeth (Betty) Bliss, as her substitute in the spotlight. Betty had recently married Zachary Taylor's military aide, Colonel William Bliss.[43]

As First Lady

Mrs. Taylor was first lady for a brief sixteen months (1849–1850), until Zachary Taylor died suddenly from an intestinal ailment in July 1850. Because she was seldom seen in public, historian Carl Anthony colorfully named her the "Phantom in the White House." Mrs. Taylor discourteously turned down a dinner invitation from the departing James and Sarah Polk the night before Zachary Taylor's inauguration. Moreover, she did not appear at either of the Taylors' two inauguration balls. She did attend the public swearing in of her husband as president.[44]

In private, Mrs. Taylor was the matriarch, but to the press and public she was a nonentity. She ran the business of the White House and focused on the maintenance of the presidential mansion. Her social activities were inconspicuous. The first lady quietly invited a few select friends to visit in the White House and also participated in the informal family dinners. A social excuse of "indisposition" to avoid tiring and frivolous—in her mind—ceremonial events was justified.[45]

It is very unlikely that Margaret took any interest in public affairs, with one exception. She may have influenced her husband to appoint Senator Reverdy Johnson, the husband of her cousin, as attorney general.[46]

Medical History

When Margaret Taylor entered the White House in March 1849, she was already sixty years old. She had previously accompanied her husband to inhospitable military commands around the United States and had borne six children, two of whom died in early childhood and a third shortly after that daughter's marriage. Medical problems did not affect this first lady's behavior or influence her husband's performance and decision making as president.

Malaria, the affliction of many Americans in the late 1700s and the 1800s, affected Mrs. Taylor. She was only one of several future and sitting first ladies of the period to be sickened by this mosquito-borne illness.[47]

Margaret Taylor, her sister, and her four daughters spent the summer and early autumn of 1820 in Louisiana, where both swamps and mosquitoes were commonplace. The entire family contracted "bilious fever," then a popular synonym for malaria, probably of the plasmodium vivax strain. Margaret was so dangerously ill that her soldier-husband rushed to her side, arriving on September 8. Upon seeing his gravely ill wife, he feared for her survival, since "at best her [prior] condition is remarkably delicate." Zachary Taylor's anxiety was merited since two of his daughters perished from the disease in Louisiana shortly thereafter. Octavia, almost four years old, died on July 8, 1820; fifteen-month-old Margaret died on October 22, 1820. Taylor's wife and his daughters Ann Margaret and Sarah Knox recovered. A cryptic remark noted that Margaret pulled through, "though with her health permanently impaired." But afterwards Margaret was healthy enough to become a mother twice more—to another daughter and the Taylors' first son.[48] Fifteen years later a third daughter died from malaria. Sarah Knox Taylor had married United States army officer Jefferson Davis and died in Louisiana shortly thereafter. Her husband also contracted malaria but recovered to lead the Confederacy several decades later.[49]

This first lady-to-be might have had recurrences. In May 1828, she accompanied her husband on a Mississippi River steamer that traveled from St. Louis to his new post at Fort Snelling, Minnesota. While aboard, she was confined to her cabin with the signature malarial symptoms of chills and fever. Other references to Mrs. Taylor's health are few. She reportedly was ill in Louisville in 1830 and was described "in feeble health" in late 1847.[50]

The identity of any physicians either before or during her time in the White House is unrecorded. The Taylors' oldest daughter, Ann, married a military surgeon, Doctor Robert Crooke Wood, who was a graduate of Columbia College of Medicine in New York. Wood was frequently assigned to Taylor's military command during the latter's military career and accompanied President Taylor on his August 1849 political trip to Pennsylvania and upper New York State. It is logical to assume that her son-in-law treated Margaret whenever she was ill.[51]

The ex-first lady's life was brief and inconspicuous to the public. She lived for a time in different locations with several of her children. Her only public appearance as a widow was at her son's wedding in 1851 in Mississippi. She died on August 14, 1852, in East Pascagoula, Mississippi, of an unknown cause. "All of the Taylor family's personal correspondence was stored at her last home which was burned by Union troops during the Civil War." The loss of this primary source material accounts, at least in part, for the dearth of material from Margaret's personal history.[52]

Abigail Fillmore: The Lame First Lady

Millard Fillmore wrote to his daughter Abbie regarding his wife's illness the previous fall and winter and called it "a lameness that may arise from the spine or rheumatic" affliction. "I almost despair of her ever enjoying health again. It is a melancholy and painful thought. I think she will not go to Washington" (January 1849).[53]

Abigail Fillmore was fifty-two years old when her husband, vice president Millard Fillmore, became America's thirteenth president on July 10, 1850. He succeeded Zachary Taylor, who died of an intestinal illness. Mrs. Fillmore was first lady for 32 months[54] and was a more active first lady than several of her predecessors.

Her social appearances, although limited, were more frequent than those of Elizabeth Monroe, Anna Harrison and Margaret Taylor. "Abigail

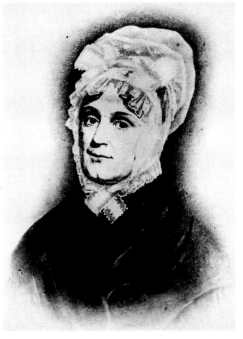

Abigail Fillmore, wife of Millard Fillmore. Her health limited her activities (Library of Congress).

is typical of those first ladies who did not give social affairs a high priority. She minimized her social calendar but still obliged the public and White House guests by offering such popular events." She held receptions on Friday evenings and Tuesday mornings and dinner parties on Thursdays. She hosted New Year's Eve receptions in 1851 and 1852. In addition to the large Thursday dinners, Abigail also hosted smaller dinners for about twenty-nine guests on Saturdays.[55]

A disabling ankle injury made prolonged standing very painful. This prohibited dancing and restrained her ability to receive the numerous guests who attended large official receptions. Sometimes, before a scheduled levee that she could not avoid, she would spend the previous day in bed to buttress her strength for the upcoming ordeal. For some social engagements she pled ill health.[56]

For these events, Mrs. Fillmore enlisted a substitute, which was a common practice of her predecessors. Abbie, her young daughter, age eighteen, became her proxy. Mary Abigail Fillmore was vivacious, well educated, fluent in French, conversant in Spanish, Italian and German, and an accomplished musician. It was an excellent choice by her mother.[57]

A second factor determining which rare public events Mrs. Fillmore would attend was its intellectual benefit to her. Therefore she presided at formal political dinners.[58] More intellectual and learned than her husband, Abigail was an inveterate reader. An intimate of hers remarked, "What Mrs. Fillmore most enjoyed was to surround herself with a choice selection of congenial friends in her own favorite room—the library." Her early reaction upon entering the White House was astonishment that it possessed no library. She immediately set out to correct that and initiated a congressional appropriation of two thousand dollars. Mrs. Fillmore's establishment of a library was a major White House innovation. Upon its completion, she conducted salons where family, friends, and those interested could converse and listen to discussions by prominent authors. These included Charles Dickens, William Thackeray, and Washington Irving.[59]

The first lady's influence upon the president was profound, and her greatest role was as a political advisor to the president, who had "been heard to say he never took any important step without her counsel and advice." She had some influence over his political appointments. However, there was on instance when Fillmore disagreed with the first lady's advice, to his own political peril. She opposed, and he supported, the Fugitive Slave Law as part of the Compromise of 1850. As a result he lost his previous northern antislavery supporters and was defeated for renomination in 1852.[60]

There is no evidence that his wife's illness or physical disability affected Millard Fillmore's conduct of his presidency or his decision making.

Medical History

Abigail Powers was born in upper New York State on March 13, 1798, the youngest of seven children. She was unique among antebellum presidential wives in that she practiced a profession, that of a schoolteacher in Sempronius, Lisle and Aurora, New York. The tall, red-headed Abigail had as one of her students the unschooled carpenter Millard Fillmore. She taught her future husband how to write and speak properly and to use a map to study geography. This first lady's intellectual curiosity never waned, as noted above. In middle age, she learned French and began piano lessons.[61]

The Fillmores' marriage was delayed until after Abigail's thirtieth birthday. The couple had two children: Millard Powers Fillmore (born April 25, 1828) and Mary Abigail "Abbie" Fillmore (born March 27, 1832). Both children lived in the White House during their father's presidency. The future first lady remained in the Fillmore's Buffalo, New York, home during part of Millard's political career in Washington. She did not attend her husband's 1849 inauguration as vice president and, except for a single brief visit to the District of Columbia, she remained in Buffalo while Fillmore was vice president. An ankle injury was a likely reason she remained in her home.[62]

Abigail Fillmore had a significant physical disability that had some effect on the completion of her social and ceremonial responsibilities as first lady. On July 4, 1842, while walking in Washington, she slipped on an uneven sidewalk and turned her foot inward. Her ankle became swollen and very painful; the problem delayed the Fillmores' return to Buffalo at the conclusion of the session of Congress. In Buffalo the injury was exacerbated by a too hasty attempt to walk. The ankle never healed completely and worsened over the months. Mrs. Fillmore was confined to bed for months and, later, for two years she required crutches in order to walk. Pain never disappeared completely for the rest of her life.[63]

Various treatments were tried and then discarded: the application of external liniments; the wearing of silk stockings; the use of oil of Origanian; trips to the sulphurous springs of Avon, New York, in 1844, and Saratoga Springs, New York. The only treatment that was completely effective was bed rest: "The more quiet I was the more comfortable my foot would be."[64] In the era prior to diagnostic X-rays, it was not determined whether the ankle injury was a fracture or a severe sprain.

The family's concern over Abigail's recovery was pervasive. In early February 1843, Millard Fillmore feared that his wife was "apprehensive that she will never be well until she keeps still." Abigail wrote her daughter in late July of the following year: "You must be a housekeeper, if I should never walk again, you are all I have to depend upon and for your own sake I wish you to undertake domestic business." Millard Fillmore did not return to the House of Representatives in 1843, possibly to tend to his crippled wife.[65]

Eventually Abigail was able to stand and walk, but with some difficulty. Her other medical complaints during the 1840s included frequent head colds and a cough. An 1842 letter written by her husband stated that Abigail had a bilious fever, the frequent contemporary name for malaria. However, the illness was not recurrent, and in the absence of a further description, a malaria diagnosis is unlikely. In 1846 she consulted a physician complaining of noises in her ear. She was informed the problem was "mainly a sensation of the nerves and no evidence of apoplexy ... no disease ... inconvenience."[66]

Unfortunately the fall and winter (1848–1849) was a period of serious illness. In a January 1849 letter the incoming vice president fretted to his daughter over "a lameness that may arise from the spine or rheumatic" affliction. "I almost despair of her ever enjoying health again. it is a melancholy and painful thought. I think she will not go to Washington." Persistent cough and headaches complicated back and hip problems, which forced Mrs. Fillmore to her bed for days. Although the family blamed a spinal disorder or rheumatism, a more reasonable explanation would conclude that a postural imbalance due to her injured ankle caused the back and hip pain.[67] Her cough progressed to bronchitis and possibly pneumonia, leading Abigail to write the following depressing sentiment to the vice president on his inauguration day, March 4, 1849: "[P]erhaps another anniversary I shall be numbered with the dead. I feel a presentiment that I shall not see many more."[68]

Abigail's Death

The first lady's health actually was quite good during her relatively brief White House tenure, at least until her last winter as its tenant. In a written letter to his sister after Abigail's death, Fillmore elaborated: "Mrs. Fillmore had not been quite as well as usual during the winter. She suffered considerable pain in her back and the back of her head, and she was restless, and often suffered from want of sleep. A slight cold gave her a cough, and she was occasionally troubled as she had before been for want of breath. The least exertion overcame her and [she exhibited] fatigue."[69]

However, despite her less than hardy health, the now former first lady Fillmore was the first in her position to attend the inauguration speech by her husband's successor. Franklin Pierce, the newly elected fourteenth president of the United States, gave a short speech under a grey sky: "A raw northeasterly wind made the thousands of spectators shiver, and snow fell continuously, melting almost as quickly as it struck the ground."[70] It was on the public stand, in the open, raw air that Abigail caught a chill which progressed to pneumonia followed by death. It was the second first family death resulting from a presidential inauguration.[71] She attended the ceremony accompanied by her literary friends, Washington Irving, the American literary figure, and William Makepeace Thackeray, the English novelist. Washington Irving, in an April 4, 1853, letter to a friend, wrote: "I almost think poor Mrs. Fillmore must have received her death warrant while standing by my side on the marble terrace of the Capitol, exposed to chilly wind and snow, listening to the inaugural speech of her husband's successor."[72]

When the Fillmores vacated the White House, they moved to a suite in the nearby elegant Willard Hotel. Mrs. Fillmore's rapid and fatal progression is best chronicled in Millard's letter to his sister, shortly after his wife's demise. (Fillmore [Buffalo] to Julia, April 12, 1853) His narrative is summarized below.[73]

Two days after the Pierce inauguration, Sunday, March 6, Abigail felt "unwell" and ran a high fever. The next day she attempted a shopping trip but became seriously ill and was forced to return to the Willard. Without any improvement by Wednesday, March 9, the renowned District physician James Crowdhill Hall was asked to make a house call. There is no record of any previous medical relationship with this doctor. Hall returned the following day and after his examination, informed the Fillmores "she had taken cold which had settled upon the lungs, or rather upon the bronchial tubes leading to and perforating the lungs, and should soon be better." He optimistically prescribed medicine and bed rest. Hall's positive prognosis was faulty, as over the subsequent three or four days the patient's cough worsened. A sitting position became necessary for comfort. Hall, alarmed, requested the consultation of a respected colleague, Dr. Thomas Miller. Abigail was subjected to cupping of her back and sides and blistering of the chest with no improvement. Thereafter Drs. Hall and Miller examined the patient once or twice daily. They noted "there was a suffusion of water in the cellular membranes of the lower part of the lungs." This is a classical description of pneumonia.[74]

The pneumonic lungs caused great difficulty in breathing. For the last two weeks of life, sleep occurred only when her head was upon a table, thus keeping the chest upright. Fever continued and fatigue worsened.[75] On the suggestion of John Kennedy, Fillmore's former navy secretary, Dr. Buckley from Baltimore was summoned. He arrived, examined the patient and consulted with the attending physicians. His astonishing conclusion was that in a few days the patient would be restored to health.

The seriousness of the illness finally was revealed in a *New York Daily Times* piece that appeared on March 23, 1853: "On account of the continued severe indisposition of Mrs. Fillmore, the ex–President's Southern tour will be postponed till next month. Perhaps abandoned altogether."[76] The medical condition remained desperate over Sunday and Monday, March 27 and 28, leading to the following letter from Millard Fillmore to his successor, Franklin Pierce, written March 28, 1853:

"She is indeed very sick and I entertain the most painful apprehension of the result. She has not been able to lie down for near two weeks but her strength holds out beyond all expectations and I hope and pray that it may continue until her lungs shall be so far restored as to enable her to take rest in a reclining posture."[77]

Another physician, Dr. Riley of Georgetown, was called to the bedside. Over the next two days Riley cupped and blistered Mrs. Fillmore and applied poultices. Perhaps as a result, her overall condition worsened greatly and the prognosis was that the illness was terminal. Only then were her physicians correct. Former first lady Abigail Fillmore died from pneumonia on Wednesday morning, March 30, 1853,

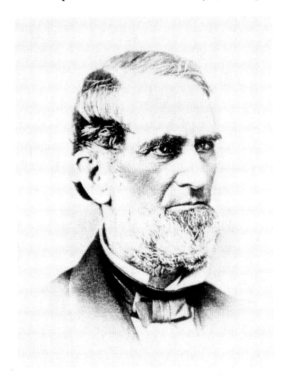

Dr. James Crowdhill Hall, prominent Washington physician. He attended the deaths of Presidents Harrison, Taylor, and Lincoln (courtesy National Library of Medicine).

Thus was the famous Dr. Crowdhill Hall on his way to assume the image of a Zelig or a Forrest Gump. He already had been present at the deathbeds of Presidents William Henry Harrison and Zachary Taylor. Now he was around when Abigail Fillmore died. Later he would be seen at the deathbed of the assassinated Abraham Lincoln.

A curious note, found years later in the Fillmore papers, accounted the payments attached to Abigail's final illness. Dr. Hall, the principal attending physician, was paid $75; his Washington colleague Dr. Miller $103; Dr. Buckley, who traveled from Baltimore, was awarded $75; Dr. Riley was paid $5 for his deathbed examination. The largest payment was to the undertaker, Mr. S. Kirby, for $116.[78]

Conclusion

These four antebellum first ladies left little mark on American history. Due either to illness or disinterest, they often employed surrogates, usually a daughter, to conduct the social and ceremonial functions of a first lady. Their illnesses varied: malaria, rheumatoid arthritis, unspecified gastrointestinal problems, a chronic foot injury, and, probably, epilepsy. Their medical problems had little effect upon the presidential performance of their husbands.

Chapter Five

Depression in the White House

The Sad Stories of Jane Pierce, Louisa Johnson Adams and Mary Todd Lincoln

Nature, Nurture or a Combination?

Jane Pierce harbored a melancholy personality that was exaggerated by her stern Congregationalist New England upbringing. Her clinical depression was fueled by her husband's political career and by the devastating loss of the Pierces' only surviving son in January 1853, just prior to Franklin Pierce's presidential inauguration. Mrs. Pierce shunned her first lady's responsibilities during the first half of the Pierce presidency, and her disposition negatively affected her spouse's performance as president.

In contrast, Louisa Johnson Adams had a happy upbringing, excellent schooling and a loving family. Her marriage to presidential scion John Quincy Adams brought her irregular intimacy, twelve pregnancies and increasing self doubt. Despite this she was a charming hostess both as the wife of the secretary of state (1818–1823) and as the first lady in the White House (1823–1827).

Mary Todd Lincoln's psychological balance was shattered during her husband's presidency. It was cracked with the death of her favorite son, Willie (February 1863), and was broken completely by the assassination of her husband (April 1865). She was diagnosed as a manic depressive and institutionalized by her son.

The diagnosis and treatment of mental disease was rudimentary during the first two-thirds of the nineteenth century. The celebrated and aforementioned Doctor Benjamin Rush was a pioneer whose "An Inquiry into the Effects of Ardent Spirits Upon the Human Body and Mind," published in 1804, earned him the posthumous accolade of Father of American Psychiatry.[1] John Quincy Adams referred this book to his wife when Louisa was experiencing an episode of emotional disturbance. Otherwise, few physicians possessed any insight into the character and assuagement of mental disease. It was not until the 1870s that specialists in psychiatry undertook the care of Mary Todd Lincoln. Previously clergy and spiritualists had attempted to fill this void.

Jane Appleton Pierce

"Mrs. Pierce found Benny lying by his side and saw that something, a seat perhaps ... had taken off the back of Benny's head and killed him instantly." "It destroyed her forever as a functional member of society during the last ten years of her life." (1853–1863)[2]

The role of the first lady in the mid-nineteenth century consisted of managing the household of the executive mansion, supporting the work of the president by maintaining a rigorous social schedule, and attending ceremonial functions. Jane Appleton Pierce fell far short in fulfilling this role. The death of her only surviving son in a train accident made the White House an unshakable burden.[3]

On January 6, 1853, President-elect Franklin Pierce, his wife, Jane, and their almost twelve-year-old son, Bennie, were aboard a train from Andover to Concord, New Hampshire. They were returning to their home after attending a family funeral. The train suddenly lurched and the Pierces' rail car was overturned. Bennie was struck on the head by a flying chunk of metal that shattered his skull. The boy died instantly. His mother saw it all. A strict Calvinist upbringing led her to see everything as the will of God. She rationalized that Bennie's sudden death must have been God's way to relieve her husband of any concern for his child's welfare so he could devote full attention to the presidency.[4] The tragedy emotionally destroyed the physically and mentally fragile Jane Pierce. She was in a catatonic state for days after the accident, unable to function or even speak. Unable to attend her husband's inauguration, she remained in Baltimore for several weeks and was completely gripped by fear. But finally she was able to take residence in the White House as first lady.[5]

Upon her delayed arrival at the White House, the first lady selected two rooms on the second floor for her suite, then closed the door and for the first year was seldom "at home" for anyone. Her depression was overwhelming. She confined herself to her rooms in the White House and became progressively withdrawn and reclusive and increasingly detached from reality. She passed her time sitting at a table almost in a trance, writing notes to Bennie, lamenting his death. Her depression was evident to everyone with whom she came in contact. A longtime friend of the Pierces, Nathaniel Hawthorne, would refer to her as "that death's head" in the White House.[6]

For the first two years of the Pierce presidency, hostess duties fell largely upon Mrs. Abby A. Means, who was Jane's girlhood friend. Abby Means consoled the distraught first lady on her journey from Concord to Baltimore and then to Washington. Abby was widowed, a lady of independent means and social experience. She was persuaded to remain in order to assist the president and first lady. She became one of the first first lady surrogates, but, unlike the earlier Priscilla Tyler, she was not a success. Means held regular receptions and a few socials, but social dysfunction and a somber tone permeated the White House, still in mourning for the president's son.[7]

Jane did not appear at the dining table when company was present. Neither did she give any attention to Washington society nor accompany the president to the customary ceremonial events. Only rare private outings with select intimate friends and her husband occurred.[8] Instead Jane spent her time either in writing to her dead Bennie asking his forgiveness or participating in spiritualist activities in attempting to communicate with Bennie's spirit. She may have held White House séances; there is an uncorroborated report that the infamous Fox sisters visited Jane to conduct a such a session. Reports also claim that she actually was successful in communicating with her three deceased children. A prior psychic premonition had warned that a tragic event would befall the family after Franklin Pierce was elected president. The death of Bennie fulfilled this prediction.[9]

Seventeen days after Bennie's death, his distraught mother wrote: "Oh! You were indeed a part of mine and of your father's heart. When I have told you dear boy how much you depended on me, and felt that you could not do without me—I did not say too much how I depended on you and oh! My precious boy how gladly would I recall all that was unreasonable—or hasty—or mistaken in my conduct toward you. I see surely and I did frequently see afterward that I had wronged you.—and would have gladly acknowledged if only that I feared it might weaken your confidence in me and perhaps on that account not be as well for you."[10]

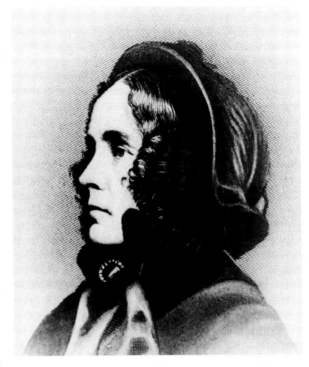

Jane Pierce, wife of Franklin Pierce. Her White House years were marked by deep depression (Library of Congress).

On New Year's Day 1855, after two years of mourning, Mrs. Pierce finally made a social debut, receiving with her husband at the annual White House reception. In August she was well enough to travel to White Sulphur Springs for a week's respite. She again received with her husband at the 1856 New Year's reception. Jane finally had assumed her first lady responsibilities, but only as much as her physical and mental heath would allow.[11]

Jane Pierce's psychotic depression while grieving Bennie's death transpired amid a life of darkness, sadness and disappointment. She suffered from poor physical health, a strict New England Calvinist upbringing, and an austere childhood. In addition, her disappointments were major, including the early deaths of the Pierces' first two sons, her marital mismatch with Franklin, and an alienation from the politics that were the core of her husband's adult lie. Mrs. Pierce was chronically ill, from her childhood through her marriage, in the White House and beyond. Family letters mention her frailty, vulnerability to winter colds, digestive and eating disorders, melancholy, anxiety and sleeplessness. At the time of the Pierce's 1834 wedding Jane was described as tubercular, frail, and in poor health.[12]

From the beginning, Jane Pierce hated the political life of Washington she was compelled to experience during Franklin Pierce's terms as a U.S. congressman and a senator. Her customary reaction was immediate retirement to her room with a bad cold upon her Washington arrival. Her Washington stays were often marked by digestive complaints, vomiting and a lack of appetite. Respiratory infections with cough and fever were frequent. For a considerable part of the 1837–1838 congressional session she was ill, confined to her boardinghouse room. Mrs. Pierce complained at the time: "Oh. how I wish he was out of political life! How much better it would be for him on every account!" She did not recover until reaching "the refuge of the New Hampshire hills."[13]

The only named physician who treated Mrs. Pierce during this Washington illness was Dr. Thomas Sewall, who, according to Jane, "did his best." Sewall had previously attended both first lady Letitia Tyler and her husband, Franklin Pierce. Neither Sewall's treatment nor his diagnosis is recorded. In retrospect Venzke proposed that Jane's respiratory symptoms suggested tuberculosis. Though not a physician, Venzke's diagnostic acumen was expert, since Jane died from tuberculosis in 1863.[14]

Away from Washington when Congress was out of session, Jane visited her sisters in Massachusetts to seek "modern medical treatments" for her physical ailments. One treatment was the application of leeches to remove her "blood toxins." The use of leeches was common during the eighteenth and nineteenth centuries as a form of bloodletting, much milder than either venesection or blistering and cupping. (Medical interest in leech therapy recurred in the 1980s with its use in reconstructive and plastic surgery.)[15]

There is no record of physicians or medical treatment during the Pierce presidency. After the Pierces left the White House they remained in Washington as the guests of William Marcy, Pierce's secretary of state. In the summer, they visited several locations in New England. The death that same summer of Jane's good friend and companion, Abby Means, added to her gloom.[16]

Back home in Concord, New Hampshire, Jane's condition grew steadily worse and a diagnosis of tuberculosis was confirmed. At the time, the only treatment for tuberculosis was a change of climate and, after consulting with her physicians, the Pierces set out in search of a cure. They sailed for Europe in the fall of 1857 and stayed for six months on the Portuguese island of Madeira. For the next few years, they sought respite in Spain, France, England, and Italy. But even the most famous European spas could not restore Jane's health and eventually they stopped in the Bahamas. "All during her travels, Jane thought of her dead children. She always carried a little box containing locks of their hair. She always kept Bennie's Bible with her wherever she went." She died on December 2, 1863, in her Concord home at the age of fifty-seven years, nine months.[17]

Jane Pierce was born into a strict Calvinist New England family. Her father was the pastor of the local Congregational church when, at age thirty-five, he was elected as the second president of Bowdoin College in Brunswick, Maine. Jesse Appleton was driven by duty, first to God, then to the students and responsibilities at the college, and only then to his family. His mission was "to cultivate moral and religious feeling, and to lead them to the knowledge and acceptance of the Savior." His life was austere, his diet sparse, and his sleep limited. He died from tuberculosis at age forty-three in 1815 when Jane was nine. Her mother, Elizabeth Means Appleton, "devoted herself solely to the severer aspects of her religion and to contemplation of the awful fate of those who died without due preparation for the judgment of God." Jane Pierce was familiar with death at a young age, as both her young brother and father died. Her Calvinistic belief in predestination may have tempered her sorrow.[18]

In 1835 Jane was pregnant with the Pierces' first child but was too frail to accompany her husband to Washington when he departed for the new term of Congress. On February 2, 1836, Franklin Pierce, Jr. was born, only to die just three days later. Congressman Pierce remained in Washington and never saw his son. On June 2, 1839, Jane's younger sister Francis

Packard died. At the time Jane, confined to a Concord rooming house, was pregnant with the Pierces' second child. On August 27, 1839, when the Pierces' second son, Frank Robert, was born in Concord, his father again was absent in Washington. Their third son, Benjamin (Bennie), was born on April 13, 1841. When Frank died from typhus at age four in Concord, Franklin was mostly absent, tied up with the U.S. Senate's business in the nation's capital. "The loss of their third and last son unquestionably caused the ultimate destruction of Jane Pierce as a functional member of society."[19]

Jane Appleton was 28 years old when she married Franklin Pierce, a marriage described as a "disaster almost from the start. The couple was completely mismatched—she, a shy reclusive sickly introvert and he an outgoing robust extrovert." The Pierce family was the polar opposite to the Appletons; the good humor of the Pierces contrasted with the Appletons' somberness: "Her husband presented quite a contrast, buoyant, vain, and social, at home in political caucus and tavern.... They were ill-mated, but for thirty years they lived together."[20]

Politics was completely incompatible with Jane's retiring personality. Over her objections, Pierce was elected to the United States Senate and began his six-year term in 1837. Her importuning to abandon politics finally had success when her husband retired from the Senate in March 1842, one year before his term's expiration. For the next ten years Jane was spared the disruption of shuttling with her children between the Pierce's New Hampshire home and Franklin's political responsibilities in Washington.[21]

Jane Pierce's hatred and fear of politics restrained her husband from accepting attractive governmental opportunities. He turned down an appointment to return to the Senate when Levi Woodbury's appointment to the Supreme Court created a vacancy. Subsequently he refused the nomination for governor of New Hampshire, a post his father had held. In August 1846, President James Polk invited Pierce to be attorney general of the United States. He took a week to think it over before he declined. At the time, Jane was in worse health than she had been when he left public life.[22]

Pierce's quest for the 1852 Democratic nomination for the presidency was a shock to his wife, who fainted when informed of his nomination. She fervently prayed for his defeat. Pierce was haunted by his son Bennie's response to the news of his nomination: "[I] hope that we won't be elected for I should not like to be in Washington and I know you [his mother] would not either." When Franklin Pierce was elected the 14th president of the United States "Mrs. Pierce could not stand it; the results were too dreadful."[23]

The presidency of Franklin Pierce (1853–1857) has been universally considered a failure, due in great extent to his inability to prevent the secession of the Confederate states a few years later. Gara, in his history of the Pierce presidency, concluded: "In light of subsequent events, the Pierce administration can be seen only as a disaster for the nation."[24] The C-SPAN rankings of presidential leadership, according to 65 historians and professional observers of 42 presidents, rated Franklin Pierce number 40 and 39 in its 2009 and 2000 polls respectively.[25] "Franklin Pierce ... was bereaved and guilt ridden. This, of course, affected his ability to perform his official responsibilities.... [I]llness, both physical and mental, at times seriously interfered with Franklin Pierce's Presidential duties and responsibilities.... As a result Pierce was a guilt ridden, vacillating and ineffective President. He was one of the least effective in our history [at a] period when strong and effective leadership was desperately needed."[26]

The full extent to which Jane's emotional and physical collapse contributed to President Pierce's inability to thwart the rush to secession and war may never be known. By blaming their son's death on her husband's presidency, Jane caused Pierce to be preoccupied by guilt and sapped of any real motivation. Throughout his administration, as a result, Pierce lost all interest in the presidency and the burning issues of the day. His term unfortunately occurred during a critical and extremely grave period of sectional crisis. By failing to act, he allowed the country to drift toward civil war.[27] "It is probable that he found difficulty dealing with many of the resulting problems, including his wife's persistent depression and almost total withdrawal, exacerbation of his long- standing misuse of alcohol." "Pierce forever had to face Jane's bitterness that his presidency had been 'purchased by the sacrifice of Benny.'"[28]

Louisa Catherine Johnson Adams

"There is something in this great, unsocial house which depresses my spirits beyond expression."[29]

Louisa Catherine Johnson, the second of seven daughters (there was one son) of a prominent American expatriate family, married John Quincy Adams, the son of a sitting American president. The wedding was at London's All Hallows Barking parish church on July 26, 1797. Louisa was twenty-two and had lived mostly in England and briefly in France. She was to set foot for the first time on United States soil in 1801 at age twenty-six. She is the only American first lady born abroad.[30]

Louisa Adams suffered severely from mental disease, characterized as dysthymia, chronic depression, and even hysteria. As one psychiatrist wrote after an analysis of her background: "While I am always hesitant to apply modern diagnostic terminology to historical data, I expect she would today be classified as one of the mood disorder categories, either dysthymic disorder or recurrent major depressive disorder."[31]

Family Matters

The naïve and sheltered Louisa married into the renowned, ambitious, but morose and troubled Adams family

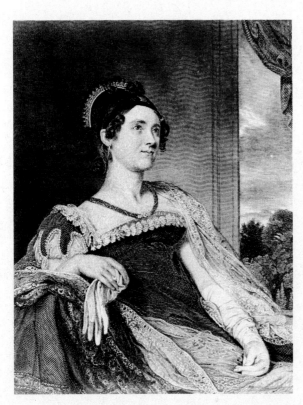

Louisa Catherine Adams, wife of John Quincy Adams. Her White House years were marked by alienation from her husband (Library of Congress).

of New England. Her father-in-law, President Adams, was bipolar. Her driven, ambitious husband, future president John Quincy Adams, suffered from chronic depression.[32] Two of three sons of both the imperious Abigail Adams and the unhappy Louisa died with mental illness. John Quincy's brother Charles died at thirty with alcoholism and chronic depression. The third brother, Thomas, was both an alcoholic and a gambling addict. Louisa's two older sons, George Washington Adams and John Adams, died at early ages. George, at 28, was a suicide, and John, at 31, was a chronically depressed alcoholic. It should be noted on Louisa's behalf that sons George and John Adams were taken from Louisa in 1809 when she went to Russia. For more than six of their formative years both were under the care of her mother-in-law, Abigail, and Abigail's sister, Mary Cranch.[33]

Many years later, reflecting upon her marriage in *Adventures of a Nobody*, Louisa wrote with regret: "I was two and twenty, accustomed to live in luxury without display, and too much beloved by my family for my good." She rebuked herself: "The faults of my character have never been corrected. owing to a happy, but also visionary education: which have made the disgusting realities of a heartless political life, a source of perpetual disappointment." As John Quincy Adams' wife, her nervous system often in turmoil, she blamed herself for the consequent emotional distress that ensnared both Louisa and her husband. She concluded that John Quincy would have been happier had he "not harnessed himself with a Wife altogether so unsuited to his peculiar character." These quotes hint at her physical reaction to stress, considered to be "hysterical" or psychosomatic. It also captures her feeling of inferiority to her husband.[34] Joan Ridder Challinor's doctoral dissertation, "Louise Catherine Johnson Adams," probed Louisa's ambivalent feelings: "The great affection and gratitude she felt because her husband had married her, and her appreciation for his great probity and high-mindedness, constantly warred with the tremendous anger he roused in her by his remote and distant personality." Louisa complained about her husband's self-centeredness and misogyny, opining how utterly tangential were women in his scheme of things: "Mr. Adams has always accustomed me to believe that Women had nothing to do with politics."[35]

The marriage of Louisa Catherine Johnson to John Quincy Adams, although it endured for more than fifty years until his death in 1848, was extremely painful for Louisa. It was a marriage of two dissimilar persons and was dysfunctional more often than functional. Mr. Adams' frequent calls to duty by his country were not matched by more mundane calls to be a devoted husband and an understanding father. A very difficult and insensitive man,[36] aloof from his wife, he either ignored or didn't ask her opinion regarding his major career moves. His acceptance in 1809 of the ambassadorship to the court of the Russian czar was a shock to his wife. Later, Adams' postpresidential election to the House of Representatives in 1830 appalled both Louisa and their surviving son, Charles.[37]

Foreign Affairs

Subsequent to their London marriage, the Adamses relocated almost immediately to the unfamiliarity of Berlin, where he served as ambassador to Prussia for four years. The succeeding nine years, spent in America, were chaotic, with many trips between Philadelphia, Washington, and Massachusetts as John Quincy pursued opportunities in the practice of the law and in the United States Senate.[38] "Louisa was ... small and quite attractive.

Dark-haired, bright-eyed and vivacious, she proved to be an outstanding hostess," not only in the Monroe administration, but also as an ambassador's wife in Berlin, Saint Petersburg, and London.[39] During John's tenure as President James Monroe's secretary of state, "John and Louisa were being applauded as hosts of some of the most successful social events in the town's memory.... The couple's victory was due mainly to Louisa's skill in planning entertainment."[40] She took great pleasure in reading and writing and loved to add spice through storytelling. Moreover, she played both the piano and the harp and was an excellent singer.[41]

In 1809, Louisa accompanied her husband to Saint Petersburg on another European assignment. John Quincy was appointed American minister to the court of the Russian czar, in Saint Petersburg. Mrs. Adams was pressured to leave her two older sons to be educated in America, and was allowed to take her only remaining child, two-year-old Charles Francis, with her.[42] She vividly recollected her departure in *Adventures of a Nobody*: "The day the news arrived of Mr. Adams' appointment ... I had been so grossly deceived, every apprehension lulled—and now to come on me with such a shock! ... Every preparation was made without the slightest consultation with me and even the disposal of my Children and my Sister was fixed without my knowledge until it was too late to change.... I having been taken to Quincy to see my two boys and not being permitted to speak to the old gentleman alone lest I should excite his pity and he allow me to take my two boys with me— In this agony of agonies! can ambition repay such sacrifice never!! and from that hour to the end of time life to me.... Adieu to America."[43]

During her nearly six years in Russia, the future first lady was depressed and self-accusatory and entertained suicidal thoughts, especially after their baby daughter, her namesake, Louisa Catherine, barely thirteen months old, died. Louisa "at times wished obsessively and overwhelmingly to die and be buried next to her child."[44] Louisa's Russian interlude ended in triumph with a forty-day, several-thousand-mile coach journey to Paris in the winter of 1815. Louisa had been summoned to rejoin John Quincy in Paris where he had successfully concluded the treaty that ended the War of 1812. Michael O' Brien's *Mrs. Adams in Winter* vividly chronicles her adventure. She was accompanied only by Charles Francis, just seven, a French-speaking maid, and two men, one a prisoner of war who was being repatriated to his native France, the second a servant. On the way, her expert French was instrumental in protecting her party from a boisterous group of French veterans who were on their way to Paris to welcome Napoleon's return from exile.[45]

John Quincy Adams served successfully as ambassador to Great Britain before his recall to the United States to become secretary of state in President James Monroe's cabinet. The two years in London (1815–1817) may have been the happiest of Louisa's marriage. A transatlantic journey had reunited Louisa's two older sons with her in 1815. From her arrival in Philadelphia (1801) to her departure from Saint Petersburg (1815)—almost 14 years— Mrs. Adams lived as a family with her husband and children for little more than a third of the time. She was with her husband but not all of her children for nearly half the time, and with her children but not her husband a tenth of the time. For three months she was alone, with neither children nor husband with her.[46]

As the American ambassador's wife in her native London (1815–1817), Louisa was "in better health than at any point in her life." Her happiness ended upon her return to the United States. She correctly feared that her husband would again immerse himself in his duties, this time as secretary of state. The marital change resulted in what the family called "fainting fits"—protestations of illness and weakness with concomitant crying: "These neurotic indispositions became Louisa's refuge…. After 1817 began a twelve-year period during which she held little importance in her husband's life and had few ways of helping him."[47]

Pregnancy and Illness

In her first thirteen years of marriage Louisa was pregnant eleven times. Her twelfth and final pregnancy occurred in 1817 when she was 42 years old. It terminated in a traumatic miscarriage in the middle of the Atlantic Ocean as the Adamses returned to the United States. In the aptly titled *Cannibals of the Heart*—Jack Shepherd's examination of this marriage—Shepherd concluded: "[T]welve pregnancies created tension between her and John Quincy, and explain her chronic difficulties and pain."[48] In the early 1800s, the possibility of obstetrical death was significant, a fact surely known by Louisa. Perhaps her mother's successful eight pregnancies provided some comfort. However, her knowledge of English history would recall that King Henry VIII's mother and two of his wives, Jane Seymour and Catherine Parr, died very soon after childbirth.[49]

In the spring of 1817, she was pregnant for the twelfth and last time. This pregnancy was both difficult and painful. Her London physician applied the remedies of the time—bleeding and leeches (see Jane Pierce), and warned that she would die if she undertook an ocean voyage. Nevertheless, she decided to accompany her husband and her three sons to America. The voyage was nearly catastrophic; her habitual seasickness contributed to yet another miscarriage. Louisa became so ill postpartum that she feared she was dying. Louisa was fortunate that Dr. Tillary, an eminent New York physician, was a fellow passenger. He bled her and prescribed laudanum.[50]

Six years earlier, in March 1811, Louisa was pregnant. John Quincy Adams had been unanimously confirmed by the Senate as an associate justice of the Supreme Court. His parents urged acceptance. But this time, Adams avoided a hazardous ocean journey for his wife and declined the appointment.[51] Louisa's pregnancies were always problematical, beginning with her first miscarriage in Berlin: "My husband's time was entirely occupied by his publick avocation. My nurse and one of my Physicians did not speak a word that I could understand, but I was fortunate in having the attendance of Dr. Brown, an Englishman and the then Queens Physician, who bestowed fatherly care and restored me to life." The expectant father was frequently absent during her deliveries. After Louisa suffered four miscarriages, a Berlin midwife was employed to support the birth of George Washington Adams in 1801. The midwife, however, was drunk; her physical technique was so rough that Louisa almost died. For five weeks her left leg was paralyzed and she could walk only with assistance.[52]

Louisa discovered in her childhood that illness brought her the attention she craved, a technique she employed throughout her adult life. During her marriage, migraine headaches and fainting spells were frequent.[53] While in Massachusetts during the interval between her husband's diplomatic missions abroad, she suffered from hysterics, with violent cramps, fainting spells, headaches, and crippling pain in her hands. The latter was treated with laudanum poultices. She also ingested laudanum to compose her nerves both during this period and when she lived in Russia.[54]

On a November 1801 trip from Washington to Massachusetts, Mrs. Adams was afflicted with a severe cough and baby George with acute diarrhea. An impatient John Quincy had to make stops in Philadelphia and New York so the patients could be treated. In Philadelphia, Dr. Benjamin Rush examined Louisa and accurately concluded: "She is under great apprehensions and still more depressed in her spirits than really ill."[55]

Laudanum—discovered by the Swiss-German alchemist Paracelsus in the sixteenth century and popularized by the eminent English physician Thomas Sydenham in the late seventeenth century—was an alcoholic herbal preparation containing approximately 10 percent powdered opium by weight. Synonymous with "tincture of opium," laudanum was used widely in England and in the United States until the twentieth century. Its original uses were as a cough suppressant, a diarrhea cure, and a pain reliever. Eventually its medical indications widened and laudanum was issued principally to produce sleep and to allay anxiety. Mrs. Adams imbibed laudanum for the latter reasons. Although the principal complications of chronic usage are drug tolerance or addiction, there is no evidence for either in Louisa's case. (However, speculation abounds that Mary Todd Lincoln, a chronic and persistent user of the drug both during and after the White House, may have become addicted.)[56]

Commencing in April 1810 and continuing through her years in the White House, Louisa Adams contracted erysipelas, a definitive organic (and not a suspect psychological) disease. Its symptoms were ear pain, deafness, fever, lassitude, and headaches. A painful, very red, and warm swelling affected the face, especially the cheeks and bridge of the nose. It may produce disfigurement. The characteristic appearance of the disease has been recognized since ancient times. Her treatment was brutal—the application of blisters to her head. During the summer of 1824, in the midst of John Quincy Adams' campaign for the presidency, Louisa fled Washington for the mineral waters near Bedford, Pennsylvania. It is not clear whether her month-long stay trying this all-purpose curative was successful. Streptococcus infection is now recognized as the cause of erysipelas and penicillin is its treatment. Unfortunately for Louisa, she was born a hundred years too early.[57]

In the 1821–2 winter the unlucky Louisa was miserable with another condition—painful hemorrhoids. Coincidentally her brother Thomas Johnson suffered from the same condition. He traveled to Washington to seek Louisa's advice since she and John Quincy knew some of the best doctors in America. That June Louisa and Thomas visited Philip Syng Physick in Philadelphia. Physick, like his mentor Benjamin Rush, makes several appearances in this story. "America's most respected and eccentric surgeon. Physick assured Louisa that he had never killed a patient in such an operation."[58]

Physick eventually operated—and then reoperated—on Thomas. Later Physick performed Louisa's hemorrhoidectomy at Mrs. Pardon's rooming house dressed, "as he always did for surgery, in his dark blue coat with bright metal buttons, white vest … and light gray pantaloons." A graphic description of the operation may be read in Shepherd's *Cannibals of the Heart*. The results of these operations, despite their occurrence in the preantiseptic and preanesthetic era, were successful. Louisa wrote in January 23, 1823: "My health is uncommonly good."[59] Mrs. Adams was also appreciative of the doctor who advised "her that sleeping with a husband who insisted on keeping the windows open was what caused most of her illnesses."[60]

When her husband was secretary of state (1817–1824), "Louisa's drawing room became a central area that notables utilized. Louisa loved beautiful music." The Adamses' residence was a "social center when John Quincy was Secretary of State ... wonderful hostess reputation ... music recitals and theater parties." Louisa's success as a hostess was not only social, but also, of more consequence, political: "John Quincy could never have become president without Louisa Catherine's efforts as campaign manager. Louisa Catherine launched what she called 'my campaign' with the political savvy she had developed during a twenty-year career in European courts."[61]

As First Lady

Louisa Adams was a depressed first lady. The contrast between her social involvement as wife of the secretary of state and that of the president was stark and harmful. She was sidelined. As the wife of the secretary of state, Louisa frequently charmed guests with her song and her accompaniment on the piano or harp. After becoming first lady, John Quincy Adams asked her to stop performing. She complied and practiced alone in the evenings, composing music and playing her harp.[62]

The absence of her children, public suspicion of her foreign birth, and limitations upon her previous social contributions made Louisa more miserable and increasingly reclusive.[63] John Quincy was neither completely obtuse nor totally untroubled by his wife's persistent unhappiness. In 1813, he suggested that she read Benjamin Rush's *Diseases of the Mind*. The result was the opposite of his intention. In Louisa's words, "I have read it through although I confess it produced a very powerful effect upon my feelings and occasion'd sensations of a very painful kind. Since the loss of my darling babe I am sensible of a great change in my character and I often involuntarily question myself as to the perfect sanity of my mind in this state of spirits a person is apt to fancy himself afflicted with every particular symptom described ... cast a heavy gloom over me which I much fear nothing will ever correct. In vain I struggle against it. Life has become so barren."[64]

Over a decade later Adams tried again. He consulted an unnamed (presumably his wife's) physician. The doctor, fortunately for him still anonymous, employed with assurance a stereotypically gendered diagnosis. Louisa was a woman who suffered from the "peculiarities of the female anatomy." It was not a dangerous condition, but it resulted in "an excited state from time to time." He implied that his patient suffered from hysteria, a now-discredited diagnosis applied exclusively to women. ("Hysteria" is derived from the Greek "hysteros" referring to the uterus.)[65]

The first family lived quietly in the White House and seldom went out. The first lady declined invitations to outside events and limited her entertaining. But Louisa did not entirely shun her ceremonial and social duties. During the season she gave dinners once a week, fortnightly levees, and an occasional ball, plus the traditional New Year's Ball.[66] Deprived of substantial ceremonial, and even of an insubstantial, political, role, how did she bide her time?

As first lady, she wrote about the demeaning role of women in America. In her experience the then accepted role of women was akin to servitude because women functioned as sexual and domestic slaves of their husbands, who subordinated women out of their own self interest. She dissuaded her niece, who wanted to marry her son John, by writing that marriage had brought her to look forward to death "where sorrow and treachery are no more." She also escaped by eating chocolate: "She spent a lot of time in her room gorging herself on chocolate."[67] During the winters she remained in her White House bedroom for days at a time. Louisa once confined herself for eight days and then again for five days without leaving her room. She preferred to spend the summers in Washington and refused to accompany the president, who summered in Quincy. In 1827, when John Quincy visited Massachusetts, Louisa chose to remain in the White House and rarely exchanged letters with her husband. Later she roamed the Hudson Valley and New Hampshire without him.[68]

In summer 1828, Louisa finally broke under the strain and became alarmingly ill. Her symptoms were mysterious but frightening enough to bring "John Quincy and her sons rushing back to Washington from ... Quincy ... recovering almost as quickly once she captured the attention of her husband and family." Louisa continued, bored, isolated, and angry, in the White House. Her husband and sons dismissed her as a hypochondriac.[69]

Erysipelas erupted again in the White House. In February 1828, Louisa became quite unwell and took to her room. Dr. Henry Huntt, the family physician, gave her an emetic and bled her three times. When his treatments were ineffective, surprisingly he returned to make three house calls. Presumably he continued his regimen of blood-letting. Henry Huntt was one of Washington's most prestigious medical practitioners and later, exhibiting no political predilection, he attended President Andrew Jackson in the White House.[70]

The Adamses' political prominence led to many perquisites that were unavailable to their fellow citizens. An important one was the availability of the best physicians of the times. Louisa was attended by Drs. Benjamin Rush, Philip Synge Physick, and, in the White House, Henry Huntt.

The effects of the presidency upon this first lady were near ruinous. She was depressed, isolated, and suffered from many physical ailments. Did her state of being affect her husband's presidency (which has been judged only modestly successful)? Probably not, as he didn't communicate with her and disparaged the opinions of women.

After the White House

Adams was soundly defeated by Andrew Jackson in the 1828 presidential election. The Adamses' oldest son, George Washington Adams, summoned to Washington to assist his parents' return to Massachusetts, committed suicide instead. In August 1829, on the trip north, Louisa's sorrow over her son's death overcame her. In her distress, she reenacted one of her successful behaviors: midway in the journey "one of those violent attacks which she is subject to with all the family and servants up and trying to assist her in her distress. She complained of coldness about the breast." The Adams party returned to Washington. Next morning she was fully recuperated.[71]

In 1835, after son John's death, "she again, as she had in 1825–8, worried about her sanity." "Louisa was so troubled by life and questioning that she rode into Boston and saw Dr. Harriot Kezla Hunt. Little is known of Dr. Hunt's impact upon Louisa, but we do know that this radical woman physician was 'a zealous little creature' and 'a very peculiar individual' who treated neurasthenic women." Dr. Hunt was trained only by apprenticeship with an English physician. She twice was refused admittance to Harvard Medical School. She opposed heroic treatments, and instead recommended diet, exercise, and regular bathing. In addition to medicine, her passions included women's rights and abolition.[72]

Louisa Catherine Johnson Adams, then a widow, died in the District of Columbia at age seventy-seven on May 15, 1852. A stroke in April 1849 affected her ability to walk and made useless her right hand. She learned to use her left. Subsequently she suffered additional strokes and heart failure. Heavy doses of opiate made Louisa comfortable.[73]

Mary Todd Lincoln

"I owe altogether about twenty-seven thousand dollars…. I must dress in costly materials. The people scrutinize every article that I wear with critical curiosity. The very fact of having grown up in the West, subjects me to more searching observation. To keep up appearances, I must have money … no alternative but to run in debt."[74]

There exist numerous books about Mary Todd Lincoln, and innumerable biographies of Abraham Lincoln, the 16th president of the United States. A thorough review of the Lincolns' marital relationship is far beyond the scope of this essay; instead it will focus narrowly on Mrs. Lincoln's mental illness, its development, progression, and effect both upon her behavior as first lady and upon the performance of Mr. Lincoln as president.

Although the severity and the time of onset of Mary Lincoln's mental illness may be in dispute, there is no disagreement that her life was buffeted by tragedy—the premature deaths of three of her four sons; the assassination of her beloved husband; the undeserved social and political scorn aimed at her as first lady; and the alienation from her Confederate step-family that paradoxically led to suspicion that she was disloyal to the Union.

Physical complaints and illnesses were unusual until later in her life, after the death of President Lincoln. The only previous significant complaint until then was headaches, described as migraine. Robert K. Stone, M.D., was the family physician to the first family, but any medical treatment is unrecorded. From her early twenties on, Mary Lincoln was plagued by headaches. These were occasionally debilitating; they persisted in the White House, and continued until her death. During the early afternoon of that fateful Good Friday in 1865, "despite her fear of an oncoming headache earlier in the afternoon, Mary decided to accompany her husband."[75] Eventually, in 1875, a Chicago jury declared that Mary Lincoln was insane and committed her to a sanatorium. With the author's apologies, this episode will be examined only briefly since excellent detailed analyses of the affair have appeared in book form.[76]

Mary Todd was born in Lexington, Kentucky, on December 13, 1818. Her mother died when Mary was six and a half years old and her father remarried. She was raised in a blended family of many birth and stepbrothers and a step-sister. Mary's birth mother and step-sister died in childbirth. Mrs. Lincoln herself had four successful pregnancies, the last of which produced future gynecological problems.[77]

A major traumatic event was the death of the Lincoln's second son, Eddie, in February 1849. Eddie struggled with tuberculosis for fifty-two days before he succumbed just shy of his fourth birthday. Mary Lincoln was "consumed by her grief—and suffered severe spells of weeping and a lack of appetite." The sorrow prostrated her and was accompanied by a refusal of water and food. Abraham Lincoln's concern over his wife's depression caused him to seek help. He chose Dr. James Smith, a cleric, not a physician. Smith proved to be an effective counselor and steered Mary Lincoln through a difficult period.[78]

For most of the Lincolns' years in Springfield, Illinois, Mary provided excellent political counsel to Abraham: "She kept Mr. Lincoln from making several mistakes that would have been fatal politically." He trusted her opinion, realizing that she was an excellent judge of people, a better reader of men's motives than himself. However, even then she was unpredictable, possessed an acerbic tongue, and exhibited unexpected rage. Gossip had it that on one occasion she chased her husband down a street with a butcher knife in her hand.[79]

As First Lady

Mary Lincoln decided on her husband's inauguration day that she would make the White House, then dismal and in disrepair, a home befitting its role as the residence of the country's chief executive.[80] She immediately accepted the social and ceremonial responsibilities of first lady and held her first White House reception within a week of the inauguration. She presided over weekly levees on Tuesday evenings. In August 1861 she hosted four thousand guests at a reception for Prince Bonaparte, the cousin of the emperor of France. Her role as hostess delighted her and made a favorable impression on most visitors. Early in the Lincoln presidency, Mrs. Lincoln functioned as a political partner, advising her husband, particularly on appointments.[81]

But her patina of prestige quickly faded, for reasons both her fault and not. Mary Lincoln was "brutalized by her husband's critics, the press, and Washington society on both personal and political levels unprecedented in U.S. politics. Her attire, hosting, family life, and friendships were all open to condemnation. The South criticized her for being pro–Union, and the North never truly trusted this former belle from a prominent Southern family. She was simultaneously accused of being pro–Union and pro–South, uncouth and too fancy. She was even accused of treason by the North and received a considerable amount of hate mail and death threats from the South." It did not take long for the first lady to unloosen her vitriolic tongue.[82]

Her political judgment, excellent in the past, became flawed and eccentric. She inserted herself into disputes over postmaster and West Point appointments. In addition, she wrongly advised the president regarding his cabinet selections. Regarding secretary of state William Seward, she opined, "I wish you had nothing to do with the man. He cannot be trusted." Her negative, eccentric, and personal judgments about politicians and others often became public.[83]

Shopping Mania and Debt

Abraham Lincoln's presidential salary of $25,000, more than five times his previous annual income, became prey in Mary Lincoln's quest to gown herself with extravagance to match her new station. In the latter part of January 1861, Mrs. Lincoln went to New York City to shop. In what was an early manifestation of her erratic judgment, she bought expensive dress goods, silks, ornaments, necklaces and earrings. These purchases, together with the inexplicable acquisition of lace curtains for the White House, "used [her] newly acquired credit to the breaking point." In addition, during the first six months of 1861, her seamstress and friend, freed slave Elizabeth Keckley, fashioned fifteen or sixteen new dresses for her.[84]

After her son Willie died, Mary Lincoln engaged in a more destructive pattern of spending. Her shopping sprees were hidden from the president, and for four years, she continued to run up debts: "She bought the most expensive goods on credit, and, in 1864, enormous unpaid bills stared her in the face." As a result, she counseled Lincoln to run for a second term. (In 1863, she owed $27,000, and at the time of the president's death two years later, $70,000.) Relieved after her husband's reelection, she continued her shopping addiction. For the second inaugural ball, she purchased a gown for $2,000 and pearl, amethyst and diamond jewelry from Washington's Galt Brothers Jewelers for almost $3,000.[85] These were enormous sums for the era.

The Death of Willie Lincoln

According to Emerson, the inflection point in Mary Lincoln's mental devolution was the death of the Lincolns' favorite son, eleven-year-old Willie. Mary, incapacitated by sorrow, remained confined to her room for weeks. The president asked Elizabeth Edwards to remain to comfort her sister. Lincoln bent over his wife and pointed to Saint Elizabeth's mental hospital seen in the distance: "Mother, do you see that large white building on the hill yonder? Try and control your grief, or it will drive you mad, and we may have to send you there."[86]

Willie became ill in February 1862. When his illness persisted, the family physician, Doctor Robert Stone, was summoned to the White House. He proclaimed that Willie was better, that he was "in no immediate danger," and that there was every reason for a full recovery. The diagnosis was "bilious fever," most likely malaria. Stone's treatment was Peruvian bark, calomel, and jalap every thirty minutes when the patient was awake. In addition, gentle blackberry cordials were provided.[87] The physician's optimism was in error—neither the first nor the last time that a presidential physician's eminence exceeded his diagnostic or prognostic accuracy. Willie's condition deteriorated, his breathing became labored, and he died. The cause of death was probably typhoid fever. Mary Lincoln was paralyzed: she retreated to her bed. Elizabeth Edwards, her sister, finally persuaded the distraught parent to get out of bed, dress, and attend church services.[88]

In December 1863, Mary's Southern half-sister Emilie visited the White House. Emilie "was alarmed by ... wide and shining eyes during rapturous descriptions of visitations from the dead.... [She] longed to communicate with her dead son Willie—not just in spirit circles, but when he came to her chamber at bedtime."[89] Emilie reported that Mary experienced hallucinations: "[Willie] comes to me every night and stands at the foot of my bed with the same sweet, adorable smile he always had; he does not always come alone; little Eddie is sometimes with him."[90] These hallucinations were probably Mary Lincoln's first truly psychotic symptoms.[91]

In the summer after Willie's death, Mary Lincoln sought the comfort of spiritualism, the belief that one can communicate with the spirits of the dead, especially through mediums. She visited mediums in Georgetown and invited them to the White House to conduct séances. Lincoln was skeptical, but in deference to his wife, he attended a few meetings. Mary claimed communication with her son during these sessions. A constellation of spiritualist stars of the nineteenth century became associated with Mrs. Lincoln. These included the Fox sisters, Charles J. Colchester, Nettie Colburn, Mrs. Laurie of Georgetown, and William H. Mumler of Boston. After the Lincoln assassination, Mrs. Lincoln continued to visit mediums and returned to their ministrations after her son Tad's death in 1871.[92]

Effect on the President

After Willie's death, Mrs. Lincoln became truly eccentric. That was a near universal assessment, by her family, by the White House staff, by official Washington, and by the country. The accepted presumption was that her presence in the president's life placed an additional burden upon him. Her inveterate bluntness and rudeness already had earned her legions of Washington enemies and detractors. After Willie's death President Lincoln no longer received much emotional support from his wife. She lost interest in receptions and refurbishing the White House. Her behavior became increasingly erratic: One day she seemed fine, the following day she would be angry for no apparent reason.[93]

A bizarre incident occurred in late March 1865, soon after the fall of Richmond to the Union army. The first couple journeyed to Union army headquarters aboard the *River Queen*. Amid a military celebration, Mary Lincoln became unhinged; she gave uncontrolled vent to her emotional insecurity and overreacted to any woman's affection for her husband. She became enraged upon learning that Mary Ord, the beautiful wife of the local commander, General Ord, rode alone with her husband. Mary, in a carriage with General Grant's wife, demanded that the carriage stop to let her out so she could upbraid the woman. When the driver refused, the first lady grabbed his arms and physically tried to force a stop. The next day Mary's jealous rage was unabated; in a frenzy of excitement she insulted Mrs. Ord, called her vile names, and stormed at her until Mrs. Ord began to cry. The same night before guests at dinner aboard the *River Queen*, Mary Lincoln "repeatedly attacked her husband for flirting with Mrs. Ord and demanded that General Ord be removed from command."[94]

In contrast to her mental health, her physical health was good while in the White House. There was a single exception. On July 2, 1863, she fell from a carriage that was transporting her from the Soldiers' Home, their summer Washington retreat, to the White House. The driver's seat detached from the front of the vehicle, throwing the driver to the ground. The frightened horses began a frantic gallop. The first lady leaped from the carriage to avoid disaster. A traumatic head injury was the result. Mary was "stunned, bruised and battered, but no bones were broken, and her injuries, which were immediately attended to by surgeons from the nearby hospital, did not appear serious."[95] Her head wound was stitched. Unfortunately, the wound did not heal properly and it suppurated. Her "injuries were now seen to be unambiguously grave, the blow to her head and the shock of the fall much worse than first believed." A physician was forced to reopen the wound and drain the pus. It took three weeks for the wound to heal.[96] The accident was not without untoward side effects. Mary's chronic migraine headaches worsened in intensity and in frequency. Fears for her sanity appeared after this episode. Her son Robert retrospectively suggested that the fall had caused mental impairment and an increasing detachment from reality.[97]

On Good Friday, April 1865, a cataclysm befell Mary Lincoln. As she sat next to her husband at Ford's Theater, a .44 caliber bullet from John Wilkes Booth's single-shot flintlock Derringer destroyed Abraham Lincoln's brain and subsequently extinguished his life. Mary was inconsolable, but cruel protocol compelled her to endure the funeral exercises in Washington and the fifty-four-hour journey of a funeral train from Washington to Springfield, Illinois. Otherwise she remained sequestered in her rooms in the White House for a month, a generosity extended by the incoming President Andrew Johnson. Her only companions were her two surviving sons, Robert and Tad, Elizabeth Keckley, the family physician, Dr. Robert King Stone, and a longtime friend from Springfield and Abraham Lincoln's former physician, Dr. Anson Henry. For the remainder of April, Mary Lincoln could manage to function only minimally, with the constant assistance of Elizabeth Keckley.[98]

Evaluation of Mrs. Lincoln's Performance as First Lady

Davidson and Connor contrasted the effects of bereavement (loss of a child) upon the presidencies of Franklin Pierce and Calvin Coolidge with that of Abraham Lincoln: "Despite Lincoln's own history of depression, his wife's psychiatric instability, attributable perhaps to bipolar disorder, and the fact that he was leading a country at war, Lincoln's overall effectiveness as president was undiminished in his grief."[99]

Mrs. Lincoln's performance as first lady has been judged harshly, albeit accurately, by historians. Watson concluded that she became a liability for President Lincoln as a result of her vanity, insecurity, impulsiveness and public outbursts of jealousy. He highlighted the Ord affair as a glaring example of the disruptions that diverted the president's focus from important matters.[100] In the ranking of first ladies, Mrs. Lincoln sits at or near the bottom. In the 1997 Watson poll, she ranked next to last, barely surpassing Anna Harrison, whose husband was in office but a month before he died. Mrs. Lincoln ranked last in the 1993 Siena Research Institute poll and at only 36 of 38 first ladies in its 2003 poll. Numbers 37 and 38 were Florence Harding and Jane Pierce respectively.[101]

Aftermath

The unhappy tale of Mrs. Lincoln's life after the White House has been more than adequately recorded. To avoid repeating what is widely known, only the highlights of her psychological deterioration are summarized.[102] Mrs. Lincoln's life from the White House until her death in 1882 was devoid of both serenity and happiness. She was nomadic, reclusive, volatile, paranoid and mentally disturbed. On one occasion she was suicidal. In May 1875, her son Robert had her committed to a mental institution, the Bellevue Place Sanatorium in Batavia, Illinois. She was released to the care of her sister four months later.[103]

With a paranoid fear of robbery Mary Lincoln carried the bulk of her net worth on her person for years. Fifty seven thousand dollars in bonds were hidden in her pocket. She accused Robert Lincoln, her sole surviving son, of falsely charging her to the sanatorium so he could steal her money.[104] Psychotic hallucinations reappeared. She admitted to her physician that "an Indian spirit was removing and replacing her scalp, removing the bones from her face, and pulling wires out of her eyes; that someone was taking steel springs from her head and would not let her rest." Additionally, Mary experienced frequent paranoid delusions, e.g., a man had poisoned her coffee on a train, the city of Chicago was burning, a "Wandering Jew" had stolen her purse, and people in her Chicago hotel would harm or kill her. Mrs. Lincoln discussed suicide with Elizabeth Keckley both in 1865 and 1867 and attempted it in 1875 by swallowing a bottle of what she assumed was laudanum and camphor.[105]

If Mary Lincoln harbored a psychiatric illness, what was its specific diagnosis and when did it commence? In appendix 3, titled "The Psychiatric Illness of Mary Lincoln," which appears in Emerson's detailing of Mrs. Lincoln's "madness," psychiatrist James S. Brust claims that she suffered from bipolar disease. He supports this diagnosis by enumerating the diagnostic features of her illness: depression, mania (episodes of compulsive buying of clothes, etc.), its relapsing-remitting course, and its regular cyclic character.[106]

The date that the disease commenced is uncertain. Many of Mary's longtime friends opined that she showed signs of insanity as early as 1860. Another view is that fears for her sanity began after the 1863 carriage accident. Emerson concluded that her intense grief over Willie's death compounded by her traumatic head injury "did not cause her to go mad but did bring her nearer the breaking point." However, Emerson did admit that signs of mental illness started before Lincoln's assassination. Evans determined that Mrs. Lincoln was insane after 1865, a result of two deaths, one violent, that occurred within three years of each other.[107]

Mary Lincoln, with her sons either deceased or estranged, died quietly in her sister's home in Springfield, Illinois, in 1882. She was sixty-four years old.[108]

Chapter Six

Julia Grant and Lucy Hayes

*Healthy, Supportive, Socially Successful
and Minimal Political Impact*

[Julia Grant] Since entering the White House she had worried considerably about her squint. She was much on display in public places. Her photographs were in circulation.[1]

[Lucy Hayes] The only drawback is her frequent attack of sick headaches. Perhaps twice a month she suffers for a day or two.[2]

Introduction

Julia Grant and Lucy Webb Hayes, the wives of Presidents Ulysses Grant (1869–1877) and Rutherford Hayes (1877–1881) respectively, had much in common before and during their years as first lady. Both were women of the American Midwest. Both enjoyed successful and loving marriages, experienced multiple pregnancies, were married to victorious Civil War generals, and frequently visited their husbands in wartime army camps.

However, the education of the two women was different. Julia Dent Grant and her three sisters "were schooled in the domestic arts by their ... mother.... They watched their mother manage her home resourcefully as they prepared themselves for the inevitable goal of matrimony."[3] In contrast, Lucy Webb Hayes graduated in June 1859 with a liberal arts degree from Wesleyan Female College in Cincinnati. She has the distinction of being the first first lady with a college degree.[4]

White House Social Success

Julia Grant and Lucy Hayes were experienced social hostesses when they entered the White House. Both were unaffected and gracious women who honed their sociability as the wives of commanding generals as they comfortably intermingled with his subordinates. The two women had previously lived in Washington, D.C. Julia was the wife of the general of the Union armies; Lucy was the wife of a congressman. She later served as hostess for her husband, then governor of Ohio. During her postwar years in the nation's capital (1865–

1869) Mrs. Grant became friendly with the diplomatic set and learned to cope with the complex social crosscurrents of the capital.[5] Her successor as first lady had alternative training. According to one biographer, "the years as the wife of an Ohio governor prepared Lucy Hayes to become one of the most effective first ladies of the latter half of the nineteenth century."[6]

Consequently both were a success in accomplishing the social and ceremonial roles of a first lady of the United States. During Julia Grant's stay, the White House was restored as the center of Washington's social life. Formal dinners took on an opulence rarely seen before or since and the first lady presided at Tuesday afternoon receptions for the public.[7] Moreover, she renovated and replaced the run-down executive mansion furnishings with enthusiasm and skill: "She not only turned the White House into a comfortable place to live, but made it the focus of the capital's social life."[8] There was even an elegant White House wedding. In 1874, daughter Nellie Grant married Englishman Algernon Sartoris.[9] Julia also was assisted at public receptions by the wives of cabinet secretaries and senators. Significant support and advice was offered by the sophisticated and socially prominent Julia Fish, the wife of Grant's secretary of state.[10]

Lucy Hayes also was a successful social hostess as first lady. Her tenure had an auspicious beginning: Mary Clemmer Ames, a popular columnist for a New York newspaper, was so impressed by Lucy's graceful appearance at her husband's March 1877 inauguration that the writer referred to Mrs. Hayes as "the first lady of the land." Following Ames, other correspondents and many social leaders began to refer to Mrs. Hayes as "first lady." The title stuck and it has adhered since to the wife of the American president.[11]

Mrs. Hayes thoroughly enjoyed her role as White House hostess, but like Mrs. Grant, she discovered that the social schedule had grown to such an extent that she required assistance. Numbers of young matrons, mostly nieces, but also daughters of friends, resided in the Hayes White House; these young, and attractive, young women were employed as social aides by the first lady.[12] After several successful receptions, "Washington reporters began to praise Lucy's competence as a hostess" and appreciate her hospitality and helpfulness. The Hayes also hosted a White House wedding; niece Emily Platt married an Army General on June 19, 1878.[13]

Lucy's most memorable contribution to White House ceremonial lore is her role in continuing the Easter egg roll. Dolley Madison had initiated an Easter egg roll for children on the grounds of the Capitol building. However, when this event on the Capitol grounds was banned for some trivial reason, Mrs. Hayes let word out on the Monday after Easter Sunday in 1877, that children would be welcomed to play egg-rolling games on the White House South Lawn.[14]

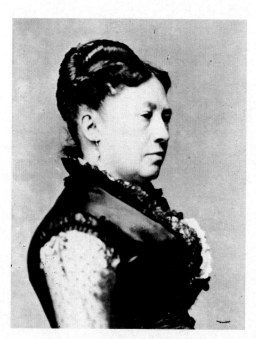

Julia Grant, wife of Ulysses S. Grant (Library of Congress).

Medical Matters and Presidential Influence

Julia Dent Grant and Lucy Webb Hayes were relatively healthy as first ladies. There is no record of either significant illness or medical treatment during their tenures and therefore no history of any difference in care from what was available to any member of the contemporary body politic. The rigors of managing the executive mansion, offering constant support to their husbands, and providing social leadership in the nation's capital did not affect their health. Finally, no illness of theirs affected the political decisions or policymaking of their husbands. But there were medical matters.

Julia Grant

Mrs. Grant experienced, as far as is known, four uncomplicated pregnancies between 1850 and 1858. She was the mother of three sons and one daughter.[15] Her major physical issue was principally a cosmetic one—strabismus. Beginning at a young age her eyes "troubled her considerably. She had a mild case of strabismus [a lazy eye, squint], a defect common enough in the early nineteenth century. She could not sew for any length of time. Moreover, it tired her to do too much reading, and she did not write if she could avoid it. All through their married life the General tried to save her eyes when he could, reading to her, writing letters that normally would fall to her and helping her in sundry small ways." Even in later years her vanity precluded her wearing glasses to improve her vision.[16]

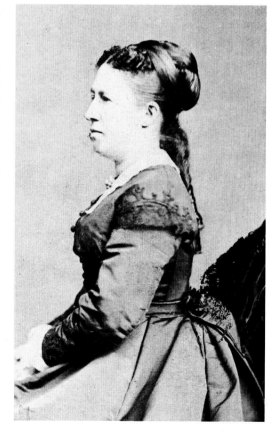

The strabismus did not bother her greatly until she became on display as a public figure. As a result, for cosmetic purposes Julia wished either to hide or to correct her squint. She began to pose self-consciously for portraits to mask any notice of the "lazy eye."[17] "During the war she had consulted Saint Louis physicians about remedying the condition but she had been advised that it was too late. [As first lady] she intended to risk a simple operation in Washington, on the chance that it might be successful. But at the last minute the General overturned everything."[18] Grant's caution may have been appropriate since, at the time in the United States, the surgical correction of strabismus was in its infancy.[19]

Mrs. Grant outlived her husband by sev-

Julia Grant. A "lazy eye" was a cosmetic problem for her. Therefore most images of her were side views of her face (Library of Congress).

enteen years. Late in her widowhood she suffered a severe case of bronchitis that was complicated by heart and kidney disorders. She died in Washington on December 14, 1902.[20]

Lucy Hayes

Mrs. Hayes was pregnant eight times and all pregnancies resulted in living children, seven sons and one daughter. However, only five of the Hayeses' eight children survived to adulthood. Three sons died before their second birthday.[21] Mrs. Hayes long suffered from rheumatism and headaches, although neither significantly affected her performance as first lady. However, these maladies occurred frequently enough for one biographer to state that "the periodic recurrences of this rheumatic condition plus the severe headaches she had throughout the years belie the impression that Lucy possessed robust health."[22]

Mrs. Hayes' most significant medical problem occurred during her eighth pregnancy. A son was born on August 1, 1873, four weeks before her forty-second birthday. This final pregnancy was complicated by severe convulsions both before and after the delivery. A diagnosis of eclampsia, the most dangerous form of toxemia of pregnancy, must be assumed. Her symptoms were so alarming that a second physician was called to attend the patient. Morphine was prescribed to relieve her pain and to induce sleep.[23]

Modern obstetrical care is well aware that an elevated blood pressure is the basis for the eclamptic convulsions. It is very likely that, in the era before hypertension could be diagnosed or treated, Lucy Hayes had long suffered from undiagnosed high blood pressure. Headaches, a common marker of high blood pressure, had bothered Lucy since her mid-twenties. On an 1857 trip to visit relatives in Chillicothe, Ohio, she wrote that her "back felt as though it would certainly give way, and [her] head was in the same condition." Headaches, frequently alluded to in her letters, would become a coda to be repeated during the rest of her life.[24] In 1875 Rutherford Hayes, the soon-to-be president, noted his wife's headaches but did not seem to realize that they were more frequent and severe than before.[25] On Election Day of 1876, when it appeared that Hayes had lost the presidential election, "Lucy retired to her bedroom with a bad headache, a physical torment with which she was on familiar terms." Before his inauguration, the president finally realized that "the only drawback is her frequent attacks of sick headaches. Perhaps twice a month she suffers for a day or two."[26]

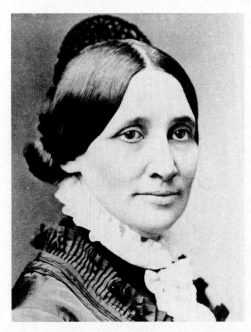

Lucy Hayes, wife of Rutherford Hayes. He commented that his wife "was large, but not unwieldy" (Library of Congress).

The most devastating consequence of high blood pressure is a cerebrovascular accident (stroke). On the afternoon of June 22, 1889, at the Hayeses' Fremont, Ohio, home, the former first lady experienced difficulty with her fingers while threading a needle. She was unable to speak and slumped back into her chair. Conscious at first, she became depressed and frightened. Subsequently she slipped into unconsciousness from which she never recovered. She died three days later; the cause of death was an "apoplectic stroke." She was only fifty-seven years old.[27]

The date of origin of Lucy Hayes' presumed hypertension is unknown, but the condition may have commenced during the early years of her marriage. Her frequent pregnancies predisposed her to this condition, and certainly her eighth pregnancy exacerbated it. Contributing to the likelihood of high blood pressure was a significant weight gain. Mrs. Hayes' weight had increased from 127 pounds in 1861 to 161 pounds in 1875. In mid–1879 her figure had ballooned to 174 pounds, fifty pounds greater than when she was a young matron.[28] It led her husband to comment, "She is large but not unwieldy."[29]

Mrs. Hayes fulfilled the classic patient profile that is a predictor of gall bladder disease: "fair, fat, female, fecund and forty." In 1883, she was unable to attend the annual meeting of the Woman's Home Missionary Society, of which she was president. Rutherford Hayes was informed that she had been attacked "by rheumatism or neuralgia of the stomach."[30] Geer commented that a "modern doctor might have diagnosed as a gall bladder disease."[31]

Lucy Hayes' other chronic and persistent complaint was labeled as rheumatism, but it was likely rheumatoid arthritis. Arthritic complaints had bothered her even before her third pregnancy in June 1858 when she was in her mid-twenties. Two weeks after the birth of the Hayeses' third son, Lucy developed a severe case of rheumatism, an attack similar to the one she had suffered prior to her marriage: "For ten days has had her rheumatism creeping over her from one place to another, giving her great pain. It began in her left shoulder and arm and in her neck." There is no treatment recorded for her rheumatism. Mrs. Hayes did not utilize baths or spas to alleviate her discomfort as others did during this period.[32]

Neither Mrs. Grant nor Mrs. Hayes required the attention of a physician while serving as first lady, although treatment by a military physician was available. Basil Norris, the surgeon general of the army, and Jedediah Baxter, chief medical purveyor, are listed as the Washington family physicians for the Grants and the Hayeses. Both of these military doctors were criticized by their civilian counterparts for providing services or pharmaceuticals to the family of the president, their commander in chief, for free.[33]

Chapter Seven

Tuberculosis

The White Plague Kills Caroline Harrison and Ravages Other First Ladies

Caroline Harrison

> [He] made a thorough examination and left at noon. He says he finds no organic trouble. We all feel much relieved.[1]

Caroline Harrison, the spouse of one-term president Benjamin Harrison (1889–1893), became the second first lady to die in the White House. She died on October 25, 1892, shortly before the voters decided the fate of her husband's reelection campaign. She was sixty years old. The cause of death was a significant infectious disease—tuberculosis. Other infectious diseases, yellow fever and malaria, that challenged the well-being of preceding first ladies, would be controlled or eliminated in the United States soon after Mrs. Harrison's demise. Tuberculosis, after experiencing a precipitous decline in incidence during the twentieth century, remains today an occasional public health concern.[2]

In contrast to the previous White House decedent, Letitia Tyler, who was an absentee mistress of the executive mansion, Mrs. Harrison prominently and effectively fulfilled the social and White House managerial responsibilities of a first lady. She imaginatively enhanced the decor and the ambience of the White House; moreover, she represented the first lady as a person of significance in public, community, and charitable affairs. Indeed, according to Watson, "Caroline Harrison may be the most underrated first lady of all time."[3]

Tuberculosis Infects a First Lady

The questions of why, when, where, and from whom the first lady contracted the infection remain unanswered. One frequent risk factor, a positive family history, was present. Franklin Gardner, the first lady's physician, confirmed "the Scott family, of which Mrs. Harrison is a member, has a consumptive vein running through its otherwise sturdy stock.... A number have succumbed, however, to the latent consumptive characteristic of the family." Both Mary Scott, Caroline's younger sister, and Capt. Henry M. Scott, a younger brother, died with tuberculosis (then frequently called consumption).[4] No other infectious contacts have been identified. However, Mrs. Harrison was active at the Garfield Hospital in Washington until 1887 while her husband was a United States senator. Consequently the possibility of exposure to a tuberculous patient cannot be excluded.

Mrs. Harrison's health was rarely robust. Her physical well-being was a frequent concern of her husband. Consequently, Benjamin Harrison accelerated the plans for their 1853 wedding: "If I marry Carrie now ... the relief it would bring to her bodily health ... would restore her health."[5] Increased anxiety over her health during the Civil War almost forced General Harrison to request a leave. Significant periods of illness persisted during his term as senator (1881–1887). However, there is no record of her symptoms, diagnosis or treatment.[6]

The medical record became clearer during her White House years. She suffered from respiratory ailments, especially in 1891. During that summer, the president informed a political confidante that he did not wish to run again, "being naturally influenced by an ailing Mrs. Harrison." Dr. Gardner was quoted in the *Indianapolis News* obituary of the first lady that the final illness began in the winter of 1891 with a cough that was assumed to be an attack of the grippe. Mary Dimmick's diary entry for December 29, 1891, was precise: "Mrs. Harrison sick with cold and too ill to go downstairs."[7]

Mrs. Harrison was well enough to preside at formal White House dinners on February 16 and April 6, 1892. The development of "catarrhal pneumonia" with pulmonary hemorrhage forced her absence from all March social events. Her presence at the April 6 dinner was marked by a frequent cough and noticeable pallor. It was the last White House social event that the first lady was able to attend.[8]

The Dimmick diary entries, although neither astute nor medically informed, are the best source of Caroline's physical deterioration. Immediately following the April 6 dinner, Mary Dimmick began her constant attendance upon her seriously ill aunt. Diary entries and a letter recorded Caroline's mental state: "suffers much from depression, the effects of malarial fever," "still very depressed and nervous," and "very nervous and ill all day." In a letter to a relative, Dimmick wrote, "She is in a state of melancholia."[9]

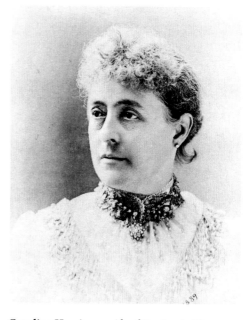

Dr. Gardner was a homeopathic physician by training and practice. When Mrs. Harrison's lung infection worsened, Gardner requested an urgent consultation on May 1 from fellow homeopath Doctor Francis E. Doughty of New York City. Doughty was considered to be an expert in the treatment of the unlikely combination of pulmonary and nervous disorders. At the time, he was serving as professor of surgical gynecology at the New York Homeopathic Medical College and Hospital.[10]

There was intermittent improvement in Mrs. Harrison. But when there was a relapse of Caroline's "bronchial trouble" both Drs. Gardner and

Caroline Harrison, wife of Benjamin Harrison, was the second first lady to die in the White House. Tuberculosis was the cause (Library of Congress).

Doughty were urgently summoned to her bedside. Despite his illustrious professional pedigree, Doughty's diagnostic and prognostic skills were missing from this case. He "made a thorough examination and left at noon. He says he finds no organic trouble. We all feel much relieved."[11]

Untreated tuberculous may be both intermittent and progressive. Caroline's condition characteristically improved over the next several weeks although she spent most of her time in bed. Finally more appropriate therapy was introduced: A special train carried the presidential party to the fresh air and peaceful rural surroundings of Loon Lake in New York State's Adirondack Mountains. Mary Dimmick continued as the first lady's constant companion. The president, Dr. Gardner, and a nurse were often present. Initially this change of scenery was salutary and her temperature, fever and cough all improved.[12]

Inevitably, the disease progressed. Pleurisy struck in early September. On September 14, a suction pump under cocaine anesthesia drained fluid from the right pleural cavity. Caroline Harrison's prominence assured high-level medical consultations even in the remoteness of the Adirondacks. Dr. Gardner was joined once again by Dr. Doughty and this time by the highly regarded tuberculosis expert, Dr. Edward Trudeau, from his nearby Saranac Lake sanitarium. It was Dr. Trudeau who finally made the diagnosis of pulmonary tuberculosis. It was nine months after Caroline's initial symptoms and five months after its serious nature became apparent. In addition, Trudeau declared her prognosis to be dire and any further treatment to be hopeless. For the first time the Harrison family became alarmed. The diagnosis of tuberculosis was announced to the public. President Harrison had previously censored all medical reports of his wife's illness.[13] "Unaware of her true condition, Mrs. Harrison often remarked that 'if they would only take her back to Washington' she would get better."[14] A special train returned Mrs. Harrison to the White House on September 20. Upon her arrival, Gardner's examination determined that her right lung was completely consolidated; later the left lung also became diseased. Her final five weeks were marked by a continuous cough, a high temperature, a rapid heart rate, and a distressed respiratory rate of 50–60/minute. Gardner was in constant attendance at the patient's bedside and issued "progress" reports several times daily. Prior to Mrs. Harrison's demise, Gardner stated defensively, "We did all that could be done, faced with the certain knowledge that will cure consumption." Caroline Harrison died in the White House on October 25, 1892, just three years after becoming first lady.[15]

Tuberculosis in the Nineteenth Century

During the late nineteenth century tuberculosis was a public health emergency in the United States. Called "The White Plague," "The White Death," and "Captain of Death," in 1900 it was the second leading cause of death, trailing only deaths caused by pneumonia and influenza. Its annual death rate was 200 individuals per about 100,000 population. A U.S. public health estimate for the 1880s indicted the White Plague as the eventual killer of one-seventh of the total population and one-fourth of the adult population. One medical historian predicted that nearly one-half of the adult population in large American cities would contract tuberculosis at some time in their lives.[16]

Before the introduction of antibiotic therapy in the twentieth century, the only accepted and useful treatment was confinement of the patient to a sanitarium, away from society, where a combination of fresh air, a good diet and rest would be salutary. The most famous and respected U.S. sanitarium was Dr. Edward Trudeau's Adirondack Cottage Sanitarium at Saranac Lake, New York, started in 1884. Trudeau, the son of a prominent and wealthy family, personally cared for his beloved older brother Francis, who was terminally ill with tuberculosis. Trudeau decided upon a medical career, graduated from Columbia's College of Physicians and Surgeons, and became a junior partner in a fashionable New York City medical practice. He was diagnosed with pulmonary tuberculosis in 1873, and "realizing that I had only a short time to live, I yearned for the wilderness I loved." Trudeau secluded himself in the Adirondack mountains of northern New York State. He discovered that resting, fishing and hunting brought a remission, and the following year he returned there with his family.[17]

Around 1880, Trudeau began to have patients referred to him at Saranac Lake by an eminent New York physician who had previously treated him. Subsequently Trudeau began to build his treatment cottages and set up a research laboratory. His fame grew. Trudeau's aim was to cure tuberculosis by diagnosing it at an early stage: "I realized that if I was to try to obtain curative results I must confine the admission of patients to incipient and favorable cases as much as possible, and refuse to take the acute and far-advanced cases."[18] Therefore Trudeau decided that any treatment for first lady Caroline Harrison would be hopeless and destined to fail. President Harrison likely understood this decision. In a March 22, 1899, letter to Trudeau, he requested that a former servant, a widow of modest means, suffering with "incipient tuberculosis" be admitted to the Saranac Lake sanitarium. The ex-president wrote: "She has not the means to seek her health unless she can exchange her services for treatment and a salubrious climate."[19]

The Homeopath Dr. Franklin Gardner

Why Caroline Harrison selected thirty-three-year-old homeopathic doctor Franklin Gardner, a native of Massachusetts, as the physician to treat her pulmonary disease is unknown. The only previous physician to be associated with her care was Dr. Thomas Addis Emmet, but Emmet practiced in New York City and his expertise was gynecologic surgery. President Harrison was in good health during his presidency. His nominal physician was army colonel Jedediah Baxter, who had taken care of him when Harrison was a senator.[20]

Most likely, the onset of Mrs. Harrison's pulmonary disease in early 1892 initiated a search for a family physician. Caroline may have preferred the gentler, patient-oriented treatment philosophy of homeopathy over the rigorous therapies of allopathy; perhaps the first lady had met Dr. Gardner socially and liked him; perhaps it was a decision by the president.

Franklin Gardner graduated from the Homeopathic Medical College of New York in 1882 at age 24 and shortly thereafter moved to Washington, D.C. His medical practice was successful, "his patrons including many persons prominent in official and social life." His professional reputation was a good one, and Gardner was identified as "the best known homeopathic physician of Washington." His reputation gained invitations for the doctor and his wife to several formal social events at the White House, a dinner on March 18, 1892, and a reception for Indiana poet James Whitcomb Riley on April 1, 1892. The first lady became seriously ill shortly thereafter.[21]

Despite his inability to either diagnose or treat the tuberculosis of Caroline, Gardner remained on good professional and personal terms with the president. The physician was summoned to the White House two months after Caroline's death to treat Harrison's granddaughter for a mild case of scarlet fever. Moreover, during 1898 and 1899 Gardner and ex–President Harrison exchanged several friendly social letters. The gracious ex-president also retained a high regard for the inept Dr. Francis Doughty. When Harrison, his second wife, and their infant daughter developed upper respiratory infections on a visit to New York City in 1897, Doughty's medical care was requested. On this occasion, the doctor was successful. The family recovered. In 1896 the widower married Mary Dimmick, his wife's companion and niece. She presented the sixty-four-year-old Harrison with a daughter, Elizabeth, a year later.[22]

The homeopath-allopath conflict was an incendiary matter that inflamed the Washington medical community during the latter decades of the nineteenth century and beyond. Gardner attempted to escape the controversy, and his cooperation with the eminent orthodox physician Edward Trudeau on Caroline Harrison's case may have been an indication. However, acrimonious contention was unavoidable. Editorials in the *Medical Mirror*, an orthodox medical journal, criticized both President Harrison and Edward Trudeau, an active member of the New York State Medical Association, for hiring, and consulting with, a member of an irregular medical sect: "I regret ... that the case ... could not have been under the care of members of the regular profession whose attainments were of such order as to command a national reputation, instead of irregulars, as irregular in this day and age is another name for mediocrity."[23]

Vesico-Vaginal Fistula

Caroline Harrison was pregnant three times. Her pregnancies in 1854 (son, Russell), and 1858 (daughter, Mary), although successful, with the delivery of two healthy children, were very demanding upon the mother. She was under close medical care during the latter pregnancy, requiring the borrowing of money to pay for medical expenses and a lengthy stay at the Harrison ancestral home in Ohio. Subsequent to Mary's birth, Caroline's father wrote her brother: "Your Ma has not yet returned, as Carrie has been dangerously ill. She is now nearly recovered." A third pregnancy, in 1861, resulted in a stillborn daughter. There were no further pregnancies.[24]

Pregnancy was a significant medical matter for America's early first ladies. Fortunately, for these women and for all their female constituents, obstetrical management and prenatal care improved markedly with time. However, even in the mid-twentieth century, Jackie Kennedy was beset with complications in four of her five pregnancies.

Twenty-two years after Caroline's final delivery, the future first lady was hospitalized for three months in a New York City hospital where she underwent an operation to correct what was probably a vesico-vaginal fistula. A vesico-vaginal fistula is a traumatic forced connection between the urinary bladder and the vagina. Patients with this condition experience unremitting pain, urinary incontinence and may also exhibit constitutional symptoms.[25] The evidence for this diagnosis is circumstantial but persuasive. Mrs. Harrison was under the care of Dr. Thomas Addis Emmet, the national expert, in the surgical correction of this problem. At that time, the principal cause of this malady was difficult or prolonged obstetrical labor. The pre- and postpartum care for both of Mrs. Harrison's live deliveries were lengthy; by inference both were difficult.[26]

Dr. Thomas Addis Emmet, an 1850 graduate of Thomas Jefferson Medical College, Philadelphia, was considered the preeminent gynecological surgeon of the last quarter of the 19th century. He was surgeon in chief to many public hospitals in New York City, including the Woman's Hospital, the first hospital in the world dedicated solely to gynecologic disorders. When he retired, Emmet estimated that he treated almost one hundred thousand women during his career.[27] An appreciative Benjamin Harrison expressed his gratitude in a June 13, 1883, letter to Emmet: "I am glad to be able to say that my wife seems to be in better health than she has enjoyed for years." The letter enclosed a draft for $415 as payment for services rendered to Caroline Harrison.[28]

As First Lady

"Caroline Harrison compensated for her dull, dour husband and charmed guests at the White House. She was intelligent, personable, and an active donor to charities. Mrs. Harrison left a legacy of accomplishments, including the redecoration of the White House, the initiation of the White House china collection, and the founding of the Daughters of the American Revolution."[29]

The diplomatic community valued her courtesy and grace, and foreign visitors appreciated her dignity. Until her illness she was active in greeting visitors almost on a daily basis; she hosted state dinners and was present during the annual New Year's receptions at the White House. Dancing was reintroduced at the Harrison White House and Caroline selected the music for the White House entertainments.[30]

This first lady was a gifted artist who lent her own design to the official state china collection. She built support for a renovation of the then decrepit White House by giving public tours of it herself and inviting members of Congress to examine the condition of the building. She was convinced that the old building was near collapse and immediately began researching architectural improvements. She set in motion plans for adding east and west wings that were implemented ten years later. Additionally, she introduced electricity to the mansion.[31]

In her zeal as mistress of the White House, Mrs. Harrison may have exposed herself to illness, and perhaps even to the tubercle bacillus. She personally examined, selected and supervised the restoration and preservation of valuable forgotten relics—furniture, silver, glass and china, many of which were stored in the unventilated basement. The kitchen in the basement was completely remodeled; plumbing was repaired and accumulated mold was removed; the attic was cleaned. The first lady personally supervised much of the refurbishment. The White House was so rat infested that ferrets were introduced to destroy the rats. "During her years in the White House, Mrs. Harrison frequently suffered from respiratory ailments that some outsiders attributed to her spending too much time in the clammy basement and dusty attic while she pursued her renovation efforts." Moreover, she painted on textiles and tapestries, a process that involved using solvents; the fumes undoubtedly contributed to her pulmonary distress.[32]

Caroline Harrison was considered by many to be an asset to her husband's political career. In 1888, Harrison received the Republican nomination for president. Thereupon he successfully challenged incumbent president Grover Cleveland and won the presidency with the majority of the electoral vote. (However, in the popular vote count he trailed Cleveland by over one hundred thousand.)[33]

In June 1892, at the Republican National Convention in Minneapolis, Harrison was renominated on the first ballot. Grover Cleveland was again his Democratic opponent. The 1892 presidential election was unique in which two presidents, former and serving, opposed each other: "Most voters seemed to agree that either candidate would fill the presidential chair with credit, as indeed each already had done."[34]

Caroline Harrison was severely, and then fatally, ill with tuberculosis during the entire 1892 presidential campaign. She died in the White House on October 25, 1892, less than two weeks before the November election. Subsequently, Grover Cleveland defeated her husband with 46–43 percent of the popular vote, and with a substantial margin in the electoral college. From July 6 until September 20, 1892, Mrs. Harrison had been treated at Loon Lake in the Adirondacks. After that, she was bedridden in the White House until her death. President Harrison was extremely attentive to his moribund spouse, making many trips from Washington to Loon Lake and then attending at her White House bedside. In a close election, every doubtful state called for Harrison's presence to make at least one speech; instead he remained at Caroline's side.[35]

An important question is whether his wife's illness significantly contributed to Harrison's election defeat. Most commentators think it did not. His opponent, Grover Cleveland, graciously limited his own campaigning upon knowledge of Mrs. Harrison's sickness. Instead, commentators ascribed Harrison's defeat to widespread labor strife and his unpopular support of the McKinley Tariff. Andrew Carnegie, the steel magnate, summed up the election results: "I fear that Homestead did much to elect Cleveland." After the election, Harrison commented, "Indeed after the heavy blow the death of my wife dealt me, I do not think I could have stood the strain a re-election would have brought."[36]

Did Mrs. Harrison's fatal illness affect her husband's decision-making? Scholars hold divergent opinions regarding Mrs. Harrison's influence in political matters and service as a presidential advisor. However, most, including this author, have classified her as the "Partner in Marriage." That is a first lady who was inactive in politics. She was a personal, not a political, advisor whose influence was limited to social, personal and ceremonial affairs. Therefore the answer is that her illness did not affect her husband's decision-making.[37]

Tuberculosis and Other First Ladies

The White Plague infected two other 19th-century first ladies, Jane Pierce and Eliza Johnson. Mrs. Pierce was chronically unwell and there were suggestions that tuberculosis was the underlying cause. A definite diagnosis was made only in 1857; the Pierces spent the last six years of her life in travel to balmy foreign destinations in a vain quest for a cure.[38]

Eliza Johnson was the wife of Andrew Johnson, who succeeded to the presidency (1865–1869) upon the assassination of Abraham Lincoln. Mrs. Johnson, pregnant with their fifth child, "developed a condition known in those days as 'consumption.' Today we would call it tuberculosis.... Eliza probably first noticed that she was coughing a great deal and feeling more tired than usual. She sometimes had a slight fever." She was forty-two years of age. A chronic persistent cough, sometimes with a bloody sputum, continued to weaken her. She tried to avoid Washington while her husband served there as a senator representing Tennessee, as "she believed that she was more likely to recover in the fresh mountain air of Tennessee."[39]

As first lady, the ill Eliza spent most of her time in her room, where she read, embroidered, sewed and knitted. She almost entirely relinquished her social and ceremonial responsibilities; her daughter, Martha Johnson, was the official White House hostess. Eliza's illness continued after the Johnsons left the White House, and she died in January 1876 at age 65.[40] (Almost a century later, in 1962, former first lady Eleanor Roosevelt developed a strange disease whose prominent features were severe anemia and a fever of unknown origin. Although suspected pre-mortem, it was only at autopsy that a diagnosis of "disseminated tuberculosis acutissima," involving the lungs, liver, kidneys, brain, and bone marrow was made. Mrs. Roosevelt was seventy-eight years old.)[41]

Chapter Eight

Ida McKinley and the Audition of the First White House Physician

Her world was dimmed by bromides, a medicine prescribed to prevent the dreaded grand mal seizures, whose side effects left her with dulled wits, skin rashes, headaches and the ever-ready petit mal seizures[1]

Navy Physician Presley Rixey Becomes the First White House Physician

Navy Captain Dr. Presley Marion Rixey was assigned to the Washington, D.C., Naval Dispensary. Out of necessity, the doctor supplemented his meager pay as a military physician by active moonlighting among the capital's civilian elite. Secretary of the navy John D. Long and his family were patients of Dr. Rixey. In autumn of 1898 Secretary Long and his daughter were scheduled to accompany President William McKinley and the first lady on a trip to Atlanta, Georgia. The young daughter of Secretary Long had recently been ill. Self-interest directed Long to ask the president whether a physician would accompany the presidential party: "Upon consideration, the President expressed himself as also of the opinion that it would be desirable for many reasons to identify a medical man with the party, and having no one in mind himself asked Mr. Long to suggest some doctor." Long's choice of Dr. Rixey was no surprise.[2]

Shortly thereafter, during a chance meeting between President McKinley and Doctor Rixey, the president inquired why the doctor had not accompanied the McKinleys on a trip to New York City the previous week. When Rixey responded that he had not received the required travel orders, "the president informed the physician that he wanted him to be his attending physician and also take care of Mrs. McKinley who had been an invalid for many years."[3] President McKinley's solicitude for his wife, Ida, was due to her long and unpredictable history of epilepsy.

Thus the serendipity of a substandard navy salary was combined with a presidential wife's need for frequent medical attention to establish the position of White House Physician. Previously the presence of a physician at the White House had been both irregular and transient except in cases of acute emergencies caused either by a dire infection or by an assassin's bullet. In contrast Rixey made regularly scheduled visits to the White House and became a customary member of the presidential party on the first couple's travels and vacations. Although this title had been conferred upon previous doctors who had attended the president,[4] it was Dr. Rixey who first fulfilled the responsibilities of the position as we recognize it today. A result of Rixey's regular attendance was his establishment of dedicated medical treatment space in the executive mansion.[5] The doctor acknowledged that the medical care of the president and first lady was his primary professional responsibility: "As to the White House physician, he must always sink his own interests in that of the health of the President and of his personal and official families. In other words, his desires, pleasures, and all other duties must be subordinated and devoted to this special service."[6]

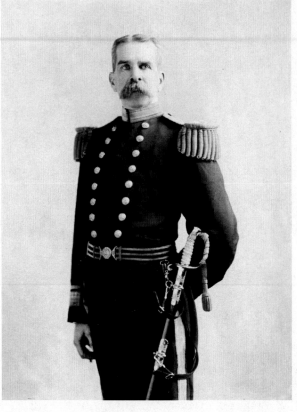

Admiral Dr. Presley Rixey whom McKinley asked to provide constant care for his wife (courtesy Bureau of Medicine and Surgery Archives).

Rixey provided the following description of his daily responsibilities: "This duty was in addition to my already large practice quite a task and comprised all that was related to the health of the inmates of the Executive Mansion, in addition to my duties as Surgeon in charge of the Naval Dispensary. My special care was the President and Mrs. McKinley. By direction of the President I made at least two visits every day, the first at 10:00 a.m., and the second at 10:00 p.m. and as many more as required.... The evening call was always in evening dress, as I would find the other guests so attired ... and I was expected to remain until Mrs. McKinley had retired with her maid."[7]

Ida McKinley was Rixey's principal patient at the White House. Before McKinley's assassination in 1901, the president was significantly ill only once. In early 1901, William McKinley developed a severe cold that evolved into influenza. McKinley was seriously ill and was confined to his bed for several days. It was another week before he was able to fully resume his work schedule. [8]

The Epilepsy of Ida McKinley

Ida McKinley was an epileptic from the age of twenty-six. This major illness struck suddenly at the conclusion of her second pregnancy. Her difficult labor resulted in the birth of the second McKinley daughter. But, shortly after the successful parturition in 1873, a

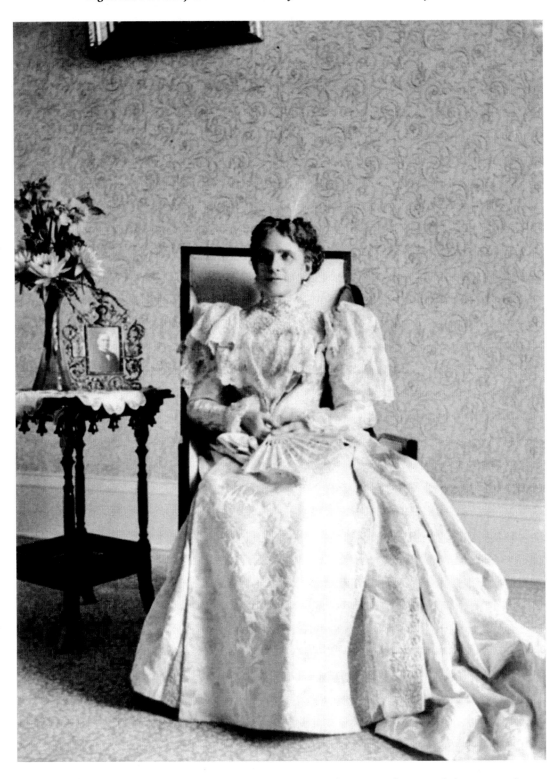

Ida McKinley, wife of William McKinley. Epilepsy and a stroke at an early age made her extremely dependent upon her husband (Library of Congress).

neurologic catastrophe felled the future first lady. She lost strength both in her right hand and in her right leg, the leg weakness impairing her ability to walk. The attack resulted in lifelong disability. Photographs of Mrs. McKinley from about this time invariably showed her right hand partially out of view. Concomitantly, seizures and severe headaches occurred, both of which increased in frequency and reappeared for many years. The convulsions were described as both large and small.[9] Unidentified "nerve specialists" consulted at the time of onset made an outlandish diagnosis of "phlebitis," i.e., an inflammation of the veins.

The tragedy was incomplete until five months later, when Ida, the infant daughter, died.[10] Unfortunately, the McKinleys' first born, their older daughter Katherine, died three years later at the age of five and a half. The McKinleys' misfortune continued; Ida was never again pregnant.[11] Ida McKinley had suffered a cerebrovascular accident (stroke) which caused irreversible damage of her left brain. The result was right-sided weakness, most noticeably of her right hand, and epilepsy. The epileptic attacks were frequent, occurred at irregular intervals, and of two different types. The most common form presented itself as a stiffening of the body, an alteration of consciousness, and a hissing sound. This clinical appearance is typical of petit mal epilepsy.[12] In contemporary medical parlance petit mal seizures are now designated "absence seizures." The characteristic clinical appearance is a vacant stare, the absence of motion without falling, and occasionally hand movements and small movements of both arms. The seizure lasts for only a few seconds and full recovery is almost instantaneous. Subsequent to the seizure, the patient exhibits no confusion but has no memory of the incident. Absence seizures are frequent and may occur often in a single day.[13]

Ida McKinley's convulsions were not all characteristic of petit mal attacks. Some were described as "big" and "prolonged and violent," but were neither specific nor diagnostic of grand mal epilepsy. Dr. Rixey elliptically referred to these as "other ailments." This situation is analyzed later in this chapter.[14]

DeToledo raised the possibility of toxemia of pregnancy as a significant precursor of her cerebrovascular accident. Studies have documented an increased incidence of stroke, especially hemorrhagic in type, in the six weeks after pregnancy. This corresponds with the time line of Mrs. McKinley's attack. The predominant risk factors are severe pre-eclampsia and eclampsia (toxemia of pregnancy), in which the systolic blood pressure measures 160 mm mercury or above. One article insisted that these pregnant women deserved immediate and special attention, intensive care, and antihypertensive therapy to reduce the stroke risk. Unfortunately, during the 1870s, there were no methods to measure blood pressure, and even if there had been, both effective antihypertensive drugs and intensive care hospital units remained far in the future.[15]

Thereafter, Ida's health fluctuated greatly, consistent only in its inconsistency and uncertainty. "Although she was never well, she was sometimes better." Five years after the death of her first child and her mother, Ida's physical condition deteriorated rapidly. Her health was variable when her husband was congressman and then senator. However, she was healthy enough to care for the Hayeses' younger children when Lucy and her husband were away from the White House. But shortly thereafter, she suffered a seizure so severe as to warrant a real fear for her life.[16]

Future first lady Ida McKinley, in the public eye as the wife of U.S. representative (1877–1883, 1885–1891) and then Ohio governor (1892–1896) William McKinley, consumed large quantities of bromides to control her epilepsy.[17] Sir Charles Locock in 1857 was the first to announce, at a meeting of the Royal Medical and Chirurgical Society in London, the anticonvulsant properties of potassium bromide. Incidentally, Locock was the obstetrician to Queen Victoria. In the latter half of the 19th century bromide was used on an enormous scale for the calming of convulsions and other cerebral disorders. Its use by a single hospital amounted to several tons a year.[18]

During Ida's years as first lady, bromides, barbiturates, lithium and other drugs were used to restrain her. She was difficult to control when in physical pain or experiencing a seizure. After sedation "she became milder, but her mind was duller. Apparently, she had to be sedated because of how much she insisted on appearing in public and how unsure they were of her behavior."[19] Bromide therapy had significant side effects: lethargy, somnolence, loss of appetite, clonic seizures, psychosis, acne and dermatitis. In 1912, phenobarbital was acknowledged as a better drug with which to treat epilepsy, and bromide is no longer approved by the Federal Drug Administration as an anti-epileptic.[20]

Epilepsy: Not a "Politically Correct" Diagnosis

McKinley's diagnosis of epilepsy was not released to the public during her husband's lifetime and newspapers avoided any hint of this diagnosis. An unctuous *Los Angeles Times* article was typical: "After the birth if their last child Mrs. McKinley was told that she might never be able to walk again. She was young then, and hope was buoyant, but the doctor's prophecies were true. For over a quarter of a century Mrs. McKinley has never walked unsupported.... For an invalid she has always displayed a remarkable constitution and will power. She always traveled with the President, if it was only for a day's journey. She has never allowed her illness to close the doors of her home to social life."[21]

William McKinley never gave a name to his wife's illness. He was consistently taciturn about her health and responded to inquiries by politely by saying that she "was not so well," or that she "was feeling better." In his autobiography, Rixey mentions no specificity regarding the first lady's chronic and acute fainting illness. It was many years later, after Ida's death, that he revealed that she suffered from "a mild form of epilepsy."[22]

Many were the euphemisms employed by contemporaries and biographers: "a condition of semi-invalidism"; "invalidism due to an irremediable condition"; "periodic attacks"; "in danger of a collapse"; "invalid"; "delicate"; and "fainting spells." Ida's niece, Kate, did not suspect her to be an epileptic and was both horrified and then resentful when, in later life, she heard the diagnosis applied to her aunt. When she heard the allusion, Kate thought it a slander spread by the Democrats: "The words, epilepsy and fits were spoken only in whispers. The press, of course, could not touch the subject."[23]

Epilepsy, a disease well described in antiquity, presently afflicts an estimated 2.2 million individuals in the United States.[24] For centuries, epileptics have been stigmatized as being possessed, usually by evil spirits or the devil. Epilepsy was linked to aggressive or criminal behavior, abnormal sexual history, hereditary degeneracy, and a specific "epileptic personality." It is only in the past half-century that epileptics' restrictions against marriage and employment have been removed. This explains the reticence about Mrs. McKinley's diagnosis. The Monroe White House may have practiced a similar reticence.[25] Rixey cooperated completely with the obfuscation: "[T]he White House Physician should clearly have it understood that he will give out nothing in regard to the health of the occupants of the White House except though the president's secretary, and then only when it is of such importance as to demand bulletins signed by the official physician and consultants.... In this way the public, which has a right to the information, is kept advised in no uncertain way and nothing is given out that might unduly alarm or affect social or business life."[26]

Rixey's Care for First Lady Ida McKinley

In 1893 McKinley sent his wife to New York City for intensive medical treatment. There she was treated by Dr. J.N. Bishop, "with whose potions she was liberally dosed for years." Bishop was an Ontario born allopathic physician who was first a teacher, then a Florida businessman, and eventually a medical student at the Long Island College of Medicine. It took him a year longer than the usual two required at that time to complete his degree since he traveled to Florida in the winters to look after his considerable business interests. His specialties were the curious combination of nervous diseases and female disorders—diseases of women.[27] Bishop continued his treatment of Ida McKinley, mainly by correspondence. Her husband willingly paid his large bills because the medicine "agreed with" Ida. Bishop's "potion" probably consisted mainly of bromide, the usual antidote for epilepsy at the time, together with various sedatives. A calm remoteness became characteristic of the first lady's mood, but the petit mal attacks continued.[28]

When Rixey assumed control of Mrs. McKinley's care, he insisted on the formula for Bishop's potion. It was compounded personally by the New York practitioner, who, unsurprisingly, wished to retain secrecy of its components. Rixey informed McKinley "he could not take any responsibility of a case which was being treated by administrations unknown to him." Consequently, the desired information was obtained. The White House physician first restricted, and then ceased completely, the administration of Bishop's compound, and Ida McKinley improved.[29]

Presley Rixey quickly gained the respect and trust of the first family: "Mrs. McKinley always had a sweet smile for Dr. Rixey, and he noticed and appreciated it. The President, too, warmly approved of his treatment. For one important thing, Rixey had cut down on the bromides on which Mrs. McKinley had formerly been so dependent. He had made a special study of her case, and was tireless in his attendance. McKinley had the utmost respect in his professional judgment."[30]

Near-Catastrophic Illness in California

After his 1900 reelection, McKinley planned a 10,581-mile transcontinental railroad tour, scheduled to begin on April 19, 1901, with a return two months later. Rixey was concerned about Mrs. McKinley's ability to withstand such a journey, but he eventually acquiesced to the McKinleys' wishes. All went well until the presidential party reached the California coast, where an abscess on the first lady's thumb led to a fever. The abscess was lanced, but dysentery followed, the fever recurred, and the patient's condition weakened precipitously. President and Mrs. McKinley abruptly left Los Angeles by special train on May 12. Mrs. McKinley was brought to the comfortable San Francisco home of Mr. Henry Scott, who had traveled westward with the McKinleys. Her physician despaired: "I soon had my patient where we could make the best fight for her life. Her strength was going fast."[31]

The first lady's condition deteriorated over the next three days. The distressed Rixey called to her bedside three of San Francisco's elite physicians—Doctors Henry Gibbons, Clinton Cushing, and Joseph Hirschfelder: "More than once we almost considered our patient hopeless, but heroic efforts prevailed." The White House physician initially released reassuring and bland statements to the press, but the consultants recognized that the first lady had developed sepsis (blood infection) from the thumb abscess. In the pre-antibiotic era, sepsis was a frightening, often fatal, diagnosis. In confirmation of the seriousness of this diagnosis, the patient's "pulse failed and she sank into a stupor. Further medical consultation was hastily called, and heart stimulants were administered." The president's West Coast relatives were summoned and tentative plans for a funeral train to Washington were discussed.[32] However, the patient rallied. Updates released through the Associated Press on May 17 were hopeful.[33]

On May 25 the patient had recovered sufficiently to start back to the White House. Rixey was careful to assure future historians of his diligence: "I had left nothing undone to make the trip safe, a special train, two trained nurses, everything that could be needed in an emergency—even a tank of oxygen was put on board. The train was to run slow or fast or be sidetracked as the patient's condition demanded." He added the following: "Her condition on arriving at the White House was as good or better than when she started."[34] Rixey's optimistic recollection is contradicted by his urgent request for expert consultation upon the McKinleys' return to Washington. Drs. William Sternberg, Walter Reed, and William Johnson were called in to advise on the case. Sternberg, after listening to Ida's heart and obtaining the results of blood cultures, made the diagnosis of acute bacterial endocarditis. An anonymous White House visitor pessimistically reported "Mrs. McKinley was in a very grave condition. There was hope of the outcome … but it was a very slender hope."[35]

The White House physician remained silent regarding Mrs. McKinley's symptoms, her diagnosis and the recommendations of the medical consultants whose expertise he had requested. Rixey's medical reputation did not suffer. "In spite of his errors in diagnosis, he remained the beloved physician and the ultimate authority on Mrs. McKinley's health." In early June, McKinley decided that he would take his wife to their Canton, Ohio, home to recover. A newspaper reporter noted both the pallor of her face and unmistakable evidence of her recent severe illness as she boarded the train to Canton.[36]

During her protracted serious illness, the first lady was the beneficiary of medical care unavailable to her peers in the public. She received VIP care both in San Francisco and in Washington, D.C. Six influential physicians, three in San Francisco and three in Washington, assisted the White House physician with her treatment. In California Rixey might have initially diagnosed Mrs. McKinley's problem as gynecological. This may account for the consultations of Drs. Henry Gibbons and Clinton Cushing, both professors of obstetrics and gynecology at area medical schools.[37] The third consultant, Dr. Joseph Hirschfelder, educated in Germany, was a specialist in infectious disease.[38]

In Washington, Presley Rixey apparently had a better grasp of his patient's condition. His consultants were principally infectious disease experts, not gynecologists. Doctor George M. Sternberg was America's pioneer bacteriologist. Major Walter Reed was a preeminent specialist in the field of infectious disease. He graduated from the University of Virginia School of Medicine at the precocious age of 17 and subsequently studied infectious disease at Johns Hopkins School of Medicine under Dr. William Welch, the preeminent American scientist of the age. Reed was head of the Yellow Fever Commission, which had just proved conclusively that yellow fever was transmitted by a mosquito vector. Dr. William Johnston was a busy and well-respected Washington medical practitioner, and a longtime professor of medicine at the District's Columbian University.[39]

The Death of the McKinleys

The first lady recovered just before President McKinley's assassination and death in Buffalo, New York, in September 1901. Presley Rixey consoled and protected Ida McKinley during a prolonged aftermath. The now former first lady was heavily sedated but was able to undergo the trials of the McKinley funeral services in Buffalo, the funeral train to Washington, the public services there, and the trip to Canton, Ohio, and his public burial.[40]

Not only did the White House physician accompany Mrs. McKinley to her Canton home, he remained there until her emotional and physical condition stabilized. Moreover Rixey, who remained the White House physician under McKinley's successor, Theodore Roosevelt, visited her occasionally by order of President Roosevelt. The visits to Canton continued until her last illness: "I was constantly in communication with her family physicians in Canton, Ohio, Dr. Phillips and Dr. Portman, and with her nurses, Miss A. Moses, and Miss Maud Healy."[41] Dr. Rixey was present at the deathbed in Canton when Ida died on May 27, 1907.[42]

First lady Ida McKinley reaped the benefits of her prominent position: The constant attendance of Dr. Rixey; VIP care both in San Francisco and Washington D.C.; and the oversight of the presidential physician during her widowhood. Such advantages were far beyond the imagination of her fellow citizens.

Her "Other Ailments": Hysteria or a Conversion Disorder

The "other ailments" ascribed to Mrs. McKinley by Dr. Rixey[43] referred to significant, often dramatic, fits and spells that exceeded both in duration and in intensity her stereotypical petit mal epileptic attacks (absence seizures). These episodes were atypical for grand mal epilepsy and most likely had no organic cause. "It is not clear whether her condition was entirely one resulting from a mild case of epilepsy or was psychologically induced, or a combination of both."[44]

Ida's dependency upon William McKinley and his reciprocal care, tenderness and constant vigilance were well known. Her dependency was brewed with a strong dose of jealousy. In the White House the first lady created logistical problems because she refused to have women companions in attendance,[45] Leech's biography related an episode from years earlier: William McKinley mentioned a good-looking woman that he had seen at the funeral of President James Garfield. His statement provoked in Ida a fit of hysterics that culminated in a severe "epileptic" attack.[46] Another episode occurred at the McKinley home in Canton in 1898. Congress was in session, which prevented the president from accompanying his wife to Ohio. She developed such violent convulsions that the doctors in attendance feared for her life. McKinley rushed to his wife's bedside to find her unconscious. William sat with her, rubbing her hands and caressing her forehead. Sometime later Ida opened her eyes, grasped his hands, and remarked, "I knew you would come." She recovered.[47]

After President McKinley's death from an assassin's bullet, Ida, interestingly enough, never again experienced the epileptic seizures that disabled her throughout her marital life. She lived for almost six years after her husband's demise. During her widowhood there was no documentation of seizures or fainting episodes. This suggested to one author "that they may have largely been emotionally and psychologically induced."[48] Her atypical fits were dramatic and usually occurred when distanced from her husband, either by geography or by transient inattention while talking to someone else, especially another woman. Mrs. McKinley's behavior is reminiscent of that of a previous first lady, Louisa Adams, who employed "hysteria" and physical outbursts to gain attention.[49]

Hysteria is no longer a recognized diagnosis. Many other diagnostic terms instead have been applied. These include hysterical epilepsy, hysteroepilepsy, nonepileptic seizure, pseudoseizure and psychogenic seizure.[50] The most applicable diagnosis, currently in use, for Ida McKinley's behavior, is "conversion disorder." It is defined as "clinically significant symptoms affecting voluntary motor or sensory function in which psychological factors are associated. The latter initiates or exacerbates the symptoms. The symptoms are medically inexplicable."[51] Moreover, conversion behavior can be superimposed upon epilepsy so that a confusing pattern results. A sustaining element for a conversion disorder is having a partner "who believes in the patient's illness and constantly supports it…. So after President McKinley died that would explain the disappearance of Ida's 'hysteria.' You'd expect there to be some secondary gain from the symptom."[52]

A First Lady Conflicted Between Her Aspirations and Her Physical Constraints

Mrs. McKinley insisted on playing the role of first lady, attending dinners, meeting with visiting dignitaries and even accompanying the president on trips outside the White House, including travel by train across the country. Her hostess activities were augmented by the helpful presence of the vice president's wife, Jennie Hobart, or one of the visiting Saxton or McKinley nieces.[53]

Previously, as the wife of the governor of Ohio, it was widely acknowledged that Ida McKinley was an invalid who was unable to discharge the ceremonial and social duties of a governor's wife. She lived in semiretirement and made only perfunctory appearances at the governor's official receptions. She spent her quiet hours crocheting.[54] The incoming first lady was unable to manage the 1897 inaugural ball. She fainted, and her husband picked her up and took her home. There was little White House entertaining in 1897. In preparation for her husband's 1901 inaugural ball Ida was heavily sedated. She was observed sitting propped up in a chair overlooking the crowd.[55]

Occasionally special visitors were permitted to call on her in her private quarters in the White House, where she sat in a wooden chair. She spent her time compulsively crocheting bedroom slippers, several thousand over a lifetime. She gave them away, mainly to charity. Another hobby was cleaning her jewelry.[56] Major adjustments to White House protocol were made to accommodate the first lady. Tradition required the president to escort the guest of honor to the dinner table at formal dinners with the first lady to sit opposite. Instead Ida sat next to William so that, if a petit mal episode occurred, the president could cover her face with a handkerchief and continue his conversation until the attack passed. Moreover, if a significant seizure took place, the president could unobtrusively escort her out of the room. Additionally, instead of standing at official receptions, she greeted people while seated.[57]

Historians have rated Ida McKinley's performance as first lady a seriously flawed one. Recent surveys listed her 32 of 36 and 32 of 38 rated wives.[58] Watson classified her as a Behind the Scenes Partner. This type of first lady is active and supportive of her spouse's political activities but is not a public participant in political or presidential affairs. Such a first lady's partnership is private and personal in nature, and, away from the public, she is a powerful, influential force in the White House.[59]

The First Lady and the President

Ida McKinley's health problems had no adverse effects upon her husband's political career. The public was kept unaware of her diagnosis. Contemporary newspapers and magazines were silent about Ida's epilepsy. The McKinleys kept her medical problems a private matter and the nature of her problems was never publicly exposed. The only descriptions of her malady were incidental observations of visitors. The country at large knew only that her health was "delicate."[60]

On the other hand, the president's devotion to his wife enhanced the public's appreciation of his character. His solicitude for her well-being became well known and met with widespread approval. "He spent his free hours sitting in stuffy rooms and driving in closed carriages because she avoided fresh air. Her headaches often required him to pass the evening in the dark. McKinley learned how to support his wife's weight on his arm, timing his quick step to her faltering pace, and how to hold her head, when her temples throbbed with the pressure of an oncoming attack."[61]

Little is known about any policy advice Mrs. McKinley may have confided to her husband, other than that General Leonard Wood should be selected to lead the military forces of the United States in Cuba and that the Philippines should be retained at the conclusion of the Spanish-American War. In both cases, he accepted his wife's advice.[62]

Chapter Nine

Strokes, Stress and Smokes

Nellie Taft and Pat Nixon

Two first ladies, Nellie Taft and Pat Nixon, who entered the White House sixty years apart, were dissimilar in ambition, family background, and political engagement. Mrs. Taft coveted the presidency for her politically unambitious husband, William Taft. However, it was Mrs. Nixon's husband, Richard, who strove inexorably towards the presidency while his wife occupied a supportive, but not a leadership, role in his political ascendancy. Nellie came from wealth; Pat's family was, at best, lower middle class. Future first lady Taft was conspicuous in political maneuvering; Pat Nixon remained in the background.

Two similarities pair first ladies Taft and Nixon in this chapter. Both suffered disabling strokes, one as she commenced her White House responsibilities, the other soon after her husband resigned the presidency in disgrace and she was attempting to reestablish her personal life. Both smoked cigarettes at a time when this habit was unfashionable for women. They were not the only first ladies to do so, but they were the ones to suffer the medical consequences of this habit.

Helen Herron (Nellie) Taft: A Formidable But Frustrated First Lady

"Given four years of good health and sustained hard work, she might have reshaped the role of the first lady decades earlier than Eleanor Roosevelt or Lady Bird Johnson did."[1]

Family Background and the Early Marriage Years

Helen Herron, born July 2, 1861, was the third of eight surviving children of the upper-middle class Herron family of Cincinnati, Ohio. Called "Nellie" almost from the start, she grew into a formidable, focused and free-spirited woman who was a determined feminist, well before that designation was birthed.[2]

Her father, although not a politician, enjoyed important political friendships. The Herron family were White House guests of President and Mrs. Rutherford Hayes during Christmas 1877. Both tradition and her biographies recount that the sixteen-year-old Nellie determined that the next time she resided in the White House, it would be as first lady.[3]

She focused her quest for marriage upon finding a mate whose qualifications matched her ambition. Her focus and talent enabled her to found and successfully manage the Cincinnati Symphony Orchestra, to become a well-loved wife of the governor of the Philippine Islands, to beautify the District of Columbia with thousands of Japanese cherry trees, and to be the first first lady to publish her memoirs.

Nellie rebelled against the cultural straightjacket imposed upon young women of economically comfortable families living in 1870s and 1880s Cincinnati. Instead of remaining at home awaiting marriageable young men to woo her, Nellie Herron slipped into taverns in the working-class district of Rhineland. During a Newport, Rhode Island, vacation in 1880, she experimented with drinking alcohol, smoking cigarettes and gambling at cards.[4] Frustrated with being an intelligent and ambitious young upper middle-class woman in late-nineteenth century middle America, with very limited prospects for furthering her education or initiating a career, she defied the constraints of her mother and taught, first as a substitute in French at Madame Fredin's school, and subsequently full time at the newly opened White-Sykes School for Boys.[5]

Photographs taken at the time depict a handsome, though not beautiful, woman of slight build. A striking feature is her constant dour, unsmiling and determined facial expression. Determined to introduce an intellectual facet to her life, she organized and led regular meetings of young upper-class men and women to discuss the political and cultural happenings of the day. In this setting she met wealthy Yale Law School graduate Will Taft. After a long audition, Nellie decided that the genial Will would provide her ticket to the White House.

William Howard Taft married Helen Herron on June 19, 1886. A few months later, Ohio governor Joseph B. Foraker appointed the new groom to a vacancy on the Ohio Superior Court.[6] Taft's preference was for the law and the courts; his wife's was for politics and the executive. For the next twenty years, Nellie campaigned to steer her husband's ultimate professional goal towards the presidency and not towards the chief justiceship of the U.S. Supreme Court. She won most of the battles with her occasionally recalcitrant husband. Ironically, for Taft, achieving the presidency was only his penultimate goal; appointment as chief justice became his ultimate career accomplishment.

The Tafts became parents of three distinguished children. Robert was born in Cincinnati on September 8, 1889, and weighed eight pounds. There were no recorded problems with either this or her two subsequent pregnancies. Helen was born August 1, 1894, and the second son, Charles Phelps, followed on September 20, 1897. Robert was a longtime United States senator from Ohio; Helen earned a doctorate in history from Yale and became dean and, later, head of the History Department at Bryn Mawr College. Charles became an attorney and, later, a prominent civic leader in his hometown of Cincinnati.[7]

Health Prior to the White House

Prior to May 17, 1909, there are few hints of any illness. According to Mrs. Taft's two biographies, her autobiography, her correspondence with her husband and contemporary newspaper reports, Nellie Taft was a very healthy woman.[8]

Nellie Herron Taft, inveterately determined and ambitious, easily became moody when bored. Anthony's excellent biography refers to Nellie's self-described "blues" during her late teenage years.[9] In the summer of 1881, she identified the roots of her dark moods: "It was simply that I was not busy…. Now when my time is not fully occupied I fall back into the same fate." In 1904 there were hints of poor health and ennui evolving into depression. After the Tafts left Washington in 1909 for New Haven, where Will taught law at Yale, both her husband and daughter worried that Nellie, without responsibility, would tend towards depression. Their solution: the first memoir of a first lady. Will worked as her literary agent; Helen "did the writing while Nellie reminisced and tweaked the narrative."[10]

The future first lady spent three years in the Philippines as the wife of Governor General Taft. The country's subtropical climate exposed her to malaria and within a year of her arrival, "medical exams soon showed that Nellie had malaria." Her symptoms and treatment are unrecorded. However, the disease may have produced debilitating aftereffects as hinted by the following: "Despite her own physical ailments resulting from malaria, Nellie took charge of arranging Will's third surgery." There was also a description of her upon the Tafts' return to the United States as "a fragile looking woman."[11] Helen Taft was not the first first lady to contract malaria but she was the first to be infected outside the United States.[12]

William Taft was recalled to Washington in 1904 by President Theodore Roosevelt with the appointment as the country's secretary of war.[13] In early 1905, his wife "felt the insidious approach of nerves, and she took immediate steps to tone herself up." Medical considerations were an underlying reason for a spring trip to Europe, where she rowed with son Robert to build up her strength. She "returned to Washington looking ten years younger and with her nerves as steady as the Rock of Gibraltar."[14] Is it possible that the allusions to " nerves" foreshadowed the cerebrovascular accident four years later in May 1909? Moreover, did Nellie, always ambitious and innately focused, use her European conditioning sojourn to prepare herself for the rigors of a first lady?

A final pre–White House medical reference was to a summer 1908 trip to Hot Springs, Virginia, to use its baths for her rheumatism.[15]

First Lady Helen Taft

William Howard Taft was elected the twenty-seventh president of the United States in November 1908. His first lady, previously goal-oriented towards the White House, ceased to be her husband's constant political prod and concentrated her energies on entertaining and the management of the executive mansion.[16]

Her emergence as the lady in the White House was welcomed by social and official Washington with the following encomiums: "immensely capable," "of exceptional learning, intelligence, and ambition," "she is probably the best fitted woman who ever graced the position she now holds and enjoys," "has brains and uses them," "an intellectual woman and a woman of wonderful executive ability." Her changes in White House custom, her ride in the inaugural parade, her civic and social reform efforts—all converged to make Mrs. Taft a presidential wife of more than the usual fascination in the national press.[17] This changed dramatically the afternoon of May 17, 1909, a mere thirteen weeks into her tenure. She had a stroke that first ended and then permanently affected her ability to speak. Although a shock when it occurred, in retrospect her cerebrovascular accident (CVA) should not have been. Her personality, family history, and history of smoking are all recognized as significant predisposing factors.

Both her parents were stroke victims. Harriet Collins Herron experienced facial paralysis in late 1886. She recovered only to be struck again in 1901. Her father, John Williamson Herron, had a cerebrovascular accident in 1902. When Nellie was recovering from her second CVA in 1911, John Herron experienced his second and became delusional.[18] A 2003 family history study demonstrated that patients suffering a stroke at 65 years of age or younger (Nellie was 48), were three times as likely to have a first degree relative with an early stroke or heart attack (Harriet Herron was 53).[19]

It is not difficult to characterize Nellie Taft as possessing a Type A personality. Her competitiveness and zeal for achievement fulfilled this designation; a consequence was chronic stress. Stressful activities during May 17, 1909, preceded the medical cataclysm of later in the day. A recent research study proved what was long surmised: Stressful habits and type A behavior are associated with a high risk of stroke.[20]

Diary entries during Helen Herron's 1880 vacation in Newport, Rhode Island, recorded early experimentation with cigarette smoking. She started to smoke cigarettes to escape depression. She began to smoke at a time when genteel women did not, and smoking became a matter of course for her. Her habit consisted of an occasional cigarette and although she never smoked to excess, she never relinquished the habit.[21] Today the dangers of cigarettes are widely acknowledged, and stroke is a recognized consequence for both men and women. The stroke risk increases with each additional cigarette. Any smoking increases the risk of a cerebral accident, 2.2 times for 1 to 10 cigarettes a day, 4.3 times for those smoking 21 to 39 a day, and 9.1 times greater for two or more packs a day.[22]

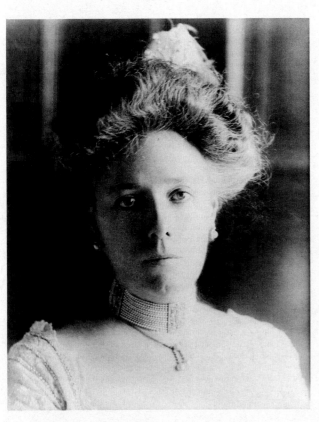

Nellie Taft, wife of William Howard Taft, was a determined first lady whose dour countenance reflected her inner drive (Library of Congress).

The First Stroke

During the afternoon of May 17, 1909, the new first lady was halfway through a more than usually stressful day. She spent the morning in a Washington hospital where Charlie, her younger son and favorite child, had undergone an especially bloody removal of his tonsils and adenoids. Continuing unease over her aging and fragile father and anxiety over her sixth congressional dinner scheduled at the White House that evening were inescapable. In an attempt at relaxation, still annoyed with her husband for his tardy arrival at the hospital, she decided upon an informal cruise on the Potomac to Mount Vernon. Aboard the presidential yacht, Nellie fainted. An aide attempted to revive her with the captain's whiskey; the boat returned immediately to Washington.

Accounts of her condition and the course of it differed, partially the result of the president's attempt to minimize the medical situation: "She made no motion and did not seem to be more than half conscious." Upon the yacht's return, military attaché Archie Butt carried the limp Helen Taft to her bedroom. For the next sixteen hours, the first lady was comatose and "utterly speechless." The president admitted in a letter to their oldest son, Robert, that the first lady had lost muscular control of her right arm and leg, and that only after three days did she begin to make audible sounds, but not words.[23]

In the early decades of the twentieth century, home care was greatly preferred over hospital care for nonsurgical emergencies. Accordingly, Nellie Taft recuperated at the White House. Dr. Matthew A. DeLaney of the Army Medical Corps was the White House physician and accordingly took charge of his patient's care. He administered stimulants, for her heart "was very weak," and put her to bed. The president wrote Robert: "The doctor soon reassured us all, and her as well … that it was a mere attack of nervous hysteria."[24]

Will Taft personally wrote the statement that was released to the press the following morning. Under the headline "Mrs. Taft's Illness Due to Social Cares," the *New York Times* reported: "Mrs. Taft's sudden and severe illness on Monday when she succumbed to the excessive heat, is yielding to rest and care, promising an early and complete recovery." The article continued: "In the ten weeks of her husband's Administration, Mrs. Taft has done more for society than any former mistress of the White House has undertaken in as many months…. This with numerous official receptions and dinners within a short time, proved too much for her." In another newspaper, it was alleged that Mrs. Taft suffered from a "slight nervous attack" and that she would be able to resume normal activities in a few days.[25] However, when the previously very active first lady did not appear during the next few weeks at scheduled concerts and White House social events, the press realized that all was not well. But the public was shielded from the severity of her disease. Nellie's sister, Eleanor Moore, served as temporary White House hostess.[26]

Within a short time, Nellie's mental faculties recovered their usual acuteness and the motor control of her right arm and leg returned. During the summer, with slow care, she could write fairly legibly. The catastrophe for this forceful and energetic woman was an inability to speak at first, and later to talk only with difficulty. Mortified by her impediment, for the first two months Mrs. Taft came into a White House corridor only when assured she would not be seen by anyone.[27]

Sister Eleanor, daughter Helen, and even the president participated in the exceedingly slow process of speech therapy. This consisted of her repetition of what was spoken to her. Each morning Dr. DeLaney checked in and tried different therapies. In early June he experimented with a machine that applied electricity to the throat.[28] Progress in restoring normal articulation was slow. Therefore Dr. Delaney sought the consultation of Dr. Lewellys F. Barker, William Osler's successor as director of medicine and physician in chief of the Johns Hopkins Medical Institutions. Barker's examination, conducted five months after the stroke, "found her practically normal except for the one trouble—articulation—and told her that that only required rest, time and the same treatment she has been receiving to restore her to health."[29]

Nellie took comfort in the Baltimore specialist, who implied that her problem was not paralysis at all but something unusual that occasionally strikes people, and so she wanted to resume her public role. However, her doctors informed the president that if she did they would release themselves from any responsibility for her care as they feared a relapse.[30] Dr. Barker again visited the White House in early 1910, and assured Taft "that she [had] made remarkable progress in the preceding two months." When the president journeyed to Panama in October 2010, his wife no longer feared a relapse while he was gone. She was comfortable enough to speak once again with strangers. Moreover, she hosted the White House debutante party during the 1910 Christmas season.[31]

With hindsight and with the medical knowledge accumulated over one hundred years, the verbal disability of Mrs. Taft is classified as apraxia of speech. It defines a disorder involving difficulty of articulation despite having intact language skills and muscular function. It occurs in about 11 percent of stroke cases and is usually minor. In the most severe cases, as in this first lady's, all linguistic motor function can be lost and must be relearned. Today's recommended treatment involves frequent one-on-one therapy with a specialist, using repetition of words or phrases. That was the therapy of her doctors and her family a century ago, and it was successful.[32]

The Second Stroke

On May 13, 1911, President and Mrs. Taft were in New York City, where the president delivered a speech at the New York Academy of Political Sciences. Two years after her initial attack Mrs. Taft's speech had improved to only a slight undetectable speech impediment. Nellie left the dinner early but collapsed at her husband's brother's home, where they were staying. Horace Taft immediately summoned his family physician, Dr. E.M. Evans. The doctor diagnosed a "nervous attack" that was mild in comparison to her earlier episode. Daughter Helen wrote: "She isn't able to articulate clearly or find the words. The doctor seems to think that the attack is similar to the first one but much less severe." The president continued to characterize it as a "nervous attack," as did the contemporaneous *New York Times* report.[33]

Five days after her collapse, Nellie Taft was well enough to return by train to Washington, D.C. Once ensconced in the White House, her condition improved. The president offered Horace reassurance: "There is nothing except the tongue which interferes with distinct enunciation, but which is improving with use from week to week. We have induced Nellie to stay in bed, so that she does not come down stairs at all, and while she resents this treatment, I think she realizes the necessity for care." The *New York Times* on May 20, 1911, under its headline "Mrs. Taft Will Rest," related that the first lady had recovered well from her attack of nervous trouble, but daughter Miss Helen Taft will preside at the White House functions for the present."[34]

The first lady sparkled at the Tafts' excessively elegant June 19, 1911, silver anniversary party held before thousands on the White House lawn. She remained on the sidelines during her husband's 1912 renomination battle, citing her physical condition as the reason. But her role on the public stage was not yet over; Mrs. Taft was the first first lady to appear at a national nominating convention of the opposing party. She attended the 1912 Democratic presidential convention in Baltimore. This gathering nominated Woodrow Wilson, who subsequently was victorious in a three-way race with William Taft and Theodore Roosevelt.[35]

Effects of Her Disability Upon President Taft

An incapacitating cerebrovascular accident, occurring so early in the Taft presidency, was a tragedy—tragic not only for the new first lady, whose determination to engrave her indelible mark upon the first lady narrative and upon the Washington social scene was thwarted, but also tragic for the president, whose closest political advisor was both stricken and unavailable for counsel and support. "During Nellie's illness Taft was a somber and stricken man, ever attentive to her needs and desires. Nellie's stroke left her very weak, with partial paralysis of some facial muscles and with a speech difficulty which took some time and considerable effort to overcome." Her condition was not only a burden for her, but also for those around her, especially her husband. He could no longer count on his wife as he had formerly since he feared for her health.[36]

Taft was stressed and his focus distracted by Mrs. Taft's condition. Gradually she took part in social situations where she could speak a formula of greeting. But dinners and socials where she had to talk were avoided.[37] Helen, the Tafts' daughter, recollected the following to a national magazine forty-five years after the fact: "Within two months of my father's inauguration, my mother suffered a brain hemorrhage which rendered her unconscious for four or five days and from the effects of which she never fully recovered. For the next two years she had, most unwillingly, to accept the role of invalid. During the whole period of my father's presidency I doubt whether she visited the executive offices half a dozen times."[38]

One Taft biographer suggested that if Mrs. Taft's health had remained good and she had been in a position to advise the president about the tariff and other matters, Taft's record might have been altogether different.[39] Another summed up: "Given four years of good health and sustained hard work, she might have reshaped the role of the first lady decades earlier than Eleanor Roosevelt or Lady Bird Johnson did."[40]

Postpresidential Years

After his reelection defeat, the Tafts moved to New Haven, Connecticut, where William was a member of the Yale Law faculty for nearly ten years. In 1921 the ex-president achieved his own, but not his wife's, professional goal when President Harding appointed Taft chief justice of the United States Supreme Court. After Taft's death in 1930, his widow continued in live in Washington, but she also developed an annual pattern of travel. She visited Charleston, South Carolina, in mid-winter, made an overseas trip until early summer, then spent several months in Murray Bay, Canada, until October, and celebrated the holidays in Washington. She lived with a cook and a maid who were Irish immigrant sisters.[41] The effects of the stroke on her articulation both lingered and persisted, but her speech generally improved after the presidency. Nellie had learned to let go of stress "that had provoked her earlier attacks, she was even calm when she fell ill."[42]

Mrs. Taft was in excellent health during her three decades as a former first lady. In 1926 she had a gastrointestinal complaint for which she reached out to her former physician in the White House, Dr. DeLaney.[43] In December 1935, she "Suffered a slight brain swelling with 'distinct paralysis on the right side.' Within twenty-four hours all such symptoms had vanished." At the time, the event was dismissed as a minor matter and not a cerebrovascular accident. However in retrospect we realize it was a transient ischemic attack, a minor stroke, and her third such event. A year later, sufficiently recovered, she left for a seven-month overseas trip.[44]

In the summer of 1941 Mrs. Taft battled a lung illness and, in addition, she fractured her right arm at her summer home. A fourth CVA followed, which led to convulsions and a slight paralysis. She recovered. Mrs. Taft was ill during 1942 and into 1943; although bedridden she was lucid. She died with "a circulatory ailment" in Washington on May 22, 1943, just shy of her eighty-second birthday.[45]

Helen Herron Taft was buried at Arlington National Cemetery. Her interment there was preceded not only by that of her husband, William H. Taft, but also by her White House physician, General Matthew DeLaney, who died in November 1926. Always the trailblazer, Nellie in death became the first first lady to be laid to rest at the storied burial ground. She preceded the much publicized burial of Jacqueline Kennedy there by half a century.[46]

Pat Nixon: A Brave and Misunderstood First Lady

Richard Nixon reported to the Nixon family physician John C. Lungren: "[T]wo days before the stroke, Pat was reading The Final Days…. Pat was extremely upset over the sections where Woodward and Bernstein portrayed us as demented alcoholics and our marriage as loveless—pure, unadulterated lies."[47]

Images: Private and Public

The public image of Mrs. Pat Nixon, first lady and wife of President Richard Nixon (1969–1974), was that of a stoic and ornamental supporter of her husband's political aspirations. She was depicted as the perfect middle-class mother and housewife, supportive and silently admiring of her politician husband. Boller compiled a list of the most critical epithets directed towards Mrs. Nixon: "plastic Pat," "antiseptic Pat," "Pat the robot," and "chatters, answers questions, smiles and smiles, all with a doll's terrifying poise."[48]

Retrospectives at the time of her death began to correct this portrayal. William Safire wrote in the New York Times: "She was politically savvy, an asset on the trail, and not just for patenting that rapt look listening to the same speech for the umpteenth time." Donnie Radcliffe, writing in a newspaper which, more than any other, was responsible for the demonization of her husband, explained: "[F]ar from a 'plastic Pat,' as some tried to portray her. She was a complicated woman, a savvy politician who was fiercely loyal to her husband."[49]

Her two biographers, Julie Nixon Eisenhower and Mary C. Brennan, portray a woman far more substantial than the mainstream media's caricature. Thelma Catherine Ryan was born on March 16, 1912, in the small mining town of Ely, Nevada, to an Irish immigrant father and a German immigrant mother. Her father insisted that she be called "Pat" and that her birth occurred on Saint Patrick's Day and not a day earlier as documented on her birth certificate.

Pat's early life was tough but she was brave, smart, and determined. Her parents were poor and when her mother died at an early age, Pat became the woman of the family, taking care of her father and brothers. The senior Ryan also passed away when Pat was young. Although an excellent student in high school, Pat gave up college in order to support her brother Tom's university studies. Other formative experiences included a cross-country drive, two years of successful performance of many technical jobs at Seton Catholic Hospital in Manhattan, New York City, graduation from the University of Southern California after a delayed start, and recognition as a much admired teacher at Whittier High School in Southern California.[50]

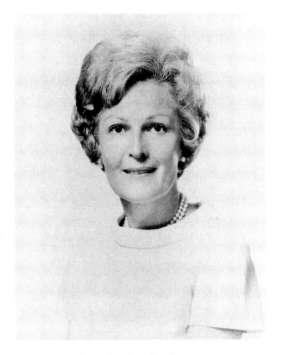

Pat Nixon, the wife of Richard Nixon, was a smoker and a stroke victim (Library of Congress).

Medical History

Pat Nixon was a sturdy and healthy wife through her husband's elective career. A single exception was a strained back in March 1958, suffered when she lifted her daughter Julie. The pain was severe and she was admitted to a hospital for the first time since her daughter's birth ten years earlier.[51]

This first lady was a smoker, although to what extent remains undetermined. But the habit was of long duration. The Watergate crisis (1972–4) obviously took its physical and emotional toll. "She got thinner, and her face appeared more puffy and lined. Her smoking, which she tried to hide from the public, increased. In fact, on several occasions, she even smoked in public." Previously she repeatedly told reporters that she did not smoke. In an interview at the time of her first cerebrovascular accident her last White House press secretary, Helen McCain Smith, recalled that Mrs. Nixon smoked cigarettes.[52]

The First Stroke

For the first time in her life Pat Nixon was confronted by her own major medical problem. On July 7, 1976, at the Nixons' retirement home in San Clemente, California, she was felled by a significant stroke.

Richard Nixon resigned the presidency in August 1974, and the Nixons moved to their California seaside retreat. But they could not escape the fallout from the Watergate political scandal. *Washington Post* news reporters Bob Woodward and Carl Bernstein, perhaps wishing to embellish a fame-enhancing narrative, wrote a follow-up Watergate tell-all, titled *The Final Days.* The book, employing no documented sources and surmising "what might have been" conversations and internal thoughts, finally appeared in print in the early summer of 1976 after several months of a prepublication advertising blitz. The book portrayed the former first lady as an alcoholic and the Nixon marriage as loveless and close to collapse.[53]

On the morning of July 7, 1976, against her husband's wishes, Pat Nixon read part of the book, which had been borrowed from one of Nixon's secretaries. Adding to her stress, Nixon had just informed his wife that New York State was about to disbar him from the practice of law. An afternoon of housecleaning added to her exhaustion. After a swim with her husband, son-in-law David and daughter Julie, Mrs. Nixon fell asleep without undressing and woke up fatigued. She recalled that she could hardly walk. At breakfast the following morning, the ex-president noted that his wife had developed left hand paresis and weakness of the left side of her mouth. Nixon immediately called Jack Lungren, the family physician, who arranged for the chief of medicine of nearly Camp Pendleton to examine Mrs. Nixon at their home. The physician diagnosed a "tiny stroke" and dispatched her by ambulance to Long Beach Memorial Hospital, fifty-four miles away.[54] Dr. Lungren admitted Mrs. Nixon with a diagnosis of cerebral hemorrhage secondary to vascular hypertension. Her blood pressure was elevated to 175/100. The physical findings were generalized weakness of the left arm and leg and slurring of speech. The brain hemorrhage was localized to the brain's right cerebral cortex.[55]

Lungren quickly reduced the blood pressure to normal and promptly asked neurologist Doctor John Mosier to monitor her recovery. Physical exercises commenced first at the bedside and later in the hospital's rehabilitation unit. Dr. Bernard J. Michela, the hospital's director of rehabilitation medicine, placed Pat on a twice-daily physical treatment consisting primarily of walking and standing exercises. Julie Eisenhower underscored her mother's stoicism during her illness: "She wanted no sympathy and no witnesses to the struggle." Pat Nixon walked six days after the stroke and was discharged after two weeks in the hospital. An around-the-clock private nurse was hired for her first weeks at home. However, in October, three and one-half months later, Mrs. Nixon became dismayed by her slow progress.[56]

At the time of the CVA, Mrs. Nixon was apparently in good health and was not taking any prescribed therapy. There was no past history of hypertension. However, "Dr. Lungren indicated today that Mrs. Nixon, by nature, had sought very little medical attention and had not had a physical checkup in the nearly two years since the Nixons left the White House. Since her examination for hypertension came at the beginning of this period, the possibility that she developed some form of the condition in recent months could not be completely ruled out."[57]

Lt. Colonel John Brennan, the ex-president's aide, speculated in an interview that "Mrs. Pat Nixon was reading Woodward and Bernstein's *The Final Days*, with its negative depiction of her character, on the June day when she suffered a stroke.... After Watergate she was in great health—she believed in her husband.... But on the day of her stroke her blood pressure was incredibly high.... I don't know if this was the cause, but she had been reading the book."[58] When Mrs. Nixon was hospitalized, a newspaper editorial sympathized: "No one knows how much such efforts [fulfilling the difficult role of wife to a public official] have cost her emotionally, although her physician has said that pressures in her life 'certainly could have been a contributing factor' in the stroke."[59]

In a hospital conversation with Lungren Richard Nixon left no doubt about whom to blame: "[T]wo days before the stroke, Pat was reading *The Final Days* … Pat was extremely upset over the sections where Woodward and Bernstein portrayed us as demented alcoholics and our marriage as loveless—pure, unadulterated lies."[60]

Second Stroke and Death

After her first stroke, Pat Nixon's health was good. Her husband elaborated in a 1982 interview: "She doesn't quite have the stamina she used to have and she doesn't like to go on faraway trips. But other than a slight, almost unnoticeable problem with her left arm, she's fine." But she suffered a second stroke in 1983, which was reported only upon her return to the Nixons' Saddle River, New Jersey, home. Her stroke was mild and she was released from New York Hospital after only five days. There was neither paralysis nor difficulty in speaking.[61]

Pulmonary problems, probably cigarette-related, troubled Pat Nixon during her last decade of life—pneumonia, bronchitis, emphysema, and, finally, cancer of the lung. She died in June 1993, at age eighty-one.[62]

In Summation

Two first ladies smoked and suffered its consequences. Both first ladies were struck by significant cerebrovascular accidents. Nellie was incapacitated just two and a half months into her husband's term. Her resulting motor disability disappeared rapidly, but she was also struck with apraxia, an inability to speak. She slowly improved but her grand plans for serving as the hostess in the executive mansion dissipated. A second, similar but milder, cerebral accident occurred two years later. She also recovered from this event. She died in her eighty-second year.

Pat Nixon had a right cerebral hemorrhage in 1976 that weakened the left side of her body. She recovered only with persistence and prolonged physical therapy. A second stroke occurred in 1983. This was followed by emphysema and lung cancer, and she died from the latter in 1993 at eighty-one.

Chapter Ten

Ellen and Edith

Woodrow Wilson's Two Wives

Ellen Wilson made a deathbed request to Cary Grayson, the White House physician: "Doctor, if I go away, promise me that you will take good care of my husband."[1]

Introduction

Ellen Axson Wilson was the third and, up to the present, the last first lady to perish in the White House. Chronic kidney disease afflicted her during her brief seventeen months as the wife of a president. She was the first of two wives of President Woodrow Wilson. Wilson's second wife, Edith Bolling Gault Wilson, would become a very controversial political actor who would expand the authority and power of the first lady beyond anything experienced either before or since.

Ellen Wilson organized the late November 1913 wedding of Jesse, the middle Wilson daughter. It was an extravagant formal affair that took place in the East Room of the White House. The Marine band played and the entire diplomatic corps, many members of Congress, together with Wilson friends and family attended. The guest list totaled five hundred.[2] However, Ellen's disease was never absent. Out of concern for his wife's health president Wilson cancelled the 1913 inaugural ball. Moreover, plans for the White House wedding of Eleanor, their youngest daughter, were left indefinite. Eleanor eventually married secretary of the treasury William McAdoo in a more restrained ceremony in May 1914.[3]

Ellen Wilson was one of the first first ladies to adopt a significant philanthropic project. Her cause was the improvement of the terrible living conditions in the Washington slums, called the Alleys. Initially she was tireless, frequently visiting the Alleys, "often taking groups of Congressman with her. She talked to the people, helped them with food and money, held numerous conferences, and insisted with her own peculiar gentle firmness that something had to be done at once." However, her illness intervened and she was forced to abandon her crusade. Congress passed the Alley Clearing Act to end these slums the same day that Mrs. Wilson passed away: "No one doubted that it was she who had brought it about."[4]

Robert Watson classified Ellen Wilson as a partial partner, i.e., a wife who is somewhat active in politics and is both interested in and supportive of her husband's political activities, A partial partner may assist with the president's speeches and appointments, and may be a public force. Such a first lady actively directs the White House social activities. Watson ranked Ellen Wilson number 10 on his list of successful first ladies.[5] Other historians ranked her somewhat lower (#16–#21).[6]

Ellen Wilson

There is no doubt that the first Mrs. Wilson suffered from chronic kidney disease and perished from its consequences. Contemporary medical textbooks and the language of the times called this condition Bright's disease. Underlying causes for chronic renal failure are multiple, but in the case of Ellen Wilson it is possible that toxemia of pregnancy was its etiology. Therefore, a close inspection of her three pregnancies is merited. Woodrow and Ellen Wilson married at the end of June 1885. Daughter Margaret was born on April 16, 1886; her sibling Jesse entered the world on August 28, 1887; Eleanor, the third daughter and last child, was born on October 5, 1889.[7]

The first pregnancy was difficult. The Wilsons were forced to hire a cook-housekeeper, as the expectant mother became miserably nauseated for the first four months. Letters from her cousin and aunt commiserated with Ellen's nausea.[8] A biographer explained: "Severe morning sickness, lasting all day, left Ellen feeling a wreck all winter long."[9] Margaret Wilson was born in Aunt Louisa Brown's home in Gainesville, Georgia, and not in Bryn Mawr, Pennsylvania, where the Wilsons resided. Ellen wanted to spare her husband the expense of a northern doctor and nurse. Ever the protective spouse, she determined to shield the anxiety-prone Woodrow from any worry that he would surely experience if he was present during her labor and delivery. Her aunt had a big house and servants; the family doctor would deliver the baby for practically nothing.[10]

Margaret was born prematurely, by two or three weeks. Naively expecting that her first pregnancy would conclude on the predicted due date, Mrs. Wilson reserved a passenger seat on the Washington to Georgia train timed to arrive well before her labor began. However, contractions commenced just as she arrived at her aunt's Georgia home.[11] Aunt Louisa's family doctor and Ellen Wilson's accoucheur fortunately turned out to be a much respected physician. Dr. George Wray Bailey had graduated 26 years earlier from the Atlanta Medical College, the predecessor of the prestigious Emory University School of Medicine. He later served as a surgeon in the Confederate army. From his rural southern practice Dr. Bailey became president of the Georgia State Board of Medical Examiners, and in 1888 the vice president of the national American Medical Association.[12]

The labor and delivery were uneventful, as reported by Aunt Louisa to the new father, distant in Pennsylvania.[13] The unfortunate absence of a birth weight in Aunt Louisa's letters to Wilson does not clarify the degree of Margaret's prematurity. Eleanor McAdoo dramatized her mother's postpartum experience: "Childbirth in the South, in those days, was considered a very dangerous undertaking. It was said that a mother, if she was fortunate enough to survive, was apt to be an invalid for the rest of her life." Aunt Louisa insisted that her niece remain to be cared for in her Gainesville house for a month postdelivery and Ellen complied. The new mother was bravely stoic throughout the entire affair, although the postpartum death of her own mother surely was not far from her thoughts.[14]

One clinical sign of toxemia of pregnancy is swelling (edema) of the eyelids. Suggestive evidence is discovered in a letter from Dr. George Howe, Jr. to Ellen: "[I] hasten to send you a prescription for your eyes. No. 1 is to be used for the lids if they are swollen at the edges…. If the lids are swollen inflamed inside, then use No. 2." Dr. Howe was Woodrow Wilson's brother-in-law, the husband of his sister. His medical pedigree is uncertain since his name does not appear on any roster of accredited physicians.[15]

In 1887, Ellen was again pregnant. This time caution made her travel earlier to Aunt Louise's home in Gainesville, leaving Bryn Mawr in mid–June well in advance of an August expected date of confinement. This arrangement was repeated "because she feared that Woodrow would become upset by her condition and she did not want to interrupt his work." Her second pregnancy was once again marked by severe nausea: "Her second pregnancy had made her more ill than the first and even she referred to it as a sickness." Her delivery and postpartum period were uncomplicated. Although undocumented, it is very likely that Dr. Bailey was again present for the delivery. Aunt Louisa once again controlled her niece's postpartum care and effected a long restful recovery.[16]

In February 1889, in Middletown, Connecticut, Ellen discovered that she was pregnant for the third time. In the interim between his wife's pregnancies, the ambitious Professor Wilson had relocated his growing family from Bryn Mawr to the Connecticut campus of Wesleyan University. Wilson had ascended the academic ladder to the rung labeled professor of history and political science.[17] For Ellen there was a repeat of the persistent nausea, and she, recalling her two previous pregnancies, became increasingly nervous.[18]

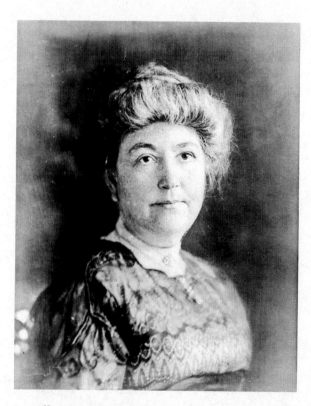

The expectant mother, "overwhelmed by the intensity of her symptoms," sought a physician's care. This time, the medical contact was earlier and the doctor was local. Ellen selected Dr. Mary-Florence Taft, a woman who was homeopathically trained, as her obstetrician. The basis for her choice can only be conjectured; perhaps the empathy of a female and the reputed gentleness of homeopathic doctors were the traits desired for Ellen's third and final pregnancy. Woodrow, expressing a widely held bias, was perturbed that a female physician would attend his wife.[19] During her seventh month of pregnancy, symptoms of toxemia alarmed the Wilsons. Headaches, unspecified eye trouble and dizziness combined with continued nausea compelled a visit to an unidentified New York specialist. Protein, another indicator of toxemia, was detected in her urine.[20]

Ellen Axson Wilson, the first wife of Woodrow Wilson (Library of Congress).

Professor Wilson, his prejudice

about the quality of female physician care unabated, wrote his brother-in-law, the afore-mentioned George Howe, for an opinion on women doctors. The uncredentialed Howe responded that female practitioners possessed a significant impediment, a nervousness occurring concurrently with menstruation, which rendered them unfit for some medical emergencies that arose during that period. But otherwise, he wrote, they were competent. Wilson was reassured by his relative's comments.[21]

Mrs. Wilson was comfortable with Dr. Taft's care. Although the pills prescribed by her were ineffective, her psychological support assisted Ellen through her third pregnancy. Dr. Mary Florence Taft was a recent medical school graduate. She received her degree from the homeopathic medical school of Boston University just three short years before she delivered the Wilson's third daughter. The doctor possessed an eminent political surname: future president and, later, an opponent of Woodrow Wilson's White House bid in 1912, William Howard Taft was her cousin. Several years later, Dr. Taft became a professor of gynecology at Hering College of Homeopathic Medicine in Chicago. Her academic research led to the publication of several articles on gynecologic practice. One, published in 1895, was entitled "Puerperal Eclampsia," which indicated that Taft was familiar with at least the most severe variant of toxemia. The specifics of Taft's care for Mrs. Wilson are not recorded.[22]

Toxemia of pregnancy is marked by the onset of hypertension and a group of associated findings including edema, protein (albumin) in the urine, headache, visual disturbances, and epigastric pain. Two forms have been identified—eclampsia and the far more common preeclampsia. The convulsions of eclampsia differentiate it from preeclampsia. Eclampsia is derived from a Greek word meaning a shining forth, in reference to the sudden appearance of convulsions, as in epilepsy. Methods of measuring blood pressure were not generally available in the late nineteenth century and therefore Ellen Wilson's blood pressure metrics are unknown.[23]

The Wilsons moved to Princeton, New Jersey, in 1890, where Woodrow received a professorship at the noted university. Six years after Ellen's final pregnancy, over a period of three and one half years (autumn 1895 to early winter 1899), the future first lady was often ill with episodic nausea and vomiting, accompanied by fever and abdominal pain. The pain was localized mainly to the area of the appendix. Ellen's enthusiasm and vitality waned, her appetite periodically vanished, and easy fatigability appeared. These symptoms occasionally forced her to her bed for days. Her medical contacts were with Dr. William Van Valzah of New York City (twice), a Dr. Wikoff, who practiced in Princeton, a Philadelphia masseuse, and possibly Dr. Edward P. Davis of Philadelphia, who was Woodrow Wilson's Princeton University classmate.

Dr. Van Valzah could find nothing organically wrong with the patient. He decided after several examinations that her symptoms were caused by the then diagnostic wastebasket for disorders of women—nervousness. He initially treated her abdominal symptoms with calomel for four nights and four mornings, but this toxic drug only increased her nausea. Finally, the doctor admitted that her "stomach and liver [were] misbehaving a little."[24]

William Van Valzah's practice in New York City emphasized diseases of the gastrointestinal tract; it was for this specialized expertise that both Professor and Mrs. Wilson sought his opinion. Woodrow consulted Van Valzah in 1898 for his own chronic digestive complaints; the professor frequently used a stomach pump as an extreme measure to treat his symptoms. Dr. Van Valzah's diagnosis and treatment were a success. He was probably the first physician who understood that Wilson's symptoms were both psychosomatic and dietary. He removed the stomach pump and regulated the patient's diet. The physician's diagnosis and treatments of Mrs. Wilson were far less successful. He was correct that her gastrointestinal complaints were not a result of pathology in either her stomach or intestinal tract. His prescription of calomel was harmful, rather than beneficial. However, Van Valzah, the coauthor of the textbook *Diseases of the Stomach* (W.B. Saunders, 1898), was unable to relate his patient's nausea, vomiting, abdominal pain and tiredness to kidney disease, a difficult correlation at the time. There is no record that he obtained a urinalysis.[25]

Van Valzah was a demonstrator in clinical medicine at Jefferson Medical College. He unfortunately became embroiled in the conflict raging between homeopathic and allopathic practitioners in the 1880s. A few years after graduation, he was hospitalized at Jefferson with "dyspepsia." Van Valzah's doctors, the orthodox luminaries of the medical faculty, finally concluded that he was "more the victim of a delusion than an actual sufferer." In other words, his complaints were psychosomatic. After a relapse the physician-patient sought an alternate opinion; he was treated by a homeopathic physician. After receiving knowledge of Van Valzah's choice of a physician, the medical staff of Jefferson demanded his resignation for crossing the philosophical orthodox/homeopath Rubicon. Dr. Samuel Gross, who was immortalized by painter Thomas Eakins in 1875, announced, "I know nothing of the particulars of the case except that he went over to homeopathy and we got rid of him. When a man goes over to homeopathy and we have no further use of him. You can't mix oil and water together. They won't unite." As a result, Van Valzah suspended his practice in Philadelphia and relocated to New York City.[26]

Dr. Wikoff is identified as the Wilson family physician during their years in Princeton. None of his professional information can be located, which casts doubt upon his medical pedigree and certification. Eleanor Wilson described him unfavorably: "He was a gloomy old soul with fierce bristling eyebrows and I shuddered every time I saw him." Wikoff's care for the future first lady is also unrecorded. It appears that he too was unable to make the diagnosis of chronic kidney disease.[27]

Ellen's health did recover for a while, leading one biographer to exclaim, "Health-wise she never felt better." However, several years later, in 1905, she was described as "pale and thin." For a period of four months the following year, Ellen was afflicted by a mysterious painful stiffness in her back and limbs. She curtailed her ordinary activities and required constant massages for any respite. Weinstein, noting that she was depressed at this time, ascribed her symptoms to a psychosomatic origin, rather than another episode of kidney disease.[28]

Unfortunately, her illness reappeared with significant and troubling symptoms. The effects of chronic renal failure, especially anemia, became apparent during the presidential election year of 1912. Her daughters Jesse and Eleanor noticed that their mother was less animated. She remained home during her husband's successful campaign for the presidency; her family and close friends became alarmed "that something was very wrong with Ellen." On inauguration day, Eleanor was shocked that the small figure "walking slowly and wearily" ahead of her was her mother.[29]

Preeclampsia (the common form of toxemia of pregnancy) increases the risk of end-stage renal disease (Bright's disease) three- to fivefold. Among women who were pregnant three or more times, preeclampsia during one pregnancy was associated with a relative risk of end-stage kidney disease of 6.3, and preeclampsia during two or three pregnancies was associated with a relative risk of 15.5. Although the absolute risk for chronic renal disease in those who have had preeclampsia is low, preeclampsia is a marker for an increased risk. The reason for the first lady's physical decline continued to be unsuspected. Colonel Edward House, Wilson's friend and political confidante, attributed her symptoms to the effects of overwork. Wilson cancelled the traditional inaugural ball, in all likelihood out of concern for his wife's health.[30]

Did Ellen Wilson's Disease Affect Her Performance as First Lady?

Chronic kidney disease, although indolent, is a sinister sickness, insidious, enervating and progressive. Despite this, Ellen Wilson for many months until her terminal decline fulfilled most of the responsibilities of a presidential wife: "Until her health began to decline, Ellen pursued the role of an active, involved First Lady."[31] Her decade-long experience as the wife of the president of Princeton University prepared her for social success in the White House.[32] Official entertaining, whether cabinet luncheons, diplomatic receptions, teas or dinners, were handled with grace and efficiency.[33] Eleanor, the Wilsons' youngest daughter, raved about her mother's skills as a hostess: "Mother carried out the usual program of dinners, receptions and musicals at the White House, gave two or three tea parties a week, and received callers almost every afternoon.... [T]here were never less than fifty people at the smallest dinner party, and often a hundred or more attended her informal teas.... She managed, however, to make even the huge receptions more homely and gracious."[34]

Doctor Cary Grayson and Mrs. Wilson's Final Illness

The Wilsons' change of residence required the selection of a new family physician. Navy doctor Lieutenant (later Admiral) Cary Grayson became their White House physician. He filled the role of the Wilson family doctor and then some, becoming confidante, advisor and intimate friend. Grayson attended William and Mary College in Williamsburg, Virginia, and received his medical degree from the University of the South in Sewanee, Tennessee. After an internship at Columbia Hospital for Women in Washington, D.C., he was commissioned an acting assistant surgeon in the United States Navy. A few years later, in 1910, he received the coveted assignment of medical officer of the presidential yacht, *Mayflower*. This billet, where Dr. Grayson got to know both Presidents Theodore Roosevelt and William Howard Taft, may have served as an audition for his prestigious appointment as White House physician and personal physician to the Wilsons.

The young navy lieutenant's career was undoubtedly abetted by the interest and friendship of a significant mentor, White House physician to Presidents Roosevelt and Taft, Admiral Presley Rixey. Rixey shared a Virginia birth and skilled horsemanship with his protégé. Moreover they were kinsmen; Grayson's half sister was married to Rixey's youngest brother. The admiral reflected upon their relationship: "I had known Dr. Grayson for many years prior to his entry in the Navy and advised him how to proceed with his medical education so as to become a naval surgeon, and in the service made good in every assignment I gave him."[35]

The circumstances leading to the installation of this thirty-four-year-old naval officer as the president's personal physician, then as his personal and political confidante, and finally as Woodrow Wilson's surrogate son, seem to be the following: The Wilsons first met Grayson on March 3, 1913, the day prior to the incoming president's inauguration. They were guests of the departing Tafts at a White House tea where they were informed that Woodrow's sister, Annie Howe, had slipped on a marble staircase and cut her forehead. Grayson, by virtue of his role as medical doctor to the presidential yacht, was both available and prepared with his doctor's bag. He sewed up Annie Howe's wound and attended her for a few days thereafter. The doctor ascribed this meeting to providence; a skeptic might attribute it to foresight and ambition.

Serendipitously, the Wilsons, in a new venue and without a family doctor, needed a new physician. Ellen Wilson probably had a significant role in Grayson's selection: "Thinking of her husband's health, she sent for Lieutenant Grayson, who had patched up Aunt Annie with such efficiency, and asked him if he would not look after the President." The doctor was informed of his appointment a few days later in a meeting with President Wilson and navy secretary Josephus Daniels. It is unknown, but quite likely, that President Taft and Admiral Rixey supported Grayson's professional promotion. As first lady, Ellen Wilson was under the care of Dr. Grayson. On rare occasions, when he finally concluded that her care exceeded his professional acumen, he sought the consultation of experts.[36]

As spring 1913 progressed, "it escaped no one's notice ... that Ellen was taxing her strength to the limit." Daughter Eleanor described her mother as "warm and white." A decision was forced. On June 20, 1913, the White House released the following statement: "Upon the advice of her physician, Mrs. Wilson has decided to abandon active participation in the philanthropic movements which have commanded much of her attention since she came to Washington. Mrs. Wilson is not seriously ill, but will remain quietly in the White House until she goes to Cornish, N.H."[37] The first lady recuperated in New England, resting, painting, and socializing with friends and other artists. Her physical strength had been restored by the time she returned to Washington on October 17, after an absence of almost four months. Wilson made only a rare visit to his wife in New Hampshire, and Ellen, whose first priority was always her husband's well-being, made one trip to Washington.[38]

Jesse was the first of the Wilson daughters to marry. Upon her return from Cornish, Ellen actively assumed the traditional responsibility of the mother of the bride, the planning of the wedding. The White House marriage of Jesse Wilson to attorney Francis Sayre on November 25, 1913, was a splendid event. In the meantime, Ellen made frequent references to being tired and the necessity of rest breaks. The president's family spent Christmas vacation in Pass Christian, Mississippi, but upon their return to the White House, the first lady began to lose weight and "the lovely color in her cheeks disappeared."[39]

On March 1, 1914, the physically failing Ellen fainted in her room. She remained confined to her room for several weeks and "she remained weak, lethargic, and anorectic, a triad of symptoms typical of chronic nephritis."[40] Finally, on March 10, Dr. Grayson realized that he needed help. He summoned Dr. Edward Parker Davis of Philadelphia to the White House to examine his patient. Davis was named for several reasons: He was a Princeton classmate of President Wilson and the two had maintained a long-term friendship, marked by frequent correspondence. He may even have treated the Wilsons when they resided in Princeton. In addition, Grayson and Davis previously had established a respectful professional relationship. Finally, the consultant's medical expertise—obstetrics and gynecology—was relevant to the ailing Mrs. Wilson's condition.[41]

After he received Grayson's request Dr. Davis attended the first lady several times in the White House. He performed minor surgery on Mrs. Wilson; the details of the operation were never made public. One biographer speculated that it corrected a chronic gynecological problem that was aggravated when she fainted. However it is known that the gynecologist brought an anes-

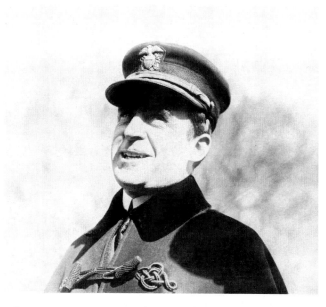

Admiral Dr. Cary Grayson, who shielded President Wilson from his first wife's illness and later covered up the policy-making of his second wife (courtesy Bureau of Medicine and Surgery Archives).

thesiologist, Dr. Widdowson, with him from Philadelphia to assist during the surgical procedure.[42]

The president was compelled to cancel a conference appearance in New York City because his wife was "distressingly weak." The Wilsons then embarked for the West Virginia resort town of White Sulphur Springs for an Easter respite. The concerned president hired a personal nurse to care for the first lady. Once again, Grayson sought the advice of Dr. Davis, this time regarding the availability of a capable local physician. Davis reassured the White House physician: "Dr. Kahlo, White Sulphur Springs, is a sensible and competent physician."[43]

Eleanor Wilson was wed in a simple White House marriage ceremony on May 7, 1914. Her husband was fifty-year-old widower William McAdoo, President Wilson's secretary of the treasury. Dr. Grayson, who by this time had become an intimate of the Wilson family, served as McAdoo's best man.[44] After the wedding, Mrs. Wilson's decline was swift. Progressive weakness and chronic indigestion were the most noticeable symptoms. At the end of June Grayson finally persuaded Ellen Wilson to spend most of each day in bed.[45]

Between mid–March and early July, Grayson was the only physician to attend the dying first lady. However, when her condition worsened decidedly, Grayson quickly arranged for professional reinforcements. He urgently requested consultations from his Philadelphia colleague Dr. Davis, Dr. Francis X. Dercum, also from Philadelphia, and Dr. Thomas R. Brown, from nearby Baltimore.

Dercum was a renowned neurologist who served as clinical professor of mental and nervous disorders at Jefferson Medical College and had authored several textbooks in this field. Five years later he would be one of the specialists Grayson consulted after Woodrow

Wilson was felled by a massive stroke. Ironically, several years earlier Mrs. Wilson had consulted Dercum regarding her husband's neurological problems. She was afraid of the effects the presidency might have upon Wilson's fragile nervous constitution.[46] The involvement of Dercum, a neurologist, at this critical stage, probably derived from the lingering misdiagnosis by Ellen's doctors, that "nerves" were the basis for her symptoms. The kidneys had not yet been implicated as the source of her troubles.

Grayson's reasons for consulting Dr. Brown are speculative; undoubtedly his medical reputation and his availability, with Baltimore's proximity to Washington, were factors. Thomas Brown was the first candidate to receive an M.D. degree from the prestigious Johns Hopkins School of Medicine. After serving an internship at the Johns Hopkins Hospital, Brown was promoted to its prestigious teaching staff. In 1912 he was selected to develop gastroenterology as a new and distinct specialty. Perhaps it was Brown's expertise with Mrs. Wilson's prominent symptoms—nausea, vomiting, lack of appetite and abdominal pain— that attracted Grayson's attention. It was an unfortunate conclusion that focused upon the secondary symptoms in the intestinal tract rather than upon the culprit organ, her kidneys.[47]

Despite the ministrations of the medical reinforcements, Mrs. Wilson continued to fail, and an alarmed Dr. Grayson moved into the White House on July 23 to be available around the clock.[48]

The Death of a First Lady and a Critique

Mrs. Wilson passed away in her room in the White House on August 6, 1914. Forewarned, the Wilson family had gathered about the dying patient. The cause of death was attributed to Bright's disease with complications. Grayson signed the death certificate that certified chronic nephritis as the cause of death.[49]

Daughter Ellen Wilson McAdoo, without any proof, stated that the underlying disease was tuberculosis of the kidneys. Perhaps she was misdirected by her friend Grayson, who was quoted some years after the death: "She was suffering from tuberculosis of both kidneys as well as from Bright's disease." Instead, Weinstein, a medical doctor, indicted damage to her kidneys that occurred during Ellen's third pregnancy. The presence of albumin in her urine indicated either an upper urinary tract infection or, more likely, toxemia of pregnancy with kidney damage: Chronic nephritis that became progressive in 1912 and lethal in August 1914.[50]

It is unknown when the correct diagnosis of fatal kidney disease finally was made, but it was not made long before her death, and it was not made by Grayson. The first mention of diseased kidneys appeared only on August 12, the date of death, in a letter from Woodrow Wilson to his younger brother, J.R. Wilson: "Ellen's condition gives us a great deal of alarm but we have by no means lost hope and are fighting hard to bring her through. The trouble centers in the kidneys."[51]

Who made the correct diagnosis and why it was so delayed are academic questions. Their answers likely would not have affected Ellen Wilson's terminal disease. Antihypertensive medications, which in present day are essential in the treatment of kidney disease, were yet to be discovered. Dubovay's biography provides this summation: "Medical malpractice or Grayson's intimate connection to the family ... a correct diagnosis would have done nothing to save Ellen's life. Prolonged bed rest and drugs to dull the pain ... would still have been advised."[52]

The ethical responsibilities of physicians to their patients are perceived differently in the early twenty-first century than during Wilson's presidency a century ago. Today's concepts of full disclosure and patient autonomy were then unknown, and a doctor was granted wide discretion regarding what he might reveal to, and what he might conceal from, a patient. It is not known, and will remain forever unknown, what Dr. Cary Grayson revealed to his patient Ellen Wilson about her medical condition.

Dr. Grayson's Responsibility to His Other Patient, President Wilson

The health of his other patient was paramount to Grayson. Not only was Woodrow Wilson the president, he was also the navy lieutenant's commander-in-chief. Grayson's words reflect his professional conflict: "My own anxiety was double for her, the invalid, and for the effects of her illness upon the President."[53]

Weinstein sympathized with Grayson's very difficult position. His close friendship with all the members of the presidential family confounded his ability to act with professional detachment: "Grayson was probably aware that she was seriously ill, but he was a military medical officer, serving under, and primarily responsible, for the health of the President. With this duty in mind, he could not risk upsetting Wilson by trying to penetrate his denial system and possibly precipitate another stroke.... This attitude may have delayed the calling in of consultants until relatively late in the illness." The White House physician became so emotionally distraught that at the end he was unable to inform the immediate family that Ellen Wilson was terminally ill. That responsibility was left to Dr. Davis.[54] Dr. Grayson rationalized his behavior in a letter to a president's advisor: "I felt it my duty to save the President from all worry, anxiety and distress as long as possible. This was an awful load to struggle under. He gradually realized the seriousness of the case and about a week before the end I told him that I thought the daughters should be here—he understood."[55]

The president was certainly confused, probably as a result of Grayson's misdirection and ignorance. His letters from late June to late July contain phrases such as the following: "...fear ... is past and she is coming along slowly but surely"; "Ellen is making good progress"; "...at present to be making little progress, and yet it still seems certain that there is nothing wrong with her."[56]

As First Lady and Beyond

The course and fatal outcome of Mrs. Wilson's kidney disease probably were not related to her responsibilities as first lady. She was ill prior to her husband's election to the presidency. When her symptoms worsened in the late spring of 1913, she temporarily retired from the White House to spend a restful summer in New Hampshire. Upon her return to Washington, she exhausted herself during the planning and organization of daughter Jesse's elaborate wedding. However, the above opinion is not unanimous. A prominent newspaper opined: that "Bright's disease ... was aggravated by a nervous breakdown attributed to the exertion of social duties and her active interest in philanthropy and betterment work."[57]

The first lady was the recipient of the continual attention and care of the White House physician. She was one of his only two patients. Moreover, Grayson was able to command when necessary the consultations of eminent physicians, e.g., Doctors Davis, Brown and Dercum. But his commitment to Ellen was muted by his prioritization of Woodrow Wilson's psychological well-being. Grayson successfully masked the seriousness of Ellen's illness; the president's connubial distractions were consequently limited, allowing him to focus on the affairs of state. Psychologically unprepared for his wife's death, Wilson became emotionally devastated and went through a severe reactive depression that lasted four or five months.[58]

Woodrow Wilson's lifelong emotional and psychological difficulties were so prominent that Sigmund Freud coauthored with William Bullitt a book that analyzed them. Regarding his wife's death, Freud and Bullitt wrote the following: "She had been a perfect wife to Woodrow Wilson: an admirable mother representative, a 'center of quiet' for his life…. [T]he loss of Ellen Axson shook the foundations of his character. He could not pull himself out of the depression caused by her death. Again and again he expressed his grief and his hopelessness … his life was unbearably lonely and sad since … death and he could not help wishing someone would kill him." In the wake of Ellen's demise, the president experienced grief, hopelessness, inadequacy, extreme loneliness, and guilt. He blamed his political ambitions for his wife's death. "He felt that his life was over, and, in the depths of his depression, he expressed the wish that someone would kill him."[59]

Did Woodrow Wilson's Bereavement Affect His Performance as President?

Mrs. Wilson died on August 6, 1914, the same day that Austro-Hungary declared war on Russia, one of the many actions that embroiled Europe in World War I. Wilson's doctor noted that his patient's attention was not upon the war, and not even upon American politics, but upon his deceased wife. Instead of exercising international leadership, Wilson was distracted, confessing to his senior advisor, Colonel House, that he could "not think straight" and "had no heart in the things he was doing."[60]

Edmund Morris, in the final volume of his three-volume biography of Theodore Roosevelt, concluded that Woodrow Wilson, during the late summer of 1914, was perhaps the only statesman who could influence the outcome of the war. But the immobilized and depressed Wilson "could concentrate only on the driest details of domestic policy…. When Wilson thought about foreign policy at all, he brooded over the still-unsettled situation in Mexico." In a grotesque coincidence, both Woodrow Wilson and his archenemy, Theodore Roosevelt, lost their first wives to Bright's disease.[61]

Grayson's efforts to pierce his patient's depression included golf, automobile drives, and trips on the presidential yacht, *Mayflower*. Any relief was only temporary. After Colonel House departed the executive mansion for a European fact-finding trip in January 1915, Wilson's loneliness became so desperate that he approached "a nervous collapse." Music and guests at the White House became additional parts of Wilson's therapeutic regimen.[62]

Although stories differ, the ever-concerned personal physician and by this time an intimate friend, Cary Grayson, was in some ways behind the introduction of the lonely president to his second wife, Edith Bolling Galt, "an outgoing, buxom, forty three year old widow, the owner of a thriving jewelry store." The wedding occurred ten months after they first met, and Wilson recovered from his inactivity and depression.[63]

Some Final Thoughts

A recurrent leitmotif in this book so far is the morbidity associated with pregnancy. This situation lasted until the first decade of the twentieth century. Louisa Catherine Adams, who experienced twelve pregnancies, may have suffered from postpartum depression. A cerebrovascular stroke felled Letitia Tyler, who experienced nine pregnancies during her reproductive years. It is not farfetched to speculate upon a nexus between her repeated deliveries, the onset of hypertension, and the hemorrhagic infarction in her brain. There is an unequivocal connection between Ida McKinley's second pregnancy and her stroke and lifelong epilepsy. Caroline Harrison's genital organs were damaged during a difficult delivery. The resultant vesicovaginal fistula required surgical repair and a long convalescence. Finally, it is probable that Ellen Wilson developed toxemia of pregnancy with chronic kidney disease.

A second recurring theme is the predilection of first ladies in the second half of the nineteenth century towards homeopathically trained physicians. Homeopathy in America increased in acceptance as the century progressed and peaked around 1900. Lucretia Garfield was treated for malaria by Drs. Susan Edson and Silas Boynton; Caroline Harrison was treated for tuberculosis by Franklin Gardner; Mary Taft delivered the third Wilson daughter. Last, Ellen Wilson's New York gastroenterologist, William Van Valzah, was expelled from the Jefferson Medical College faculty because he was treated by a homeopath instead of an orthodox-trained physician. This theme will be expanded in the following chapter, as two homeopaths became White House physicians in the 1920s.

Edith Bolling Galt: The Second Mrs. Wilson

"[T]he practice of calling the President's wife the 'First Lady' was always a disagreeable one to me. I think that if some clever person would start a little crusade against it in the newspapers it could be ridiculed to death."[64]

Political Role as First Lady

Edith Bolling Galt married the widower President Woodrow Wilson on December 18, 1915, a mere fifteen months after Ellen, his first wife, died. He was introduced to the widow Edith in March and impetuously proposed marriage in May 1915, two short months after they first met and eight months after his wife was buried. The president's dependency and requirement for a woman's emotional support were well-known.[65]

Edith Bolling Galt became Wilson's policy and governmental confidante even before their December wedding.[66] Their close partnership continued during his reelection, his second presidential term, America's role as a combatant in World War I, the Paris Peace Conference, and most controversial, during the president's dangerous disability from a cerebrovascular accident that struck in October 1919.[67]

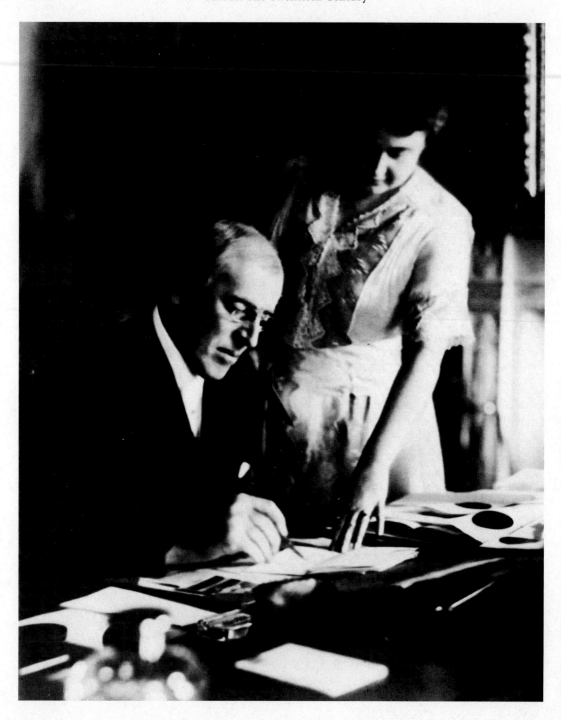

Edith Bolling Gault Wilson, the second wife of Woodrow Wilson (Library of Congress).

Mrs. Wilson's behavior during this period, extraordinary and extra-constitutional, is both well-documented and extremely controversial. Excellent expositions of this period abound, therefore an extensive narrative will not be included here. Many important accounts of Wilson's disability and Edith's commandeering role already have been written. In the words of one of her biographers: "Edith made a crucially important decision— Woodrow Wilson should remain in office. In making this and subsequent decisions, she almost certainly tried to do what she believed he would have wanted her to do."[68] As a result of her intrusion, another biographer referred to Edith Wilson as "the Unintended President."[69] Others have referred to this episode as "petticoat government" and "regency."[70]

Medical History as First Lady

Edith Wilson's health as first lady was excellent. Her endurance and tirelessness invigorated Wilson's presidency and her determination managed to keep Woodrow Wilson president. Her excellent medical condition possibly saved the Wilson presidency at the time when many were counseling resignation.

Only two relatively minor illnesses occurred. In September 1917, the first lady was felled by a high fever and a generalized aching sensation. Her condition was serious enough that her husband postponed an important policy meeting. Meanwhile, Dr. Grayson, the White House physician, was out of town. Consequently Dr. Sterling Ruffin, previously her doctor, was summoned to the White House. His diagnosis was "the grippe" and Mrs. Wilson was bed-bound for two weeks.[71]

"The grippe" is a synonym for influenza according to Dorland's medical dictionary. A viral disease, it may have many clinical presentations and variable outcomes and has been around for centuries. It is very tempting to connect the first lady's isolated attack of the grippe with the great 1918–1919 worldwide influenza pandemic. McCallops was convinced that Mrs. Wilson had contracted "the virulent strain of influenza that would kill millions of people around the world the following year." However, this claim cannot be substantiated. The influenza pandemic probably commenced in Haskell County, Kansas, four months earlier, in late January 1918 and exploded among army recruits in Camp Funston, Kansas, in late March 1918. If Edith was not felled as part of the pandemic, her husband was. Woodrow Wilson contracted the pandemic influenza on April 3, 1919, when in Paris during the protracted negotiations to conclude World War I.[72] It was also in Paris in May 1919 that Edith's other physical problem occurred. An infected foot required that Mrs. Wilson hobble about with crutches for a time.[73]

Cary Grayson continued as the personal physician of the Wilson family for the entire two-term presidency. It does not appear that he was called upon to treat the second Mrs. Wilson at any time during her more than five years as first lady. But Dr. Sterling Ruffin did. Ruffin was "well-known as a diagnostician," "one of the city's better physicians," and "a man of distinguished appearance, of great dignity of manner, and of outstanding ability."[74] Grayson was on good professional terms with Ruffin and requested his advice during the period of Wilson's disability. Later Ruffin was asked to consult during the illness of Edith Wilson's successor as first lady, Florence Harding.[75]

Sterling Ruffin was Edith Bolling Galt's personal physician prior to her becoming Mrs. Woodrow Wilson. She described Ruffin as an old friend and the physician was an invitee to her 1915 wedding. Ruffin, a lifelong bachelor, was rumored to be romantically linked to Edith both prior to her second marriage and after Woodrow Wilson's demise.[76]

Significant Personal and Medical History Before the White House

Edith Bolling was a ninth-generation direct descendant of Pocahontas, the fifteenth-century Native American princess. Pocahontas was the daughter of the Virginia Algonquian chief Powhatan, who befriended the English colonists when they landed in Jamestown in 1607. She married the English settler John Rolfe and bore him a son named Thomas Rolfe. Thomas's granddaughter wed Robert Bolling. The first lady's heritage was through the Bollings of Virginia. There was much publicity about Edith's Indian heritage at the time of her marriage to the president.[77]

Edith Bolling was a widow when she met President Wilson. She previously was married to Norman Galt for almost twelve years (April 1896–January 1908). Galt died, leaving to his widow the well-known Galt Jewelry Store in Washington, D.C. The future first lady smartly selected a capable manager who provided for the store's continued operations and a reasonable income for the owner. Mrs. Galt gave premature birth to a baby boy on September 23, 1903. The infant lived only three days; the delivery was said to render the mother unable to bear more children. Thus, this was her only pregnancy. In 1906, Edith required an emergency appendectomy.[78]

A third, intriguing and ultimately significant, story line from Edith's pre–White House biography was her very close relationship with Altrude Gordon and Ms. Gordon's future husband, Dr. Cary Grayson. Edith was a friend of James Gordon, an elderly millionaire. James Gordon died in early summer 1911, but before his death he extracted a promise that Edith would look out for his motherless seventeen-year-old daughter, Alice Gertrude (Altrude). Subsequently the widow and the orphan became close friends and traveled together to Europe and Maine. A few years later Altrude was introduced to Dr. Grayson, fourteen years her senior, at a dance. They soon became a romantic couple; Edith encouraged the romance and often acted as their chaperone. She stood up for Altrude at the Gordon-Grayson wedding in New York City in May 1916.[79]

The relationship between the first lady and, later, widow and the presidential physician was supportive and ultimately consequential. Edith referred to Grayson as "my dear boy" and called him "long a valued acquaintance of mine." She successfully lobbied President Wilson to promote "my dear boy" to Rear Admiral ahead of many senior medical officers.[80] There is no report that Dr. Grayson provided medical care to Mrs. Wilson. More significant was his allegiance to the first lady's successful plot to retain the presidency for her husband.

Social and Ceremonial Roles as First Lady

The second Mrs. Wilson was a successful White House hostess and enjoyed the pomp, notice and attention afforded by the ceremonial aspects of her position. She did well during Woodrow Wilson's triumphal tour of European capitals in 1918 and 1919. Her presence as social mistress of the executive mansion was but a brief interlude. The United States' entrance into World War I, the Wilsons' protracted presence at the Paris Peace Conference and Woodrow Wilson's medical disability prohibited significant Washington entertaining.[81]

Health as Caregiver to the Ex-President (1921–1924)

President and Mrs. Wilson retired to a Washington, D.C., home where Edith was an almost constant caregiver for her disabled husband. Her physical endurance and strength held up until late 1923. At that point she became tired and exhausted, and Cary Grayson, who had remained Woodrow Wilson's physician, prevailed upon her to take a brief vacation. When she returned, she was confined to bed for five days with a high fever.[82]

Health as a Widow

Edith Bolling Wilson was again a widow, upon the death of President Wilson in 1924, and lived as one for nearly thirty-eight years. When she died in Washington on December 28, 1961, at 89 years of age, she was at the time the longest living former first lady.[83] Her role as a widow was to shape Woodrow Wilson's history for posterity, similar to the mission of that of a successor, first lady Jacqueline Kennedy, forty years later.[84] Despite chronic cardiac disease and episodic congestive heart failure, Edith remained active. She sat on the platform during John Kennedy's January 1961 inauguration. But less than a year later Edith was dead from a respiratory infection and the complications of heart disease. She passed away on Woodrow Wilson's birthday.[85]

Homeopathic Physicians and the Kidney Disease of Florence Harding and Grace Coolidge

Charles E. Sawyer ... was suspicious of anyone—particularly medical experts—whom he perceived as threatening his status as close friend and homeopathic physician to the Hardings. The Duchess said Doc was the only person who could keep her alive. He was, Alice Longworth later said, the first lady's own Rasputin.[1]

Calvin turned to Mrs. Hills and said: "Hillsey, I'm afraid Mammy will die."[2]

Introduction

After the death of Ellen Wilson from chronic kidney (renal) failure, the spouses of the two presidents who succeeded Woodrow Wilson, Florence Harding (1921–1923) and Grace Coolidge (1923–1929), were both stricken in the White House with acute renal failure. In both patients the disease was centered in the drainage system of the kidneys and not in the kidneys per se.

Mrs. Harding died as a consequence of her disease one year after her departure from the White House. In contrast, Mrs. Coolidge's illness was transient; she survived for another thirty years, leading an active and productive life. A second contrast was the degree of transparency accorded their illnesses. Florence Harding's symptoms, medical course, treatment and attending physicians were the stuff of newspaper headlines. Grace Coolidge's illness would not be revealed until many years after she left Washington.

Another similarity was their treatment by homeopathically trained physicians, Charles Sawyer and Joel Boone. Previous chapters have addressed the influence of this medical philosophy upon first lady care during the apogee of homeopathy in America during 1880–1900. Lucretia Garfield's malaria was diagnosed first by Susan Edson, a homeopath. The primary care of Caroline Harrison, dying from tuberculosis, was administered by homeopathic doctor Franklin Gardner. Future first lady Ellen Wilson engaged Susan Taft as the obstetrician during her third pregnancy. Taft's treatment is unknown, but she was able to guide her patient through the very difficult pregnancy and delivery. Interestingly, Woodrow Wilson's concern about his wife's physician selection was based on gender, not on training.

Homeopathy

Homeopathy was developed in Germany by Dr. Samuel Hahnemann (1755–1843) and was introduced to the United States in the 1840s. Its minimalist treatment regimen attracted many patients, which resulted in a protracted and vituperative conflict with the dominant orthodox, or allopathic, medical culture as promoted by the American Medical Association.

The practice of homeopathy was based on the principles of similia and infinitesimals. The principle of similia held that a specific disease would be cured by remedies that produced in a healthy person the same or similar symptoms as those produced by that disease. The law of infinitesimals proposed that the smaller the dose, the more effective it became in stimulating the body's vital curative force. Therefore arose a paradox: The more dilute the dose of medicine, the greater its potency.[3]

The homeopathic principles of similia and infinitesimals, while perhaps ineffective, at least did no harm. In contrast, the hallowed treatments of nineteenth century orthodox medicine—cathartics, emetics, scarification and bleeding—often did. This kinder, gentler form of medicine attracted many patient-adherents, especially in urban areas and among the well-to-do. Orthodox-homeopathic strife was kindled with the transplantation of the

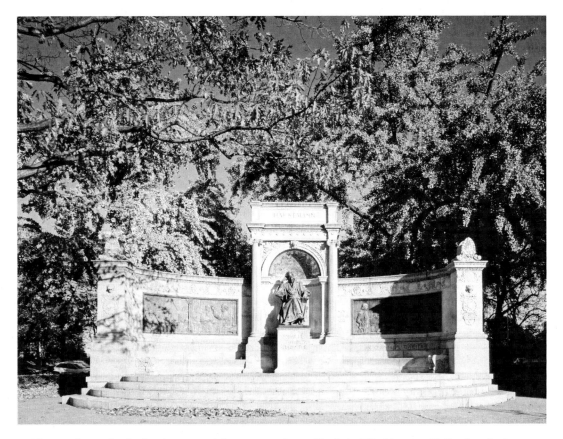

The much-overlooked 1901 memorial statue on Scott Circle in Washington, D.C., that depicts Samuel Hahnemann, the founder of the homeopathic medical discipline (Library of Congress).

unorthodox philosophy in America, smoldered while homeopathy increased in popularity, and burst into flames during the 1880s and 1890s. The American Medical Association forced its members to avoid all contacts with all practitioners of the Hahnemann school. If this prohibition were violated, the transgressor was punished. An example was that of Ellen Wilson's New York gastroenterologist, William Van Valzah, who was chased out of Philadelphia by his orthodox medical colleagues because he preferred the personal care of a homeopathic physician. Whether the AMA's motivation was primarily philosophical or financial is unknown.[4]

At the turn of the twentieth century, American homeopathy peaked in influence and adherents. In 1900 between 8 and 10 percent of physicians were homeopaths. Twenty-two homeopathic medical schools were extant in 1900, and in 1898 American homeopathy hosted nine national medical societies, thirty-three state medical societies, eighty-five local societies, sixty-six general homeopathic hospitals, seventy-four specialty homeopathic hospitals, fifty-seven homeopathic dispensaries, and thirty-one medical journals. Towards the end of the nineteenth century, orthodox doctors discovered a need to cooperate with homeopaths in order to effect meaningful state licensure laws. Both groups of physicians realized that unity was required to ensure a system of quality health care, The coalition's goals were twofold: To drive incompetent doctors from the practice of medicine and to limit the prerogatives of newer medical sects—chiropractors, osteopaths and Christian Scientists.[5]

Drs. Sawyer (62 years old) and Boone (32 years old) were trained during different eras; both were involved in the care of first lady Florence Harding, and Boone treated first lady Grace Coolidge. Their White House tenures provided opportunities to contrast their medical knowledge and degree of homeopathic parochialism.

Charles Sawyer and the Harding Family

Dr. Charles Sawyer was an 1881 graduate of the Homeopathic Hospital College of Cleveland. Sawyer was very prominent in homeopathic circles, as president of the Ohio State Homeopathic Medical Society and the American Institute of Homeopathy. In addition he authored articles that appeared in the *Journal of the American Institute of Homeopathy*.[6]

His connection to the Harding family dated to July 1897. Future president Warren Harding's mother, Phoebe Harding, was a practicing homeopathic physician who was accused of negligence in the death of a patient. Sawyer, then a prominent physician in the same Ohio town, was called in as a consultant in the legal controversy. His testimony supported Dr. Harding's professional performance, saving her practice from ruination. The local newspaper commented, "This statement, from a man of Dr. Sawyer's ability and standing in the community, relieves Mrs. Harding from all responsibilities in the affair."[7]

Subsequently "Doc" Sawyer and his wife became very friendly with Warren Harding and his wife, Florence. Their friendship was possibly due to the homeopath's beneficial intervention in the Phoebe Harding malpractice case, or perhaps it was a natural result of social companionship between two "power couples" in a small mid–America town. Both Hardings became increasingly dependent upon Sawyer for their medical care, Florence, almost obsessively so. Sawyer's medical responsibility for Mrs. Harding lasted until his death in 1924.[8]

Florence (The Duchess) Harding

Two Decades of Kidney Disease

Florence Kling DeWolfe, a determined and independent single mother of one, married up-and-coming Warren Gamaliel Harding, a man five years her junior, in July 1891. Called the Duchess by her husband and many others,[9] she was forceful, competent and smart. The Duchess effectively managed Harding's career as a newspaper publisher and a politician. Her thirty-three-year marriage with Harding produced no children.

Florence Harding's first recorded battle with kidney disease forced the cancellation of the Hardings' planned cruise to Cuba. In early 1905 Florence was admitted to Grant Hospital, Columbus, Ohio, with acute renal failure. The diagnosis was a "floating kidney" with obstruction of its ureter. "Floating kidney" was then a somewhat popular diagnosis; it referred to an abnormal descent of a kidney from its normal position when the patient was recumbent upon the patient's standing upright. More common in women, it rarely produced sufficient ureteral kinking or bending to cause an obstruction to the normal flow of urine into the bladder. Complications included infection of the affected kidney with severe cramping pain, and more serious, the retention of toxic products, so-called uremic poisoning.[10]

Unfortunately for Mrs. Harding, severe ureteral blockage had occurred and uremic poisoning ensued. On February 24, 1905, Dr. James Fairchild Baldwin elected to wire the affected kidney in place. He did not perform a nephrectomy because of previous "heart damage." Heart disease, without any specificity or documentation, became a frequent allusion during the rest of the Duchess's life.[11] Her postoperative convalescence was lengthy, requiring hospitalization for eight months. The surgical wound required dressings twice daily. Her surgeon, Dr. Baldwin, a graduate of Jefferson Medical College, was considered "in his day ... the equal of any surgeon in America." He was the founder of Grant Hospital, then the largest hospital in the United States.[12] A minor relapse of Mrs. Harding's kidney ailment occurred in spring 1908. It placed the Duchess once again under Doc's care: "As the summer wore on, she grew increasingly dependent upon his homeopathic concoctions for all her physical problems, real and imagined, believing Doc was the one man who could keep her alive.... It was the beginning of her complex emotional yet unromantic entanglement with him."[13]

Four years later, in 1912, the Duchess made frequent visits to the Sawyer-owned

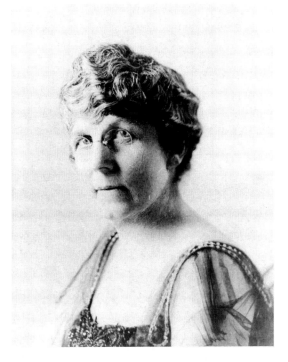

Florence Harding, the wife of Warren Harding. She was a strong believer in homeopathic medicine (Library of Congress).

White Oaks Sanatorium for physical and psychological respite.[14] The entrepreneurial Sawyer moved his health care facility from downtown Marion, Ohio, to the rural White Oaks Sanatorium, where he constructed fourteen bungalows placed around a central courtyard. An enclosed hall called the Cloister encircled the courtyard and connected all of the buildings. Sawyer promoted White Oaks "as a haven from the cares of the world, a place where patients could relax and reap the full benefits that nature's bounty and modern medicine could provide." His enterprise was advertised as a respite for those afflicted by nervous diseases and mental disorders. Treatments included "rigorous outdoor exercise, light therapy, hydrotherapy, massage and electrotherapy."[15]

Sawyer's son, Carl, a 1906 graduate of the allopathic Rush Medical School in Chicago, joined his father at White Oaks, and thereby became involved in the care of Florence Harding. The younger Sawyer eventually was certified by the American Board of Psychiatry and Neurology. Carl Sawyer's transition from homeopathy to orthodoxy reflected the friendly coexistence of the two branches of medicine that began around 1900.[16]

Another serious kidney attack occurred in December 1912 and persisted into 1913. The Sawyers treated the Duchess with unspecified measures at White Oaks. The gravity of the attack was underscored by the senior Sawyer's prognosis that his patient was not expected to live. Doc attributed its onset and severity to an underlying cardiac condition. References to Mrs. Harding's diseased heart abound, but its nature was never clarified.[17] An episode in autumn 1915 was treated by the elder Sawyer. This was considered mild, since Mrs. Harding insisted in journeying to Washington, D.C., to witness her husband take the oath as the new United States senator from Ohio. This proved to be unwise, as a relapse occurred.[18]

In January 1916, the then-senator's wife became ill with heart palpitations, acute indigestion, pain, abdominal swelling and severe "flu." Residing in the District of Columbia and distant from the amenable ambience of the Sawyers and their White Oaks Sanatorium, the Hardings elicited the services of the esteemed Washington practitioner Dr. Sterling Ruffin. The doctor was nonpartisan, treating both the Democratic Wilsons and the staunch Republican Duchess. Ruffin's examination detected no evidence of renal dysfunction. However, in Florence's opinion, Ruffin did not measure up to Sawyer's talents. In a dismissive tone she opinion: "This Washington doctor … I never want to see him." Sawyer, summoned from White Oaks, arrived in Washington and dosed his loyal patient with his homeopathic regimen of "dark pellet," "green medicine," "flat white tablets," and "yellow pellets." Mrs. Harding recovered.[19]

Another severe attack occurred in November 1918, the most menacing since the initial episode in 1905. The kidney had swollen to ten times its normal size and, in the words of her husband, was "far more painful than you can imagine." The diagnosis was hydronephrosis secondary to obstruction of the ureter. Carl Sawyer, then stationed as an army doctor at nearby Fort Meade, attended, together with Dr. Bernard Hardin, who practiced in several District hospitals. Surprisingly, Mrs. Harding liked Hardin. Four years later, she sent him flowers and also a letter of concern over the doctor's ill health, possibly as a reflection of her satisfaction and appreciation for his earlier service to her. Despite this, she took only the pills prescribed by the senior Dr. Sawyer.[20]

Since Mrs. Harding was convinced that only Doc Sawyer could keep her alive in the White House, her husband insisted that Sawyer become the White House physician. However, the inducements of a brigadier general's appointment and additional bureaucratic titles were required to lure Sawyer from his lucrative White Oaks practice to Washington, D.C.[21]

Doc Sawyer kept the first lady alive during a near-fatal medical emergency during August and September of 1922. While on an August 25–27 cruise aboard the presidential yacht the Duchess developed indigestion. Fortunately, Sawyer correctly suspected a recurrence of kidney disease and confined his patient to her White House bed.[22] Initially the illness was described as "an ailment neither alarming nor serious ... due to the effects of a cold complicated with a recurrence of a hydronephrosis." The patient's condition gradually worsened until September 7, when great pain caused President Harding to summon Dr. Joel Boone, then Sawyer's assistant, to her bedside. The following day Florence Harding developed uremic toxicity and nearly died. The alarmed president said to a friend, "I am afraid that Florence is going."[23]

Sawyer, frightened as his patient's condition worsened, relied heavily on Dr. Boone and, in addition, urged both his son Carl and the president's cardiologist brother, George Harding, to hurry to Washington from Ohio. In this VIP's medical emergency Doc sought both safety and solace in numbers. He enlisted expert surgical consultations from the renowned Rochester, Minnesota, surgeon, Dr. Charles Mayo, who in turn brought in Dr. John Finney, chief of surgery at Baltimore's Johns Hopkins.

President Harding insisted on full transparency for his wife's medical condition. This was one of the few times that the seriousness of a first lady's illness was presented to the country in complete detail. Harding was mindful of the recent political controversy attached to the secrecy of President Woodrow Wilson's stroke.[24] On September 8, Sawyer released the following statement to the press: "Mrs. Harding, whose illness is a recurrence of attacks before coming to the White House developed complications Thursday and Thursday night which made her condition critical. These complications are so serious that recovery is not yet assured. Doctor John Finney of Baltimore was called in consultation tonight and Dr. Charles Mayo is en route from Rochester, Minnesota. Doctor Carl W. Sawyer and Doctor Joel T. Boone have joined in the attendance of Mrs. Harding today." After this announcement, twice daily medical bulletins were released until the first lady was out of danger. A Philadelphia newspaper editorialized that such disclosure was "striking in comparison with the attitude of the previous Administration as to compel notice."[25]

When Dr. Finney arrived at the bedside from Baltimore on September 8, he: "found her very ill, suffering from an acutely infected cystic kidney. Her pulse and temperature were high, and she appear[ed] very toxic." The consultant confirmed Sawyer's diagnosis of hydronephrosis of the affected kidney. This diagnosis, literally "water inside the kidney," refers to distention of the affected kidney's urine collection and excretion system with destruction of its ability to function. Finney advised as treatment the comparatively simple procedure to surgically drain the kidney by incision. Finney's autobiography continued the story: "This course, however, did not appeal to Dr. Sawyer.... I insisted on seeing the president before going and stating the case to him as I saw it. Dr. Sawyer again objected, and so the matter was up to the President who sided with Dr. Sawyer. I returned to Baltimore."[26]

Dr. Charles Mayo arrived on September 9 and insisted that Finney return to Mrs. Harding's bedside. The patient's condition remained dire. Finney resumed his lively narrative: "Dr. Mayo ... strongly advised drainage of the kidney by incision.... [O]ne had to be a bit dogmatic. Perhaps nature would come to the rescue, perhaps not. If not, the chances of recovery were practically nil.... Dr. Sawyer again disagreed and said that he did not believe much in operating anyway. The question was once more put up to the President ... [who] again decided in favor of Dr. Sawyer and against the operation both Dr. Mayo and I advised. It was a new experience, I am sure, for Dr. Mayo, coming from the Mayo Clinic, to have his opinion and advice summarily disregarded. I was more accustomed to it in the East."[27] Shortly thereafter, nature did take its course. The urine flow occurred and the first lady recovered, albeit very slowly. Letters written as late as February 1923 indicated that Florence Harding's convalescence was protracted.[28]

Thus a poorly educated homeopathic doctor was able to stare down two of the most illustrious and respected surgeons in America and have his decision "to watch and wait" vindicated.

Dr. Charles H. Mayo founded and led the renowned Mayo Clinic with his older brother, William, in Rochester, Minnesota: "The names of William and Charles Mayo are famous throughout the world wherever surgery is practiced." Upon entry of the United States into World War I, the brothers Mayo were made joint chief consultants in charge of all the surgical services in the United States Army.[29] John Finney was a graduate of both Princeton University and the Harvard School of Medicine. He was second in rank on the surgical staff of Johns Hopkins Hospital until Dr. William Halsted's death in 1923, and for two years served as acting professor of surgery and chief of service at Johns Hopkins Hospital and Medical School. Finney was much admired for his public spirit and as an educator.[30]

John Finney met Mrs. Harding socially several times thereafter at the home of Mrs. Evalyn McLean. He further wrote: "I was called on the telephone from the White House by Mrs. Harding herself, who cordially invited me to join the presidential party as a member of the medical group. She said that, as I already knew, she had not been very well and neither had the President, and they would appreciate it if I would join them on their trip to the West Coast and Alaska." Although the surgeon regretted that he could not accept, Finney maintained contact with the presidential party by telegram.

President Warren Harding died from a heart attack in San Francisco on August 2, 1923, almost one year from the onset of his wife's near-fatal illness.[31] In stark contrast to his deft handling of the Duchess's kidney disease, Sawyer seriously misdiagnosed and mismanaged the heart disease of her husband.[32] After President Harding died at age fifty-seven, the widowed first lady went back to Marion, Ohio. In January 1924 former first lady Florence Harding returned to Washington. She was accompanied by the wife of Dr. Charles Sawyer, and upon her arrival she took up residence in an apartment at the Willard Hotel.[33] Dr. Joel Boone offered to care for Mrs. Harding after the senior Sawyer resigned as White House physician. However, Doc was determined to retain his position as Florence Harding's personal physician. Six months after Mrs. Harding took up residence in the nation's capital, her kidney disease recurred. Sawyer immediately traveled to Washington and refused to leave until Mrs. Harding accompanied him back to his Ohio sanitarium. There she remained under the watchful care of the Sawyers.[34]

On November 3, 1925, Carl Sawyer released a bulletin that Florence Harding was again suffering from nephritis and had severe abdominal pain. The younger Sawyer was quoted at the time: "She has developed a number of symptoms that were present in her serious attack in 1922 in the White House. Other complications have arisen which were not present at that time, and her condition now is rather serious." Sawyer requested outside surgical consultation. In a strange addendum he identified the death of his father as a factor contributing to the deterioration of his patient.[35]

On November 8, Drs. Wood (of Cleveland) and Carl Sawyer performed an exploratory operation at White Oaks. James Craven Wood was a pillar of the Midwest Homeopathic community and specialized in obstetrics and gynecology. Their surgery report stated there was "an almost complete contusion of the right ureter, necessitating an exploratory puncture, which is hoped will afford temporary relief." The patient survived the palliative operation, but her respite was brief. She died on November 21, 1924. Sawyer listed the cause of death as chronic nephritis and myocarditis, with evidence of hydronephrosis.[36] Charles Sawyer had died suddenly, at sixty-four years of age, at his White Oaks Sanatorium on September 23, 1924, outliving his famous patient, the president, by just over one year. Florence Harding, then residing at White Oaks, was the last person to see Doc alive.[37]

Grace Goodhue Coolidge

Grace Goodhue Coolidge, Florence Harding's successor as first lady, was a stark contrast to her flamboyant predecessor, dissimilar in personality, in political influence, in controversy, and in longevity. However, there were two similarities. Both women nearly died in the White House from a similar kidney infection. Both were under the care of the assistant White House physician, navy doctor Joel Boone.

Boone was the naval presence in the White House during three presidential administrations. He was the naval medical bridge between Admiral Cary Grayson, who served Woodrow Wilson, and Admiral Ross McIntire, who was Franklin Roosevelt's personal physician. Dr. Boone was admitted directly into medical school after high school and graduated from the Homeopathic Hahnemann Medical College of Pennsylvania in 1913. In contrast to Sawyer, he completed a year of postgraduate training as an intern at Hahnemann. Thereupon he immediately enlisted in the U.S. Navy. After 1900, American homeopathic and orthodox physicians compromised on their differences; similarities in diagnosis, treatment and patterns of consultation emerged. As a result, Boone's professional philosophy and practice were indistinguishable from that of a member in good standing of the American Medical Association.[38]

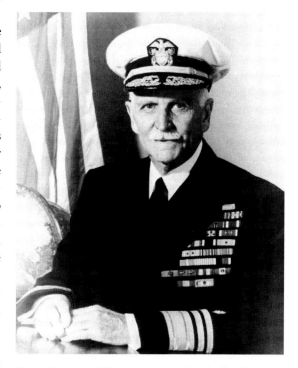

Navy doctor Joel Boone treated first ladies Florence Harding and Grace Coolidge (courtesy Bureau of Medicine and Surgery Archives).

Professional, Family and Early Medical History

Grace Coolidge was a professional woman. At a time when it was unusual for a woman to even enter a university, whether because it was not the norm or affordable, she graduated from the University of Vermont in 1902. Furthermore she commenced upon a career of teaching the hearing impaired. After graduation she entered teacher training at Clarke School for the Deaf in Northampton, Massachusetts. She taught at Clarke for three years until her marriage to Calvin Coolidge. Her support for Clarke and the hearing impaired was lifelong and unwavering.[39] Born Grace Anna Goodhue in Burlington, Vermont, on January 3, 1879, she was an only child. In adulthood Grace measured five feet four inches and had "masses of lustrous dark hair." Her biographers credited her eyes as being her most remarkable feature, which were described as "gray-green ... wide set and grave, even when her face was alight with laughter." It was her habit to focus them with close attention on anyone she was addressing.[40]

The future first lady possessed lifelong good health, with the exception of a clandestine kidney crisis while she was living in the White House and several obscure illnesses during her early years. She initially enrolled at the University of Vermont for the 1897 fall semester, but withdrew fewer than three months later because "she needed to improve her health," and, in an opaque reference, "an oculist [eye physician] had recommended she take time off." Biographer Isabel Ross noted that Grace "had trouble with her spine as a child but vigorous exercises had strengthened her." Grace definitely liked long walks and made them a lifelong daily habit.[41]

Marriage to Calvin Coolidge

At age 24 Grace Goodhue married attorney and ambitious politician Calvin Coolidge in Burlington, Vermont. The groom was 32. It was a marriage notable more for its dedication to duty and responsibility than for its joy and happiness. Eleven months later John Coolidge was born; twenty months after that, Cal Jr. made his appearance.[42]

Grace Coolidge's autobiography, written many years later, contained this retrospective: "The wedding ceremony has seldom united two people of more vastly different temperaments and tastes than on the fourth of October 1905, when Mr. Coolidge and I made our marriage vows standing in the bay window in the parlor of my father's home."[43] Coolidge biographers underscored the personality contrast: "They made an uncommon pair—the girl with the wide smile, fine eyes and friendly manner, and the spare, tight-lipped lawyer.... His mouth was his most forbidding feature—a thin slash sweeping down at the corners with a suggestion of perpetual gloom. He seemed aloof because of his remote and frosty manner, plus his declarative chopped-off statements, as sharp as exclamation points." The groom was characterized as notable for his "shy disposition, somber demeanor, and conscientious devotion to duty."[44]

First Lady Grace Coolidge

In 1920 Massachusetts governor Coolidge, whose political star was burnished by his successful handling of the Boston police strike, was selected as the vice presidential nominee for Warren G. Harding's successful presidential candidacy. Coolidge was an inconspicuous vice president. Grace Coolidge gracefully bore both the traditional obscurity of her position and the hostility of first lady Florence Harding. Everything changed when Warren Harding died from a heart attack. In the early morning of August 3, 1923, Calvin Coolidge was sworn in as the nation's 30th president by his father, a Vermont justice of the peace. The ceremony took place in John Coolidge's remote farmhouse in Plymouth, Vermont. The quaint domicile was without a phone, central heating, electricity or indoor plumbing.[45]

As first lady, Grace was underappreciated, especially by her husband, the president. The 45-year-old Mrs. Coolidge fulfilled the social, ceremonial and supportive roles of her position with great charm, poise and grace. Her personality was her strongest point; it brought spontaneity and joy to the White House. Grace had an eye for style; she became a fashion leader during the Coolidge presidency.[46] One biographer summed up her White House tenure: "She was comforting and nurturing to her partner, her husband, the president. Yet she was not a presidential partner since she did not get involved in politics. In addition, her management of the White House menus and staff was often overruled by her husband. With a change in housekeepers in 1926, she had more control over the budget and her husband was pleased with the arrangements."[47] However, for a while the penurious and controlling Coolidge examined all household bills and personally initialed the payment checks.[48]

Three events shaped Grace Coolidge's experience as America's first lady: Her near fatal kidney attack in 1928; the death of her younger son, Calvin Jr., in 1924; and the estrangement from her husband during most of his presidency.

Kidney Disease While First Lady

The first lady nearly perished from renal failure in early 1928. Her prominence elicited the medical services of six physicians: four consultants and the two White House physicians, Charles Coupal and Joel Boone. The professional relationship between the latter two was fractious. Although army doctor Coupal, as the President's personal physician, was senior, navy lieutenant commander Joel Boone was a prolific and opinionated writer. His diary entries provide most of the historical narrative of this episode and form the core of the following discussion.

On February 2, 1928, Grace Coolidge was fortified with both bromides and codeine to get her through an evening White House reception. When she left the social engagement, a physical examination revealed exhaustion and a weak but rapid pulse. The patient's condition improved over the succeeding two days. However, on the second day Boone judiciously sought advice from two eminent private internists, Drs. Walter Bloedorn and Paul Dickens. They advised an emergency cystoscopy, a visualization of the lower urinary tract.[49]

It was not until two days later, February 6, when both staff doctors, very anxious and dissatisfied with the first lady's progress, actively considered their consultants' previous advice. Coupal urged a referral to the prominent Johns Hopkins urologist Dr. Hugh Young. The following day, February 7, Boone traveled to Baltimore to discuss Mrs. Coolidge's medical problem with Dr. Young. The possibility that tuberculosis was the cause of the disease was discussed. Boone brought tuberculosis to the president's attention in a private conversation.[50] Young and his assistant, Dr. W. Scott, also from Johns Hopkins, examined Grace Coolidge at the Washington Naval Hospital on February 8. Strict secrecy was the desire of Mrs. Coolidge. Therefore neither the examination nor its results were announced. Consequently Boone drove the patient to the hospital in his own car without the customary accompaniment of a Secret Service agent.[51]

The president's wife was three hours on the examination table. Young's cystoscopic visualization and urinary tract X-rays disclosed an abnormal right kidney that was both enlarged and misplaced. Its drainage tube, the right ureter, was kinked. As a result of this blockage, the drainage system—closest to the kidney—of pelvis and calyces were swollen. As a result, the first lady was vulnerable to both uremic poisoning and a serious kidney infection. Both complications had occurred in the case of Florence Harding six years earlier. In contrast, surgery was performed in this case: the passage of instruments with irrigation of the kidneys was a successful treatment. An X-ray of Mrs. Coolidge's chest was negative for any disease, including tuberculosis.[52]

Drs. Young and Scott subsequently retired to the secrecy of Coolidge's private White House study, where they were joined by Boone and Coupal. Young informed the president that Mrs. Coolidge had a kidney infection. He also advised Boone to sleep at the White House in order to monitor Mrs. Coolidge' condition. The patient's symptoms worsened over the next two days as she suffered severe pain spasms from her diseased kidney. The frightened president became so distraught that he confided to a long-time friend, "Hillsey, I'm afraid Mammy will die."[53]

Dr. Coupal was worried about Mrs. Coolidge's heart and urged the administration of digitalis, a heart stimulant. His colleague Boone disagreed and was supported by Walter Bloedorn ("No! Don't let them stampede you. Use your own judgment.") and by the president ("You know best"). An electrocardiogram performed two days later confirmed Boone's opinion.[54] As a result, President Coolidge increasingly relied upon Boone to manage his wife's care. He judged that the navy physician's abilities were superior to that of his titular superior, Charles Coupal, a conclusion shared by Boone, who disparaged Coupal's ability, considering it to be that of a family physician of the sort that one might have discovered at that time in towns and small cities in the United States.[55]

Almost two weeks after the disease's onset, the patient continued to battle terrible pain. Coupal urged the administration of benzyl benzoate as a pain killer, then in use as an antispasmodic to halt intestinal, biliary and ureteral colic. Boone, continuing his intellectual feud with his colleague, administered it " against my better judgment." When there was no improvement, Boone decided that codeine was the appropriate remedy. In a peculiar display of professional one-upmanship, the doctor complained to Coolidge about Coupal's therapy and phoned Dr. Young, who agreed "with my deductions and treatment of Mrs. C, congratulates me on my conduct of the case."[56]

Due to insufficient rest, and despite her adherence to Boone's admonition to avoid walks, Grace Coolidge remained both weak and tired through the early part of the Coolidges' 1928 summer vacation at Brule, Wisconsin. The kidney attacks finally subsided during the summer, and there was no recurrence thereafter. In this pre-antibiotic era, rest and supportive care were sufficient to overcome the infection.[57]

Near-identical Kidney Disease in Two Successive First Ladies

Several comparisons are appropriate with Mrs. Harding's illness in the White House six years previously. The disease was the same, but Mrs. Coolidge's recovery was permanent, while Mrs. Harding's outcome was eventually fatal. Both received VIP medical care from many physicians, both military and civilian, who were among the most illustrious in their field. In both situations, Boone was involved, and in both professional disagreements arose. However, the complete secrecy in the Coolidge White House was in stark contrast with the transparency in the Harding's executive mansion.

Four years after the comprehensive media coverage of her son's fatal illness (see below) all news of Grace Coolidge's condition was suppressed. This may have been at the first lady's request. Grace had complained earlier about her lack of privacy, especially after having endured the death of her younger son in the public eye.[58] The society sections of contemporary newspapers noted Mrs. Coolidge's absence at events where her presence was anticipated, but there was no significant clarifying comment.[59]

Dr. Hugh Young abetted in placing a shroud over publicity by his semi-clandestine appearances at the Washington Naval Hospital and in Calvin Coolidge's study. His respect for his patient's confidentiality was reflected in his 1940 autobiography. Grace Coolidge was not listed in its subject index. (The urologist had previously treated the disabled Woodrow Wilson in the White House. Young wrote about this episode at length in the same volume.)[60]

Fatal Illness and Death of Calvin Coolidge, Jr.

The Coolidges were not the only presidential couple whose child died immediately before, during, or shortly after their term in the White House. The tragic deaths of young Benjamin Pierce and Willie Lincoln were discussed in a previous chapter and a more recent example, the demise of newborn Patrick Kennedy, is considered later.[61]

During the first half of the twentieth century, White House physicians, with a very short list of patients to follow and only an occasional acute illness to treat, often interacted socially with members of the first family. Both Drs. Coupal and Boone connected with the Coolidge sons, John and his younger brother, sixteen-year-old Calvin Jr. They rode horseback, played tennis, shot pool, went sightseeing and had lunches aboard the *Mayflower* together. Boone acted almost as an older brother.[62] A tennis foursome between the two Coolidge sons and the two physicians was the setting for the subsequent Coolidge family tragedy. Cal Jr., late and in a rush to join his companions already on the court, donned his tennis shoes without wearing protective socks. A blister appeared on his toe afterwards. The boy was reticent about the lesion, took a bath and applied iodine. Symptoms arose over the next few days; he became tired and listless; pains shot up his leg, which became stiff.

On July 2, 1924, Cal was absent from a scheduled tennis foursome. Boone quickly sought out the president's son to determine whether he was ill and located the boy in the Lincoln bedroom, lying down while the first lady played the piano. Boone's examination noted a fever and swollen lymph glands in his groin. In addition, red streaks ascended his leg and a blister, darker and larger than usual, was located "on the third toe just behind the second joint on the anterior surface."[63] Boone, alarmed by signs of a significant systemic infection, called Coupal to the bedside. The two physicians operated in tandem during the entire tragic episode, in sharp contrast with their disagreements four years later during the illness of Grace Coolidge. Antiseptic dressings were applied and a blood culture was obtained. Boone personally took the specimen to a military laboratory for analysis. The physicians disclosed their apprehension to Grace Coolidge and the president. Mrs. Coolidge was calm, resourceful and an efficient asset throughout her son's illness.

The president's son was sicker the following day, more febrile and very restless. Colonel William Keller, the chief of surgery at Walter Reed Army Hospital, and Charles W. Richardson, a noted Washington physician, came to the White House to consult.[64] The military physicians thought it wise to enlarge the medical team with more civilian consultation. John B. Deaver, professor of surgery at Philadelphia's German Hospital, arrived on the next train. He joined Keller in suspecting appendicitis as the cause of the illness but was insufficiently certain to operate immediately. However, Calvin's condition continued to deteriorate and the blood culture from two days earlier disclosed a systemic infection due to staphylococcal aureus bacteria.

Drs. Boone and Coupal were aware that the situation was grave and that some sort of notification to the public was necessary. "President's Son Is Seriously Ill; Foot Is Poisoned" was the headline in the July 5 edition of the *Atlanta Constitution*. The bulletin was informal in nature and not signed by the doctors. It was explained that no formal bulletins would be issued, the White House taking the position that the patient was "not a public character, and should be treated with no more dignity than any other upstanding American boy."[65] A far lesser degree of transparency was practiced by these same doctors four years later.

On July 5, Deaver returned, accompanied by a pathologist, Dr. Kolmar from the University of Pennsylvania School of Medicine. Deaver decided hospitalization was necessary; an operation was performed at Walter Reed Hospital. Assisted by Keller, Deaver made an incision over the left tibia and chiseled some of the bone for culture to determine whether the infection had traveled. It had. "It was their belief ... that the poison in the system had centralized sufficiently to warrant an effort at draining it from the body before the youth's strength was further wasted in fighting the infection."[66] This was a peculiar notion since a prior culture of the blood had already disclosed a generalized infection.

The patient's decline was precipitous. Calvin Coolidge, Jr. died on July 7, 1924, from staphylococcal septicemia, only four days after the severity of his illness was recognized.[67] Many prominent American newspapers remarked on Mrs. Coolidge's courage and endurance during this ordeal.[68]

Grace Coolidge: Estranged Wife and Widow

In *The Tormented President* Gilbert analyzed Calvin Coolidge's depression after his son's death: "not believing that death had occurred, of missing his young son, of not being happy without him, of seeing him playing tennis on the WH courts every time he glanced out the window, and of soon joining his son in death." The president's behavior in office underwent a remarkable change: he became indifferent instead of engaged, listless instead of alert and in control, passive instead of actively engaging with his cabinet and Congress.[69] Coolidge's major depression resulted in a pronounced propensity to sleep. He slept eleven hours a night. His accustomed post-lunch naps lengthened to between two and four hours. His presidential work schedule was reduced to four and a half hours a day.[70]

In sharp contrast, his first lady reacted with hope and acceptance. She spoke of her son's smile, of his happiness in heaven, of her sense of nearness to him, and of allowing her to glimpse God's faith and the glory of his grace. She handled the loss of a son far better than her predecessors, Jane Pierce and Mary Lincoln. Grace wore all white at that August's Republican National Convention and throughout the summer. She immediately returned to entertaining and presented a cheerful demeanor in the White House.[71] And she discovered that the "Summer Game" was a source of fun and enjoyment. Mrs. Coolidge regularly attended the Washington Senators' baseball games. She became a rabid fan, sat by the Senators dugout, was known by all the players, and refused to leave the ballpark even when her dour husband left during the early innings. In later years, when she retired to Massachusetts, she became a loyal supporter of the Boston Red Sox.[72]

Grace discovered Dr. Joel Boone to be an intelligent, attentive and available listener, and she came to rely upon the physician as a counselor and friend. She requested his advice on the selection of a boarding school for her sons. He recommended his alma mater, Mercersburg Academy in Pennsylvania, which the boys subsequently attended.[73] Grace befriended not only Boone, but also Boone's wife and daughter Suzanne. Suzanne was often asked to spend nights at the White House and the Coolidges took her to the circus. The first lady, becoming estranged from her husband, enjoyed her discreet talks with Boone as a way to unwind. The Coolidges' proximity during their long 1925–7 summer vacations led to increased marital unhappiness. No word of these problems got out, only in Grace's conversations with Boone.

During an Adirondack summer vacation, Grace and Boone had a long conversation about John, her remaining son. She confided to the doctor that she and Coolidge were not "at all in accord on John."[74]

If she challenged the president on John's upbringing, he would retaliate and not speak to her for three days.[75] Calvin Coolidge's concept of the relative positions of a husband and wife may be a reason for any marital discord: "Marriage is the most intricate institution set up by the human race. If it is to be a growing concern it must have a head. That head should be the member of the firm who assumes the greater responsibility for its continuance. In general this is the husband…. In my humble opinion the woman is by nature the more adaptable of the two and she should rejoice in this and realize that in the exercise of this ability she will obtain not only spiritual blessing but her own family will rise up and call her blessed."[76]

Ex-president Coolidge's health declined in retirement and he died quietly on January 5, 1933. His widow lived for another twenty-four years and enjoyed a long and productive retirement in Massachusetts.[77] Perhaps her daily exercise regimen of six to eight hours of walking was a reason for this. In 1952, when her health began to fail, the first sign of it was her disinclination to walk.[78] Mrs. Coolidge had heart trouble during the last five years of her life and became very stooped.[79] She died of congestive heart failure at age seventy-eight; the death certificate listed as the cause of death kyphoscoliotic heart disease.[80] The former first lady had remained friends with Dr. Boone and his wife, and Joel Boone attended her funeral.

Chapter Twelve

Mamie Eisenhower and Menière's Disease

In early November 1973, TV host Barbara Walters asked Mrs. Eisenhower the following: "I am going to ask you something, because it's been a rumor for years, and I want to finally put it to rest. You know what the rumor is." The former first lady responded: "Oh yes, that I am a dipsomaniac."[1]

A First Lady Dogged by Rumors of Alcoholism

First ladies, as the wives of prominent men, are frequent objects of scrutiny by the press, by personal enemies, and by political opponents. The political station of a husband may cause pain, anxiety and even scandalous aspersion for the wife. No first lady experienced more defamation than Mary Todd Lincoln.[2] But Mamie Eisenhower suffered her own aspersions. She was long troubled by a lack of balance and an unsteadiness of gait. For three years during World War II the Atlantic Ocean separated General Dwight and Mamie Eisenhower from each other. Mamie resided in an apartment in Washington, D.C., and experienced profound loneliness. After she awkwardly stumbled and spilt gravy down the uniform of a soldier while volunteering at the District of Columbia Soldiers Club, the Washington rumor mill concluded that Mrs. Eisenhower was drunk. The Washington wags conjectured that Mamie had sought the solace of the bottle to combat her marital isolation.[3]

A suggestion of alcoholism, once whispered, is never silenced. During the 1952 battle for the Republican presidential nomination, the campaign of Robert Taft, Eisenhower's rival, spread stories about Mrs. Eisenhower's drinking habits. Their credibility may have been amplified by an event at a Washington embassy party. Eisenhower requested that Mamie's dinner partner take her by the arm since she was unsteady on her feet. During a subsequent transcontinental political railroad trip, "Mamie was acutely conscious throughout the trip of rumors circulating since the war that she drank too much."[4] A Republican convention delegate from Nebraska boldly broached the subject to the candidate: "General we're not worried about what you stand for.... But we are worried about your wife.... We hear she's a drunk."[5] Ironic indeed that the campaign of senator of Ohio Robert A. Taft would circulate these rumors. Senator Taft was the oldest son of former first lady Nellie

Taft. An entry on the first ladies' personal interests page of the National First Ladies' Library recorded the following regarding the drink preferences of Robert's mother: "Helen 'Nellie' Taft, lager beer and champagne cocktail (perhaps the one who imbibed the most)."[6] The rumors persisted during Ike's (General Dwight Eisenhower) 1956 presidential campaign. Paul Butler, head of the Democratic party, intimated that the first lady's recent illness was perhaps a result of drinking.[7] The allegations finally reached print, fortunately in a less than reputable source. The *National Enquirer*, a supermarket checkout tabloid, published the rumors in its June 7, 1959, edition.[8]

The Eisenhowers retired to their Gettysburg, Pennsylvania, farm in 1961, where the rumors of alcoholism persisted. Dr. William Sterrett, Mamie's primary care physician in Gettysburg recalled: "When the Eisenhowers first moved to Gettysburg, the story was all over Adams County that she was an alcoholic." As an example of the extent to which tales of Mamie's drinking were embellished, Sterrett recounted this rumor: The velvet rope atop the stairs of the Eisenhowers' previous house in Denver did not signal that the couple had retired to bed, but rather was to protect a drunken Mamie from falling down the stairs.[9] Neither Ike nor Mamie publicly confronted these allegations until the Barbara Walters interview in late 1973.

Unlike several other first ladies, notably Sarah Polk, Lucy Hayes, and Rosalynn Carter, Mrs. Eisenhower did drink alcohol.[10] A January 4, 1946, notation in her medical record written by Dr. George Robb reads, "uses alcohol moderately." During the war years in Washington, she drank no more than anyone, which was usually one cocktail. Her favorite was an Old Fashioned. Many testimonials over her career attested that she never drank to excess and was never seen drunk. Her Gettysburg doctor asserted, "Mamie's drinking had virtually ceased many years earlier."[11]

A Chronic Medical Condition

The rumors were false but they abetted scandalous gossip among the political and media classes. It was not alcohol but a chronic disease that produced Mrs. Eisenhower's dizziness and unsteadiness. In Dr. Robb's medical history, he noted that a diagnosis of carotid artery hypersensitivity had been made previously. Robb could not confirm this diagnosis.[12] Unfortunately Dr. Sterrett used the old Walter Reed records to perpetuate an unsubstantiated diagnosis. The practice of continuing to attach a disproved historical diagnosis to a patient out of courtesy to a physician predecessor, or out of habit, has long vexed the practice of medicine. Mamie continued to harbor the misdiagnosis given her decades earlier. In a 1972 interview the widowed Mrs. Eisenhower responded: "For twenty-five years or more than that I carried this equilibrium problem, which is carotid sinus."[13]

The carotid sinuses are pressure receptors adjacent to the major arteries on both sides of the neck. An exaggerated reflex of the carotid sinus (hypersensitivity) produces a sudden loss of blood pressure, dizziness, and fainting. A practical method of diagnosis is the reproduction of these symptoms by manual massage of the patient's neck. Mamie tested negative when this maneuver was tried on her in 1946.[14]

Menière's and Mamie

A far more likely diagnosis to explain Mrs. Eisenhower's symptoms is Menière's disease. A firm diagnosis allegedly was established at Walter Reed Hospital in 1953.[15] Other biographers assert only that Menière's disease was diagnosed sometime after World War II.[16] The symptoms of this condition stayed with her until the end of her life.[17]

Menière's disease is a diagnosis of exclusion, characterized by episodic spells of vertigo that usually last a few hours and are associated with fluctuating, unilateral ear fullness, tinnitus (ringing or buzzing sound), and hearing loss.[18] Prosper Menière was a prominent mid-nineteenth century French physician who connected deafness in a young woman with an excess of fluid in her inner ear. He presented his discovery in a paper titled "On a Particular Kind of Hearing Loss Resulting from Lesions of the Inner Ear" to the Imperial Academy of Medicine in Paris. Menière died a year later in 1862 with his significant discovery unrecognized.[19] For over seventy years, Menière's disease was not defined as a specific entity; nor were effective treatments identified to alleviate its symptoms. Only in 1972 did the American Academy of Ophthalmology and Otolaryngology Committee on Hearing and Equilibrium finally publish a clear definition of Menière's disease.[20] Effective therapies for the disease were discovered earlier; in 1934 a low-salt diet and diuretics were first recommended to alleviate the "water-logged" condition of the inner-ear labyrinth. Surgical techniques were introduced in the 1950s and have improved significantly since.[21]

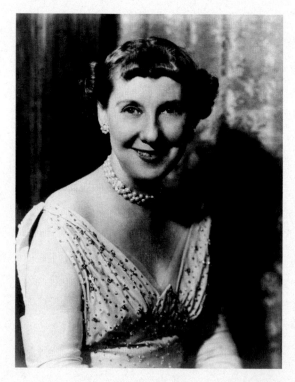

Mamie Eisenhower, the wife of Dwight "Ike" Eisenhower. The consequences of Menière's disease led to scandalous press speculation about her (Library of Congress).

Mrs. Eisenhower had a long history of vertigo (a spinning sensation with disorientation). In 1929 after a descent down the Alps, her husband noted her dizziness and "stomach upsets." These symptoms subsequently recurred in other situations. Later, while stationed in the Philippines, she developed an equilibrium problem described as a "pitching sensation."[22]

During the war years, while the Eisenhowers were in Washington, D.C., the attacks became more acute than those previously experienced in the Philippines. The symptoms were devastating and frequently disabling. When a sudden attack occurred, Mamie "couldn't stand steady for any length of time without assistance, and even the simplest tasks could become unfortunately complicated. Sometimes ... she couldn't even hail a taxi without someone lending her an arm." Although she had a car, she was afraid to drive it. The unsteadiness forced her to curtail her volunteer work with the American soldiers. "I crawled on my hands and knees from my bathroom to the kitchen. I didn't dare to walk …. I couldn't walk." Her antidote was smelling salts, which she always kept in her possession when she left her apartment. Her husband, concerned about her problem, wrote from Versailles, France, in September 1944: "It would be wonderful if the medicos could find out what is the reason for your lack of balance."[23] The Eisenhowers lived in New York City while Ike was the president of Columbia University (1948–50). Mamie could not walk the block from their apartment to the university without someone holding her arm.[24]

The anatomical cause of Menière's disease is well established. Its symptoms are produced by the accumulation of excess fluid within the semilunar canals (labyrinth) of the patient's inner ears. Less certain is what provokes the excess fluid. Many associations have been postulated: diet, allergy, autoimmune disorders, and psychological distress. Anxiety, stress and depression have been linked with Menière's symptoms. Whether these are a cause or a result of the disease remains a conundrum.[25]

Mamie Eisenhower's long marriage to an ambitious army officer was often beset by worry and nervousness. Gastrointestinal symptoms were a frequent accompaniment and may have resulted from her anxiety. During Ike's 1922–24 assignment to the Panama Canal Zone, Mamie repeatedly suffered from digestive complaints. Her symptoms were significant enough to require a transfer to Walter Reed Army Medical Center in the District of Columbia. After several months of hospitalization she was released, feeling better but without a definitive diagnosis.[26]

The Eisenhowers' next army post was Fort Leavenworth, Kansas. Once again there was a hospitalization, this time at the Leavenworth base hospital in 1926. The diagnosis is unrecorded, but the treatment was sedatives. Her gall bladder was removed in Pueblo, Colorado, in July 1931 (Mrs. Eisenhower's parents lived nearby in Colorado). Preoperative history at the time recorded six years of flatulence and pain and years of emotional distress. The concomitant physical examination revealed a very irritable and easily upset patient who was described as the thin, nervous type.[27]

Eisenhower was stationed in the Philippines as General Douglas MacArthur's adjutant from 1936 to 1940. During this chapter of Mamie's life, gastric complains coincided with "a pitching sensation," most probably an early symptom of Menière's. A specific diagnosis escaped her physicians until an upper gastrointestinal ulcer began to bleed profusely. Mamie collapsed, became comatose for days, and barely survived. She lost thirty pounds and went to a weight of 105 pounds after the near-catastrophic event.[28] Gastrointestinal complaints would persist until her death.

During the war years, Mamie, separated from General Eisenhower, lived alone in a Washington apartment. Digestive complaints and Menière's attacks kept her bedridden much of the time. Anxiety for her husband's safety led to insomnia and recurrent significant weight loss. Unsurprisingly, she suffered from depression.[29]

Episodes of Menière's continued in the White House, and curtailed some of Mrs. Eisenhower's ceremonial appearances. She did not accompany President Eisenhower to his May 1960 Paris summit with Nikita Khrushchev or on his 1959 and 1960 overseas goodwill trips at the conclusion of his presidency. The first lady feared for her balance.[30] Serendipitously, medications prescribed for her other maladies probably controlled the Menière's symptoms of vertigo and unsteadiness. Phenobarbital was given to control anxiety and a diuretic together with a low-salt diet were proposed for her heart disease.[31]

Rheumatic Heart Disease

Mamie Doud contracted rheumatic fever at her parents' Colorado Springs home when she was about eight years old. The acute symptoms included abnormal involuntary movement of her muscles (St. Vitus Dance) and leg pains. As a consequence she was kept home from school for the better part of a year. Complications resulted due to the inflammation of her mitral and aortic valves. Rheumatic scarring of her mitral and aortic heart valves would be a medical problem for the rest of Mamie's life. In the pre-antibiotic era, significant valvular disease frequently resulted from untreated rheumatic fever.[32]

Mamie's cardiac symptoms worsened during the war and contributed to her fatigue. As a result, military doctors restricted Mrs. Eisenhower's physical activity and forbade her to fly.[33] Surprisingly, the wife of the Supreme United States Commander in Europe was not evaluated by a cardiologist until her 1946 examination by Lt. Col. George Robb at Walter Reed. Robb diagnosed inactive rheumatic valvular disease with mild mitral insufficiency, aortic valve insufficiency and aortic stenosis. Mamie was not in congestive heart failure at this time. . Further cardiologist examinations were made in 1950 that detected a progression of her valve disease. General Eisenhower became alarmed. He worried that in the face of a gradual deterioration of his wife's heart condition whether further harm would occur if she accompanied him to Europe as he became the first commander of NATO.[34]

When Mamie was in Washington in November 1951, the chief of cardiology at Walter Reed, Colonel Thomas Mattingly, assumed control of her cardiac care. He closely monitored Mrs. Eisenhower's heart condition until his retirement from the army in 1958. He observed that the heart disease gradually worsened during his watch; her heart enlarged and shortness of breath after exertion appeared. Mattingly thereupon restricted the first lady's physical activity. The cardiologist was consulted one last time, in 1978, by Dr. Julius L. Bedynek when the widowed Mamie Eisenhower's heart failure progressed alarmingly. The question was whether heart surgery was indicated. Mattingly concurred that surgery was not appropriate and agreed with the medical regime of digitalis, diuretics and a low-salt diet.[35]

One year later, on November 1, 1979, Mrs. Eisenhower died. She suffered a stroke on September 25, 1979, and died five weeks later.[36]

First Lady Mamie Eisenhower

As first lady (1953–1961), Mrs. Eisenhower worked from the bedroom she shared with the president. She routinely sat up in bed to plan her day and direct her staff, most likely an adjustment to her physicians' advice to rest when she could. The onset of her inner ear symptoms was often unpredictable, so her behavior was precautionary. One biographer detailed her daily morning routine. Mrs. Eisenhower read the morning newspapers before breakfast and meeting her staff. She paid close attention to advertisements for sales of food and other items useful in the White House. When the head usher came in with her breakfast tray, the two discussed menus for the day and details for any upcoming social events. The usher was followed by the executive mansion's housekeeper and Mamie's secretary. The first lady then dictated letters for two or three hours and afterwards planned her daily schedule.[37] Thereby Mrs. Eisenhower was able to minimize the symptoms of Menière's and chronic rheumatic valvular heart disease and to enhance her effectiveness as manager of the executive mansion. Critics of the Eisenhowers, ignorant of her physical disabilities, concluded that the first lady was either inactive or incapacitated.[38]

As the wife of a career army officer, Mamie understood hierarchies and was skilled in commanding and directing staffs. She handled the White House finances. Its staff appreciated her clarity in direction and her effectiveness.[39] This first lady handled her social responsibilities very capably and, for the most part, succeeded in her ceremonial duties. However, medical issues did limit her overseas travel. She excelled as a supportive wife for her president husband. She had long seen her role as the provider of emotional support to Ike and had endured thirty-four moves decided by the army. She summed up her White House years by declaring, "I never pretended to be anything but Ike's wife."[40] Mrs. Eisenhower, a successful military spouse, eschewed politics. She neither participated openly in this activity nor selected a public volunteer cause during her eight-year tenure. On only a single occasion did President Eisenhower solicit her political opinion: Whether to run for a second term after he had suffered a major heart attack.[41]

As a result of constant and very good medical care, intelligent monitoring of her physical activity, and the cross-over benefit of medications prescribed for her heart and her anxiety, Mamie Eisenhower played an important supportive role for the president. Moreover her responsibilities as first lady did not affect her health. She was hospitalized once during this period when a hysterectomy was performed in August 1957.[42]

Two physicians shared responsibility for her medical care as first lady: General Howard Snyder and Colonel Thomas Mattingly. In November 1945, Snyder held a job in Washington as assistant inspector of the War Department. He previously had examined Mrs. Eisenhower and had some familiarity with her medical history. Then, at Mrs. Eisenhower's request, Snyder's commanding officer, General Eisenhower, directed the doctor to travel to Boone, Iowa, where she was hospitalized with bronchopneumonia. Snyder performed as ordered and upon arrival he was asked to also take care of Eisenhower's sinus and bronchial problems. By mutual agreement, Snyder, a trained surgeon, became Ike's as well as Mamie's personal physician and had his military career extended for fifteen years, until January 1961. In 1953, at age seventy-one, he became the White House physician. Thus the first lady's doctor, as in the cases of Presley Rixey and Ida McKinley, and Charles Sawyer and Florence Harding, was promoted to the position of the president's personal physician.[43]

Colonel (later Brigadier General) Thomas Mattingly was chief of cardiology at Walter Reed Medical Center and became the U.S. military's most renowned cardiologist. Dr. Snyder asked the cardiologist to monitor the first lady's heart condition, which he followed on a regular basis. However, during the Eisenhowers' tenure, these physicians expended far more time, care and energy upon her husband's medical problems. The president suffered three near-catastrophic medical emergencies: A severe heart attack, obstructive Crohn's disease of the intestine, and a transient ischemic attack of the brain.

Even so, it is curious that with all the available specialized medical care consultation with an otolaryngologist to evaluate Mamie's Menière's disease was never requested.

Chapter Thirteen

Obstetrics in the White House:

Jackie Kennedy, Frankie Cleveland, Edith Roosevelt and the Second Mrs. Tyler

Only two first ladies bore living children while a first lady. Both Frances (Frankie) Cleveland and Jacqueline (Jackie) Kennedy married older men. Frankie became first lady at only twenty-one, and Jackie, at thirty-one. Both were college-educated,[1] presented a stunning appearance, and excelled at their expected social and ceremonial responsibilities. The press and the public were fascinated to excess with Mrs. Cleveland and Mrs. Kennedy during both their White House and their post–White House years.[2] Both women remarried after the deaths of their husbands and were the only two former first ladies to do so.

The fecund Edith Roosevelt, birth mother of five and stepmother of one, allegedly suffered two miscarriages in the White House. These episodes escaped public knowledge at the time, and were only hinted at in retrospect.

Julia Tyler was twenty-four years old when she married the widower President John Tyler, thirty years her senior, in 1844. John Tyler was prolific and his young bride was fecund, but Julia Tyler's short eight-month White House reign did not produce any offspring. The Tylers' post–Washington marriage was far from barren; five sons and two daughters began arriving in the Tyler home fifteen months after his Presidency.

Jackie Kennedy's Obstetrical History

"The infant, an unnamed girl, died before drawing her first breath ... When Jackie regained consciousness following the surgery, the first person she saw ... was Bobby Kennedy."[3]

Jacqueline Bouvier married John Fitzgerald Kennedy on September 12, 1953, when she was twenty-four. After Kennedy's death she married Aristotle Onassis, on October 20, 1968, when she was thirty-nine. She was a widow again in 1975 after the death of Onassis and lived until the age of sixty-four. (Interestingly, Jackie Kennedy was the first first lady to be born in a hospital.[4] It was not until the mid–1920s that hospital births became the standard obstetrical venue; previously home deliveries were the norm.[5]) Jackie Kennedy was married to John for ten years and two months; she served as first lady of the United States for a brief two years and ten months. As Mrs. Kennedy, Jackie was pregnant five times; first lady of the United States, she was pregnant once.

As a fascinating person in an admired marriage, Mrs. Kennedy has been the subject of more than a score of biographies. Many of these have covered her neuroses, her amphetamine usage, and the Kennedys' conjugal difficulties. These will be noted here only as they relate to Mrs. Kennedy's difficult obstetrical history.

First Pregnancy

Her first pregnancy ended in a miscarriage in 1955. She was three months pregnant; the event received no media coverage at the time. Heymann recorded Senator Kennedy's flamboyant womanizing during this period and postulated a link with marital anxiety and the ill-fated pregnancy: "Her doctor told her that if she remained so high strung she might have trouble bearing children."[6] Political columnist Jack Anderson summarized how Jackie prepared for her first baby at Hickory Hill in the Virginia hunt country, but was often left alone in the huge house while her husband was off politicking. "After her miscarriage, she couldn't bear to enter the nursery she had so lovingly designed."[7]

Second Pregnancy

Jackie's failed second pregnancy in 1956 was far more traumatic, both physically and emotionally. Senator Kennedy narrowly lost the Democratic vice presidential nomination at the 1956 August convention. His subsequent behavior has been severely condemned by biographers Thomas Reeves and C. David Heymann.[8] Within a few hours, Kennedy left his eight-month-pregnant wife to fly to a carousing vacation on a yacht on the Mediterranean. Available young women joined the senator and his lusty chum, Florida senator George Smathers, aboard the party-yacht.[9]

Jackie was warehoused at her parents' estate in Newport, Rhode Island, while her husband was away. Following the excitement of the convention she was beset with considerable discomfort, which was compounded by rumors of her husband's infidelity. Severe stomach cramps and hemorrhaging necessitated an emergency ambulance trip to Newport Hospital, where doctors performed an emergency caesarian section. An infant baby girl was stillborn on August 23, 1956. Arabella Kennedy was named by Jackie Kennedy posthumously. Arabella and her brother Patrick are buried with their parents at Arlington Cemetery.[10]

The *Washington Post* reported that the senator finally arrived at his wife's side five days after the stillbirth.[11] A Newport Hospital spokesman attributed the stillbirth to "nervous tension and exhaustion following the Democratic Convention." A friend attributed it to lack of sleep. Rose Kennedy placed the blame on Jackie's nicotine addiction, while Janet Auchincloss, Jackie's mother, implicated Jack's absence. After leaving the hospital Jackie remained at her parents' Newport estate, a considerable distance from Washington, and from her husband.[12]

Jackie's mother-in-law had a point. The future first lady was a secretive but habitual smoker. Rose Kennedy was prescient; recent medical studies have reported that smoking during the first trimester of pregnancy doubles the risk of miscarriage.[13]

Third Pregnancy

Mrs. Kennedy's third pregnancy was successful; her postpartum recovery was both uneventful and a very happy interlude. On November 27, 1957, Caroline Kennedy entered the world at New York Hospital after a normal nine-month gestation. Caroline weighed seven pounds, six ounces. The delivery was once again by caesarean section. Her mother was twenty-seven and her father forty.[14] Jackie Kennedy's fourth and fifth pregnancies, in 1960 and 1963, bookended both President Kennedy's brief presidency and her own abbreviated reign as America's first lady.

Fourth Pregnancy

Mrs. Kennedy's fourth pregnancy coincided with JFK's successful campaigns for the 1960 Democratic presidential nomination and for the presidency of the United States. Her obstetrician, John Walsh, advised his pregnant patient to "curtail her activities for about six months." The physician's directive justified Mrs. Kennedy's frequent absences from the presidential campaign.[15]

After the election, the president-elect spent most of his time planning policy at his father's Palm Beach, Florida, estate while Jackie remained in their Georgetown, D.C., home. A caesarian section was planned for Georgetown University Hospital on December 6; the

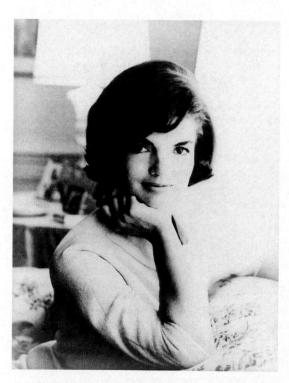

baby was due on December 27.[16] Kennedy flew to Georgetown to spend Thanksgiving with Jackie, but he dismissed his wife's plea to remain in Washington until the birth. He flew back to Palm Beach and his wife went into premature labor two hours after his departure.[17] Mrs. Kennedy was rushed to the hospital, where Dr. Walsh delivered a healthy, 6-pound 3-ounce, John Fitzgerald Kennedy Junior. The doctor informed the press that the infant was premature only chronologically. The soon-to-be first lady required a transfusion of two units of blood. The president-elect immediately flew back to Washington in a desperate, but unsuccessful, dash to be present at the birth. Jack Kennedy was absent from all of Jackie's deliveries, except perhaps for the birth of Caroline.[18]

Mrs. Kennedy and her son were discharged from Georgetown Hospital two weeks after her C-section. The plan was to fly immediately to Palm Beach to recuperate. However, a political responsibility intervened—a social visit at the White

Jacqueline Kennedy, the wife of John Kennedy. Her obstetrical history was an arduous one (Library of Congress).

House with outgoing first lady Mamie Eisenhower. Jackie's nurse warned the physically and emotionally exhausted new mother that "if she got up on her feet she might die." After walking up the White House steps and greeting Mrs. Eisenhower, Mrs. Kennedy looked desperately for a wheelchair that was not there. "If she was not ill before, she was ill now, and she took John John and the nurse and flew down to Palm Beach." There she remained for six weeks until just prior to the inauguration.[19]

Secret Service agent Clint Hill observed that as soon as she arrived from Washington, "Mrs. Kennedy immediately went to her bedroom to rest, and rarely emerged for the next week."[20] This comment may be the first notice of a severe postpartum depression. Frenzied political and family activities at Palm Beach provided the opposite of a necessary recuperation. Jackie returned to Washington shortly before her husband was inaugurated president.

The inauguration and the inaugural balls were a nightmare. Anxious, exhausted and depressed, the new first lady awoke "alone and terrified.... [H]er legs were gripped by painful muscle spasms [and] to her horror, she realized she was unable to stand." She summoned Dr. Janet Travell, the White House physician, who gave her a Dexedrine (amphetamine) pill to get through the inaugural balls. By midnight the pill's effects had dissipated, and an exhausted Mrs. Kennedy insisted that she be returned to the White House.[21]

During a post-assassination conversation with Arthur Schlesinger, the widow talked about her near-catatonic state during the January 1961 inauguration ceremonies: "I left after a couple of hours because again, I was really so tired that day.... And about 9 o'clock or something. when it was time to start getting dressed, again I couldn't get out of bed. I just couldn't move. And so I called Dr. Travell just frantic and she came running over. And she had two pills, a green one and an orange one, and she told me to take the orange one. So I did and said, 'What is it?' And then she told me it was Dexedrine, which I'd never taken in my life—But thank God, it really did the trick because then you could get dressed.... I guess the pill wore off because I just couldn't get out of the car."[22]

The first lady stayed in bed for a week after the inauguration. Dr. Travell became concerned about her depression and overall physical condition and prescribed an immediate return to Palm Beach, where Mrs. Kennedy remained secluded in a bedroom.[23] In retrospect it is clear that a postpartum depression commenced almost immediately after John's birth and was still present six months later. Jackie's symptoms were extreme fatigue, sadness, withdrawal, and lack of motivation.

Ceremonial and social events that required Mrs. Kennedy's grace and style began to appear on the 1961 "New Frontier" calendar. The president increasingly worried that his wife's depression would mar state visits to Canada, Paris, and Vienna. Since neither time nor Travell had lifted his wife's mood, he took the desperate and dangerous step of inviting Dr. Max Jacobson, also known as Dr. Feelgood, due to his happy and invigorating potions, to Palm Beach. Kennedy and a close friend had been injected previously by Jacobson with positive results. The general reaction to Feelgood's injections in the arm, hand, hip, buttocks, or solar plexus, was "a sense of being lit up from within."[24] Eventually Robert Kennedy, JFK's brother and closest advisor, apprehensive over Jacobson's treatments, had five of Feelgood's therapeutic vials analyzed by the FBI's laboratories. Analysis revealed high concentrations of amphetamines and steroids in all five vials.[25] Counseling, antidepressants, and hormonal therapy are the usual treatments for postpartum depression. Instead, the first lady, whose position could command the best medical care in America, was subjected to the amphetamine shots of Dr. Max Jacobson.[26]

Max Jacobson may be the most fascinating of all the physicians who medically ministered to America's first ladies. A Jew from Berlin, Jacobson fled the Nazis to establish a medical practice on Manhattan's Upper East Side. His treatments consisted almost exclusively of injections of his potions, which contained amphetamines as their principal ingredient. His patients were a "Who's Who" of the entertainment industry and included Eddie Fisher, Alan Jay Lerner, Tony Curtis and Milton Berle. Later he treated Jack and Jackie Kennedy. The Secret Service agents that guarded JFK code-named the physician "Dr. Feelgood."[27]

When beckoned by the new president, Jacobson flew to Florida, interviewed the first lady, noted her depression, and injected her. As a result her mood changed completely. Her presence during the subsequent state visits charmed both the Canadians and French president Charles DeGaulle. The only annoying side effect was a dry mouth.[28] Max Jacobson continued to treat both Jackie and Jack. Mrs. Kennedy was injected on at least six occasions, and undoubtedly more, in Palm Beach, in the White House, and in Paris.[29] After her husband's assassination, Jacobson flew from New York City to the White House at Jackie's request. On the night of November 23, 1963, he injected the first lady with his medicinal cocktail. Afterwards, Mrs. Kennedy told her brother-in-law, "I have no idea what the shot contained. All I know is that my nerves have finally begun to settle."[30]

Fifth Pregnancy

In 1963, Jackie Kennedy was pregnant for the fifth time. She summered at Cape Cod near the Kennedy Hyannis Port estate, but planned to return to Washington to deliver by the inevitable C-section at Walter Reed Army Hospital.[31] Previously Dr. John Walsh, her obstetrician, Dr. Janet Travell, the official chief White House physician, and Mrs. Kennedy's Secret Service agent Clint Hill, auditioned several Cape Cod area hospitals to determine the one most suitable if once again premature labor would occur. The trio selected the hospital at Otis Air Force Base. Dr. Walsh offered to remain at Hyannis Port for the remainder of the summer to monitor the first lady, an unusual obstetrical perquisite specific to the wife of a United States president. Moreover, the air force spent nearly five thousand dollars in refurbishing the hospital's eight-room suite should the first lady become a maternity patient there.[32]

Columnist Jack Anderson wrote of a different situation: "It will take a major crisis to keep President Kennedy from his wife's side when their baby is born. For his presence, say confidants, has become an issue in their marriage."[33] Kennedy was certainly apprehensive over the upcoming birth. In mid–July, Jackie awoke with an uncomfortable feeling. A frantic search for Dr. Walsh ensued and Mr. Kennedy became "very upset over the doctor's absence." The physician had been on a walk, but Kennedy insisted that he "always tell someone where you are, how you can be reached immediately." The discomfort was a false alarm.[34] Despite JFK's admonition to the obstetrician, it was Kennedy who was once again absent for the delivery.

On August 7, Mrs. Kennedy experienced sudden labor pains, and Walsh and his patient boarded a helicopter for Otis. A four-pound, 10.5 ounce baby boy, named Patrick Joseph

Kennedy, was born there shortly after midnight, once again by C-section. The infant was five and one-half weeks premature and almost immediately had difficulty in breathing. The diagnosis of idiopathic respiratory disease syndrome was established and the chief resident of Boston Children's Hospital, Dr. James E. Drobaugh, was summoned to transport the baby to Boston by helicopter. Despite intensive therapy and the expertise of prestigious physicians (Drs. Stephen Clifford, William Bernhard of Harvard and Dr. Samuel Levine of Cornell), Patrick died after a life of 39 hours and 12 minutes.[35] Unfortunately, Patrick was born too soon. Fifty years later medical advances have allowed neonatal intensive care units to save babies born at thirty-two weeks of gestation. A senior neonatologist at Boston's Beth Israel Deaconess Medical Center was quoted in a recent article: "We hardly worry at all about a baby like the Kennedy infant."[36]

Mrs. Kennedy was discharged from the hospital after a week (at the time a seven-to-ten day postpartum hospital stay was routine). Once again she required two units of blood.[37] Kennedy press secretary Pierre Salinger announced the first lady's recuperation plans: "Mrs. Kennedy has made a very satisfactory recovery. However, in order to assure her complete rehabilitation and continuing good health, it will be necessary for her to curtail her activities and not undertake an official schedule until after the first of the year." The plan was to recuperate at Cape Cod until mid–September, then to go to her parents' home near Newport for several weeks, and then to Virginia. Lady Bird Johnson and the Kennedy sisters-in-law were expected to fill in for Jackie at social and ceremonial activities.[38]

The plans were soon changed by Mrs. Kennedy. She remained on Cape Cod only until September 6 and at her parents' estate at Newport until September 23. On October 1, she commenced a vacation on the luxury yacht owned by Aristotle Onassis that cruised the Aegean Sea. She returned to Washington by way of a stop in Morocco.[39] Life aboard the yacht was apparently very restorative, as she had the following conversation with her Secret Service agent: "Mr. Hill … the president is going on a trip to Texas next month, and he wants me to join him. I had told him I didn't want to go—I didn't think I was ready. But now I feel so much better and I really want to help him as much as I can. Maybe I will go after all."[40] Thus on to Dallas and the legend of Camelot.

Mrs. Kennedy's obstetrician boarded Air Force One when it returned from Dallas with Mrs. Kennedy, the body of her dead husband, and the new president, Lyndon Johnson. The doctor was available to console the grieving first lady. He injected her with sodium amytal, a barbiturate, and Vistaril for anxiety that night and the following evening.[41] Walsh was an army physician in Europe during World War II. After the war he established a private practice in Washington and Bethesda, Maryland. Additionally, he was a clinical professor of obstetrics and gynecology at Georgetown University Medical School. It is unknown why Mrs. Kennedy chose Walsh to be her obstetrician, but she became his patient in 1957.[42]

Frances (Frankie) Cleveland

"On Friday, September 1, after long weeks at Gray Gables, the President, Mrs. Cleveland, and Baby Ruth returned to the White House in the midst of a rain. Eight days later Dr. Bryant ushered into the world the second Cleveland child, another daughter—the first child of a President ever born in the White House."[43]

Marriage to Grover Cleveland

Grover Cleveland was both the twenty-second (1885–1889) and the twenty-fourth president (1893–1897) of the United States. His tenure was interrupted by the election of Benjamin Harrison (1889–1893). When first elected, Cleveland was—and remains—only the second bachelor to be president. On June 2, 1886, in the first and only presidential wedding in the White House, the forty-nine-year-old Cleveland married twenty-one-year-old Frances (Frankie) Folsom. The groom had known his new bride from her infancy; she was the daughter of his deceased law partner. Cleveland was the administrator of the Folsom estate and the unofficial guardian of Frances, Folsom's daughter.[44]

As First Lady

Frankie Cleveland was very healthy during her two tours as first lady of United States. She soon discovered that she was a popular icon in the eyes of the press and the public. Moreover, she was a quick study in adapting to her social responsibilities: "Frank demonstrated every ounce of her poise and skill," clearly no longer the inexperienced schoolgirl of the previous year.[45] During the second Cleveland administration, "Frances now devoted her energies to her family."[46]

However, Mrs. Cleveland's most significant contribution to her husband's presidency may have been her conspiratorial role in assuring the secrecy of his cancer operation on July 1, 1893. Almost a third of the president's upper jaw was excised during surreptitious surgery upon a yacht sailing along New York's East River. The entire episode was clandestine in order not to spook the political and financial communities during the economic panic of 1893.[47]

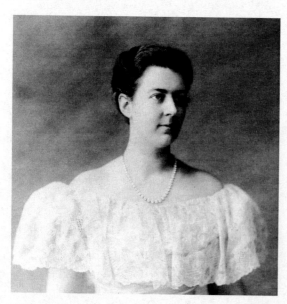

Frances "Frankie" Cleveland, the young wife of Grover Cleveland and the only first lady to become a mother in the White House (Library of Congress).

The president recuperated at Grey Gables, the Clevelands' summer home in Bourne, Massachusetts. There he joined his wife, who was in the third trimester of her second pregnancy. The upcoming birth helped to divert attention from the future father's medical status: "Her obvious condition gave the press something to focus on in reporting about the Clevelands.[48] On September 1, 1893, three months after his surgery, the president, Mrs. Cleveland, and their young daughter returned to the White House.[49] On September 9, 1893, Dr. Joseph Bryant managed the successful and uncomplicated birth of the second Cleveland child, another daughter. Esther Cleveland is so far the only presidential child ever born in the White House. Esther was named after the biblical Esther and lived for eighty-seven years.[50]

Dr. Bryant of New York City practiced medicine in the days before medical specialization. Not only was he an expert surgeon who removed the president's cancer aboard a boat, he also delivered the first two Cleveland children. The cancer surgery was a complete success; the tumor neither recurred nor spread during Grover Cleveland's lifetime. Bryant was the longtime family physician and friend of the Clevelands. After the death of Ruth, their first daughter, in January 1904, from diphtheria, Dr. Bryant subsequently cultured all the members of the family. Antitoxin was administered but possibly too late.[51]

Frankie had five successful pregnancies between 1891 and 1903—three sons and two daughters. The first child, Ruth, was born after "rather a long labor—but not at all severe." Except for Ruth, all the children were long-lived. The youngest, Francis Grover Cleveland, died in 1995 at the age of ninety-two. Perhaps Frankie wished that her much older husband would be able to enjoy his offspring. Her third pregnancy, with Marion in 1895 while Cleveland was still president, evoked this comment: "I feel that it is only fair to their father to have them as young as he can." Marion was born at Grey Gables and not in the White House.[52]

After the White House

The Clevelands retired to Princeton, where the ex-president died in 1908. His widow remarried; on February 10, 1913, she wed Princeton professor Thomas Jex Preston in the home of the Princeton president, John Grier Hibben, who officiated. Frankie was the first presidential widow to remarry, succeeded only by Jackie Kennedy. To minimize any disapproval, the wedding plans were kept clandestine. But disapproval occurred nevertheless. Mrs. Cleveland, like Mrs. Kennedy after her, was a national monument and it distressed many people that the base was of clay.[53]

The former first lady was in good health for many years. She died in her sleep in Baltimore, Maryland, fifty-one years after leaving the White House.[54]

Edith Roosevelt

"Edith continued to find her identity in motherhood." In a letter to her sister, she wrote, "The baby trunk made me rather sad.... I shall keep the little things another year in the hope of using them"[55]

Edith Kermit Carow was the second wife of Teddy Roosevelt (TR). On October 27, 1880, the twenty-two-year-old future president married nineteen-year-old Alice Hathaway Lee in Brookline, Massachusetts. Three and a half years later Alice Roosevelt died, two days after giving birth to a daughter, named Alice after her mother. The cause of death was toxemia of pregnancy with acute kidney failure.[56]

Edith Carow, both a childhood playmate and the teenage sweetheart of Theodore Roosevelt, became his second wife at Saint George Church, in Mayfair, London, on December 2, 1886. He was twenty-eight and she twenty-five. The wedding took place in England as TR was sensitive that a second marriage soon (two and one half years) after Alice's death would be viewed as a social faux pas by the Roosevelts' New York circle of friends.[57]

As First Lady

Edith and TR were married for thirty-three years, the marriage a happy, supportive, and successful one. Edith was a strong and healthy woman whose physical endurance in no way hindered or obstructed Roosevelt's political career. She was a strength as first lady (1901–1909); conversely the responsibilities of being first lady in no way were a burden to Edith. She was a success both socially and as the manager of the White House. She was credited with "a brilliant social regime, even creating a 'social cabinet' composed of the wives of cabinet members." Another reporter summarized the first lady's tenure: "[S]he presided as mistress of the White House (1901–1909) with grace and distinction.... She was an excellent conversationalist and a musician of more than ordinary attainments." However, her primary responsibility continued to be the role of mother to her children.[58]

Medical History

Only three significant medical events occurred before Mrs. Cleveland's death at eighty-seven years of age. The first was an abdominal abscess subsequent to the birth of her fifth child. The second event took place in September 1911. While riding at Sagamore Hill, the Roosevelt's Long Island home, Edith was knocked senseless after falling from her horse.

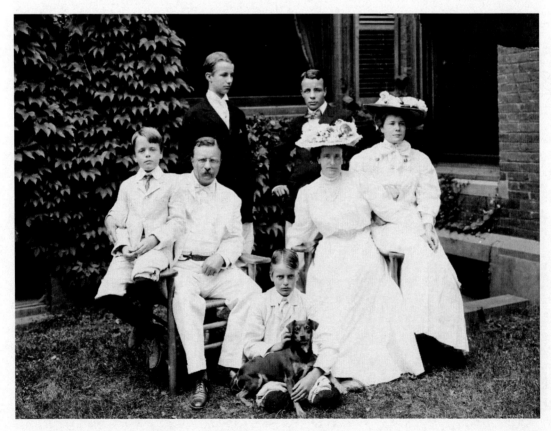

Edith Roosevelt with Theodore Roosevelt and their five children. She had at least one miscarriage in the White House (Library of Congress).

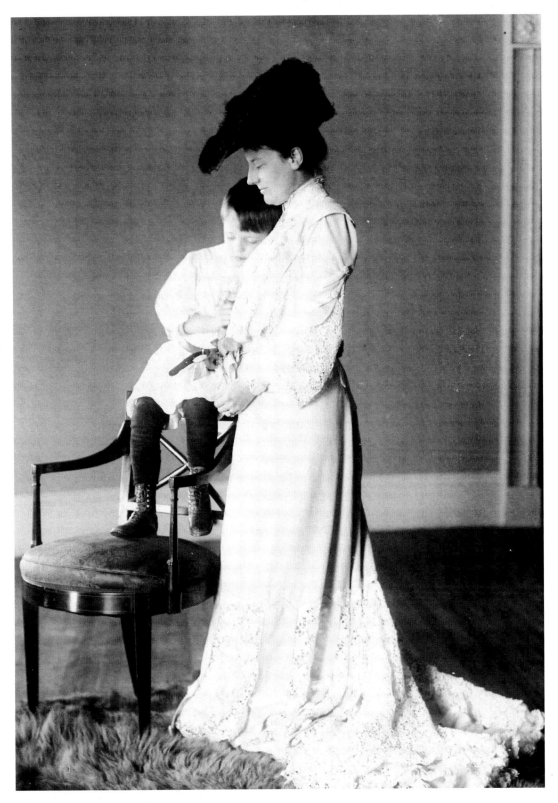

Edith Roosevelt, the wife of Theodore Roosevelt, holding Quentin, their youngest son (Library of Congress).

She remained comatose for 36 hours before gaining consciousness, and she became lucid only at intervals during the next nine days. Mrs. Roosevelt did not remember the accident and continued to suffer from bad headaches. It was many weeks before she was well enough to go outside.[59]

In 1935 Edith broke her hip after a fall and was hospitalized for four months. After twenty-nine years as a widow, Edith Roosevelt died with congestive heart failure and arteriosclerosis.[60]

Obstetrical History

Edith Carow Roosevelt gave birth to five healthy children, four sons and one daughter, within a ten-year period (1887–1897). All labors but one were quick. The exception was the 1891 parturition of her third child, Ethel, her only daughter. This was described as a long and difficult labor. Two births may have been premature. All the babies were born at the Roosevelts' homes, in New York City, Sagamore Hill, or Washington, D.C. It is likely that a physician attended all the deliveries.[61]

Mrs. Roosevelt's first postpartum period was problematic, partially due to postpartum depression and partially because of contemporary postnatal practices. Edith remained in bed for two weeks wrapped up like a mummy.[62] A second postpartum event was more serious. On January 17, 1898, four months after the birth of Quentin, Edith's youngest child, she was stricken with fever, pains and "sciatica." These symptoms persisted for five weeks until the patient noticed a lower abdominal swelling. Between 1890 and 1930 prominent Washingtonians frequently depended upon the expertise of staff physicians from Johns Hopkins Medical Institutions in Baltimore. The renowned Dr. William Osler, chairman of its Department of Medicine, was asked for his opinion. After his examination, Osler declared that Edith was critically ill from an abscess of the psoas muscle. He recommended an immediate operation. A gynecologist confirmed Osler's diagnosis and operated on March 6. The abscess was drained through an open abdominal wound. Weeks passed, until April 4 when the patient was well enough to go for a carriage ride. On April 11, 1898, TR volunteered for military service in the Spanish-American War. He left Edith and his children behind in Washington to ride up San Juan Hill and into the annals of history.[63]

First lady Edith Roosevelt, raising five children as well as a stepdaughter, Alice, from her husband's first marriage, still desired to increase the size of her family. She previously had suffered at least one miscarriage, in August 1888, and perhaps more.[64] As a resident in the White House she continued to think about motherhood and expressed her desire to Admiral Presley Rixey, then the White House physician. However, Rixey did not find Edith's desire to become pregnant at forty-one reasonable.[65]

"[A]s First Lady, Edith twice became pregnant, although miscarriage intervened." In spring 1902, the first lady was most likely pregnant. Rumors circulated in Washington that Mrs. Roosevelt was expecting. A joyful letter to her sister Emily Carow seemed to confirm her physical state: "I have the most enormous appetite, though I loathe anything sweet, can't touch wine and care but little for tea and coffee! Meat seems to appeal to me!" A disappointed and cryptic May 9 entry in her diary signaled a miscarriage: "Was taken sick in night."[66] A year later, a second White House pregnancy was suggested. During the pre–Lenten social activities in 1903, while arranging the dinner before her last musicale, Edith felt faint and had to retire upstairs. She was confined to bed for two days. *Town Topics* mused that it was the stork.[67]

Julia, the Second Mrs. Tyler

"The lovely lady Presidentress is attended on reception-days by twelve maids of honor, six on either side, dressed all alike…. Her serene loveliness receives upon a raised platform, wearing a headdress formed of bugles and resembling a crown."[68]

Julia Gardiner became the second-youngest first lady. In 1844, at age twenty-four, she married the widower president, John Tyler. Her reign also was distinctive, as her White House residence was the briefest of that of any other first lady, a mere eight months.

David Gardiner, wealthy and the father of two vivacious and very pretty daughters, Julia and Margaret, became, with his daughters, part of President John Tyler's social family. Julia Gardiner was born into wealth and enjoyed a pampered and affluent lifestyle, one without significant responsibilities. The unmarried Miss Gardiner was very attractive, socially adept and flirtatious.[69]

The invalid first lady, Letitia Tyler, whose marriage to John Tyler produced eight children, died on September 10, 1842.[70] The president proposed marriage to the vivacious Julia fewer than six months later.[71] Miss Gardiner demurred until a calamity killed her father. On February 28, 1844, an explosion aboard the navy cutter *Princeton* killed David Gardiner and Tyler's secretaries of state and the navy. President Tyler and Julia Gardiner were aboard but were uninjured. Dolley Madison was also on the ship; the presidential widow would become Julia's mentor in adapting to Washington's social decorum.[72] The Tyler romance accelerated and Miss Gardiner married the fifty-four-year-old president in a quasi-secret ceremony in the Church of the Ascension in New York City on June 26, 1844. The wedding plans were so clandestine that many characterized their marriage as an elopement.

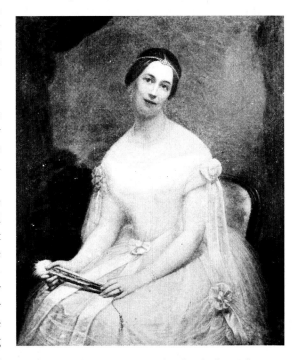

A beautiful young bride in the White House was certain to attract attention and popular favor, as did the young and elegant first ladies Frankie Cleveland and Jackie Kennedy years later. Julia Tyler was determined to make her social mark in the few months available to her. She succeeded by very active and elaborate entertaining. The new first lady also was clever in soliciting favorable coverage by the press. The appellation "The Lovely Lady Presidentress" resulted from her efforts.[73]

Julia Tyler, the young second wife of John Tyler, bore her husband seven children after the White House (Library of Congress).

Her residency in the White House may have been too brief for her thirty-year-older husband to demonstrate his virility or Julia her fecundity—but not for long. The first offspring from Julia's wedding to John appeared on July 12, 1846, fifteen months after the Tyler's departure from the White House. Six additional baby Tylers graced the ex-president's second family.[74]

The widow Tyler survived until July 10, 1889, outliving her husband by 28 years. There were no significant medical issues reported by historians.

Chapter Fourteen

Twentieth Century Stalwarts

Lou Hoover, Eleanor Roosevelt, Bess Truman and Lady Bird Johnson

These four women, except for the two terms of Mamie Eisenhower and the truncated tenure of Jacqueline Kennedy, occupied the White House from 1929 to 1969. Each of the four brought significant strengths to the White House. Moreover their good health was an asset and not an inconvenience; neither sickness nor physical difficulties encumbered their presidential husbands. Responsibilities as first lady did not impair their health. At least one, Bess Truman, neither desired nor especially enjoyed her time in the executive mansion. Therefore, the discussion of each will be brief and their histories will be economical but pithy.

Lou Hoover

"Few political wives were alike as Lou and Eleanor. Both addressed controversial issues, did magazine writing, vigorously advocated that women become active in politics, and were political advisors to their husbands."[1]

Mrs. Hoover was smart, accomplished, physically fit and adventurous. She graduated from Stanford University with a degree in geology, one of the first, if not the first, American woman with a degree in that field. Soon after graduation she married Herbert Hoover, who became a very successful and wealthy mining engineer. They spent their first years together in China and

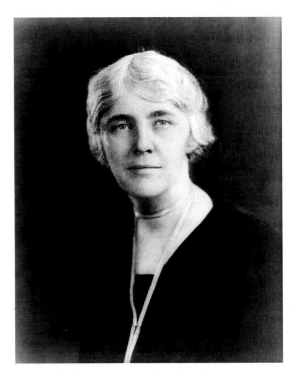

Lou Hoover, the wife of Herbert Hoover, was a very healthy first lady (Library of Congress).

later visited and worked in many parts of the world. Lou became more than Herbert's mate; she was an equal partner and an invaluable political advisor in the White House.[2] Among her numerous volunteer activities, the Girl Scout organization was preeminent.[3]

Mrs. Hoover was healthy until her sudden death from a heart attack in New York City on January 7, 1944, when she was 69 years old.[4] Her *New York Times* obituary observed: "Mrs. Hoover brought to the White House as cosmopolitan a background as a woman could have, one which commentators have found hard to parallel without going back to Mrs. John Quincy Adams."[5] The Hoovers raised two sons: Herbert Hoover Junior, born March 1905, and Allan Henry Hoover, born July 1907.[6]

The medical gadfly Joel Boone became the chief White House physician and personal doctor to the Hoover family. He had enjoyed previous social interactions with the Hoovers while the future president served as secretary of commerce in both the Harding and Coolidge administrations. Dr. Boone's voluminous writings provide a quotable source for Lou Hoover's doings in and around the White House. When the Hoovers accompanied President and Mrs. Harding to Alaska aboard the USS *Henderson*, "Mrs. Hoover ... asked Boone to teach her to dance." Later, in the White House: "[Boone] recently had had a conversation with Mrs. Hoover about a preparatory school for her nephew that led to enrollment at Boone's beloved Mercersburg Academy."[7]

In the autumn of 1930, Herbert Hoover, Jr. returned to Washington, D.C., suffering from a rapid twenty-pound weight loss. Boone was asked by the president to examine his son. A subsequent chest X-ray looked suspicious for tuberculosis. To avoid publicity (Boone was good at this) the doctor assigned a fictitious patient name to Herbert Jr. and asked Dr. Louis Hamman, "who had been chief of tuberculosis work at Johns Hopkins," to meet with the patient, not at the White House, but at Boone's apartment. After an examination, Hamman reviewed his chest X-rays at the Washington Navy Hospital and concluded, "There is absolutely no question that this is a tubercular infection." Boone prescribed a several-month regimen of rest, diet and isolation.[8] His supervision of young Hoover's care continued; in October Boone announced that Herbert Hoover, Jr. would be taken the following month to Asheville, North Carolina, for treatment. Asheville's climate was sound and it was also proximate to Washington.[9]

This event documented Boone's medical competence, his sensitivity to patient confidentiality, and a predilection to employ experts from the Johns Hopkins Medical Institutions as consultants. In summation, Boone wrote: "Mrs. Hoover enjoyed good health—certainly better than Mrs. Harding's—but was such a busy person and so caught up in activities of her husband that her health could suffer."[10]

Eleanor Roosevelt

"Claiming that her wheelchair-bound husband, crippled by polio, needed her as his eyes and ears, hands and feet, she became the most ubiquitous First Lady in history."[11]

Eleanor Roosevelt was a very different type of first lady, one who doffed the social and ceremonial roles previously deemed essential in a first lady's job description. Also absent were the traditional wifely activities of companion and protector. Mrs. Roosevelt, psychologically damaged by an earlier affair between her husband and her own social secretary, embraced an exaggerated political role, often tinged with hostility towards, and frequently disruptive and distracting for, President Roosevelt.[12]

Mrs. Roosevelt remains the longest-serving American first lady (twelve years, two months), and is the most admired. Polls consistently rank her as the nation's most successful first lady.[13] Her public persona, if anything, increased after her husband's death in April 1945. She was a dominant actor upon the national and international stage for the remaining seventeen years of her life as she energetically pursued goals of peace, civil rights, and women's enrichment.

Excellent health, with few exceptions, was her companion before, during, and after her White House years, Her maternal grandmother, Mrs. Hall, entrusted with Eleanor's upbringing after the early deaths of both parents, alerted the headmistress of London's Allenswood finishing school that the teenage Eleanor was in delicate health. Mlle. Souvestre disagreed: "She does not any more suffer of the complaints you told me about. She has a good sleep, a good appetite, is very rarely troubled with headaches and is always ready to enjoy her life."[14]

Mrs. Roosevelt was pregnant six times. Her first child, Anna, was born after a difficult nine months, and the pregnancy was marked by nausea. All the other children were boys. The third child and second son perished from heart disease before his first birthday.[15]

A rare exception to her good health occurred in 1912. Both Eleanor and Franklin were downed by typhoid fever. Its usual symptoms are high fever, abdominal pain, weakness and loss of appetite. The future first lady's symptoms are unrecorded other than that it was a week before her temperature began to subside.[16]

Eleanor Roosevelt lived for seventeen years after FDR's death and died at age seventy-eight in December 1962. She was prodigiously active well past her seventieth birthday; her energy began to wane only in early 1960. She was knocked down by a driver who "carelessly backed a station wagon into her as she was crossing a Greenwich Village, Manhattan street to a charity meeting. David Gurewitsch taped up her leg, but despite torn ligaments she continued with her engagements for the day."[17]

Dr. David Gurewitsch was "Eleanor Roosevelt's friend, confidant, personal physician, housemate, and traveling companion during her post–White House years." She met the doctor in 1944 in New York City. After she relocated to New York from Washington, she asked Gurewitsch to become her personal physician. Their

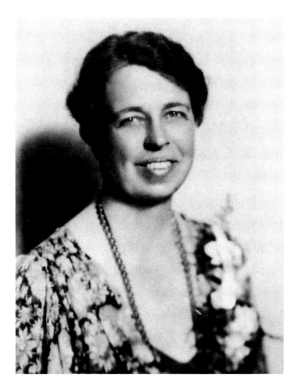

Eleanor Roosevelt, the wife of Franklin D. Roosevelt. To date she is the longest serving first lady (Library of Congress).

relationship was briefly interrupted when the doctor required overseas treatment for tuberculosis.[18] In early 1960 David Gurewitsch diagnosed aplastic anemia as the cause of his patient's decreased energy. "The illness would flicker and subside—infections, fevers, chills, and aches. She dealt with them by ignoring them."[19] The cause of aplastic anemia is often unknown. Approximately six months before her demise, Mrs. Roosevelt was treated with steroids because the anemia had worsened to affect platelet formation. The platelet count decreased to such an extent that internal bleeding became a possibility. Steroid therapy has frequent side effects, and it reactivated an old tuberculosis scar in Mrs. Roosevelt's lung. Tuberculous bacilli spread throughout her body. She realized that death was imminent and demanded release from the hospital to die at home, which she did three weeks later.[20]

It is fitting that one of the final decisions of this most political of presidential wives be placed in a political context. Dr. Barron H. Lerner, writing for the liberal *Huffington Post*, used Mrs. Roosevelt's resistance to very expensive terminal care within a hospital as an argument in favor of the Affordable Care Act (ACA), aka Obamacare. Lerner wrote in October 2012: "Hospitals remain full of elderly patients as or more ill than Eleanor Roosevelt receiving aggressive and expensive medical interventions ranging from ventilators to hemodialysis to intensive care. Even when they prolong life, they often cannot reverse terminal conditions. The ACA is a wonderful opportunity for us to reassess the true value of medical treatments…. There is something to be said for dying at home like Eleanor Roosevelt did—unattached to any machines."[21]

Bess Truman

Upon hearing from her husband, the vice president, that President Roosevelt had died, "Bess put down the telephone and began to cry. She made her way down the hall to her daughter's bedroom, sobbing so hard that she could barely speak."[22]

On June 28, 1919, 34-year-old Bess Wallace married 35-year-old Harry Truman in the small Trinity Episcopal Church in her hometown of Independence, Missouri. It was the first and only marriage for both; the Trumans embarked on a happy and very successful partnership that terminated with Harry's death fifty-three years later on December 26, 1972.[23]

Bess experienced two miscarriages, in 1920 and in 1922 when she was 35 and 37 years old. Unhappy about the losses, she feared that she had waited too long for a pregnancy. However, nearing the advanced maternal age of forty, "Bess gave birth to Mary Margaret Truman in an upstairs bedroom at 219 North Delaware and made a bed for her in a bureau drawer."[24] Margaret's happy delivery on February 17, 1924, concluded her mother's obstetrical history.

Excellent health, Midwestern common sense, and a deeply respectful and honest relationship with her husband permitted the first lady to be a reliable and effective soundingboard for President Harry Truman (1945–1953). The president publicly referred to his wife as "the boss." Although she had a passion for anonymity, Bess was a full partner in Harry's presidential decisions.[25]

Bess Truman had no great affinity either for Washington, D.C., or her role as first lady in the White House. She cried when informed that her husband would succeed Franklin

Roosevelt as president.[26] She assiduously avoided attention: "She never made a speech. She never gave a personal interview and never held a press conference. She was determined to keep her private life private.... Mrs. Truman never gave an opinion on a public issue—except once.... [S]he thought that the historic walls ought to stand."[27] Mrs. Truman much preferred to live in Independence, Missouri, and, more particularly, to reside in the Gates Mansion, the home she had known all her life. During her husband's presidential tenure, Bess Truman spent as much time as possible there, including the summer months and holiday seasons.[28]

As Harry Truman's presidency was drawing to an end, her cheerfulness was much remarked upon, and most political reporters acknowledged that the first lady, although proficient in fulfilling her social and ceremonial duties, would rather be dwelling somewhere else.[29]

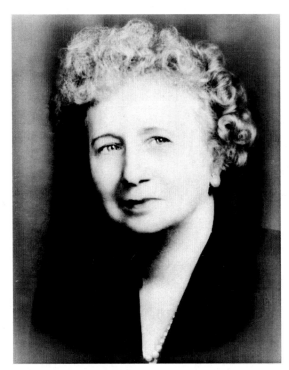

Bess Truman, the wife of Harry Truman. At this writing, she is the longest-lived first lady (Library of Congress).

Mrs. Truman's medical history while first lady was uneventful. Only a single episode of ill health is recorded. In early December 1948, the first lady traveled to Norfolk, Virginia, for a presentation aboard the battleship USS *Missouri*: "In the middle of the ceremony she developed a severe nosebleed. Back in Washington, Dr. Wallace Graham ... took her blood pressure and discovered it was extremely high." Graham, the Trumans' White House physician, first applied pressure to control the hemorrhaging. When this procedure was unsuccessful, the doctor cauterized the bleeding site. He then treated the patient's hypertension by prescribing an unknown antihypertensive drug and instituting a no-salt diet. His treatment worked; Bess Truman's blood pressure reverted to normal and she shed twenty pounds of weight.[30]

The Trumans had a long personal and professional relationship with Dr. Graham. Wallace Graham was the son of Dr. James Walter Graham, a military colleague of Harry Truman from the First World War. The president looked up Graham's military physician son when in Germany for the 1945 Potsdam Peace Conference and brought Wallace back to the White House to serve as the Trumans' personal physician. Graham's excellent medical care for the first family was rewarded by promotions first to brigadier general and then to the temporary rank of major general in the air force reserves. Graham departed both the White House and the air force when the Trumans returned to Missouri, where he entered private practice. The doctor continued as the Trumans' physician for the remainder of their lives.[31] Doctor Graham attended Harry Truman's death on December 14, 1972.[32] He also attended the ex-first lady's multiple hospitalizations in her later years: hypertension[33]; breast tumor surgery[34]; right hip fracture[35]; and stroke.[36]

In late 1958 Bess Truman discovered a lump in her left breast. She decided to delay any medical evaluation, using Harry's 75th birthday celebration and the birth of their second grandchild as rationalization for her procrastination. Finally on May 16, 1959, after the tumor had grown to grapefruit size, she was admitted to the Kansas City Research Hospital. A mastectomy was performed; the tumor turned out to be benign. It was an "unusual type of tumor known medically as a benign myxoma." Mrs. Truman was discharged on her eighteenth hospital day. It took Bess a long time to recover from the operation.[37]

Graham made house calls to the Truman home and was quoted in Mrs. Truman's obituary: "The Trumans' family doctor, Wallace Graham, said Mrs. Truman, who was hospitalized for 22 days in September with a bleeding ulcer, had been battling pulmonary congestion since that hospitalization and had been in a coma-like state since Friday."[38] Bess Truman remains the longest-living of the first ladies. She died at 97 years of age.

Lady Bird Johnson

"She was a stoic, rarely admitting pain, a trait her husband characterized as perhaps her only fault. She had four miscarriages but never indulged in self-pity."[39]

Lady Bird Johnson was gifted with the three essentials for survival, and success, in the White House: Strength, courage and excellent health.[40] And she was indeed very healthy, before, during and, for many years, after her residence in the White House. She suffered several miscarriages during the pre–World War II era, but delivered healthy daughters in 1944 and 1947.[41]

Mrs. Johnson died in 1997 at age 94 and is the second longest-lived first lady.[42] Four years earlier, in the summer of 1993, there was a slight stroke which later caused recurrent episodes of dizziness. Subsequently, macular degeneration impaired her vision and eventually made her legally blind. In 2002, a second cerebrovascular accident destroyed her ability to speak. Another consequence was an inability to swallow; a nasogastric feeding tube was inserted to provide nutrition.[43]

Lady Bird and Lyndon Johnson were married for thirty-nine years and formed a very effective political, social, and financial team. This first lady was well prepared for her expected social and ceremonial duties, as she had acquired a quarter-century of Washington political experience. Moreover, as the wife of the vice president, she often substituted at events for first lady Jacqueline Kennedy, who was not at all interested in attending political or routine social affairs.

"To a greater degree than Eleanor Roosevelt, Lady Bird Johnson devised and developed the staff, procedures and tactics that subsequent First Ladies have employed when they entered the public arena."[44] Her success as the wife of the president has been acknowledged consistently in polls that assess first ladies. She is always ranked in the top ten wives for effectiveness.[45]

Chapter Fifteen

Breast Cancer and Other Maladies

Betty Ford, Rosalynn Carter and Nancy Reagan

Introduction

Two first ladies, Betty Ford and Nancy Reagan, the wives of Presidents Gerald Ford (1974–1977) and Ronald Reagan (1981–1989), suffered in public through the diagnosis, treatment, and aftermath of breast cancer, the most emotionally and physically frightening disease for females, which eventually strikes one in eight American women.[1] It is stunning that it was not until the third century of the American Republic that cancer became a part of the conversation about the first ladies' health. It is especially a surprise since in 2010 cancer was the second leading cause of death of American women.[2]

Cancer (except for innocuous skin cancers—mostly basal cell carcinomas—in several, and lymphoma and lung cancer as the causes of death in two others—Jackie Kennedy and Pat Nixon respectively—long after their residencies in the White House) did not attack a first lady until September 1974. The shadow of a breast malignancy twice previously had darkened the mood of a president's spouse. Abigail (Nabby) Smith, the only daughter of John and Abigail Adams, died from breast cancer, despite a mastectomy. Ex-first lady Bess Truman had a large benign mammary tumor removed with no further ill effects.[3]

Mrs. Ford also suffered from a second severe ailment—painful osteoarthritis of the neck that compounded her chronic depression. Alcoholism and drug dependency resulted from the pain and the depression. Her heroic recovery and its benefit to the public is presented at the end of the chapter. First lady Betty Ford was the first of the first ladies to publicize the problems in her medical history for the public good.

Betty Ford

"Two weeks after her admission to Long Beach, Betty Ford admitted she was an alcoholic."[4]

This first lady was born Elizabeth Ann Bloomer in Chicago on April 8, 1918, the youngest, and the only girl, of three siblings. At the age of twenty-four she wed salesman Bill Warren. They divorced after five years of marriage. Betty became the third first lady, after Rachel Jackson and Florence Harding, to previously have been divorced.[5] She married the rising politician Gerald Ford in 1948. Four healthy children arrived in the following nine years.[6]

Breast Cancer

The Ford White House endorsed complete transparency in its reporting on the first lady's breast cancer—its diagnosis, treatment and recovery. Mrs. Ford believed that the public would benefit from a frank discussion about this dread disease. A second compelling reason was an attempt to recover from the widespread alienation attached to the Nixon presidency. Nixon's resignation a few months earlier made the unelected Gerald Ford the 38th President of the United States (1974–77).[7] Florence Harding, a predecessor as first lady, allowed full medical disclosure of her illness to dissipate the political cynicism that resulted from the secrecy of Woodrow Wilson's disability.

The diagnosis of Betty's breast cancer was serendipitous. On September 26, 1974, the first lady accompanied her personal assistant, Nancy Howe, to Bethesda Naval Hospital for Mrs. Howe's previously scheduled breast examination. On the spur of the moment Betty Ford decided to undergo an examination as well.[8] There is no record when she last had a complete physical examination. The *New York Times* reported that a gynecological check-up, probably a limited exam, six weeks previously was normal. The first breast mammogram machine was introduced in the 1960s and it was only in 1976, two years after Mrs. Ford's diagnosis, that the American Cancer Society recommended annual mammograms for women over the age of fifty.[9]

Navy captain Douglas Knab, the chair of Bethesda's Department of Obstetrics and Gynecology, was the first to examine Mrs. Ford at Bethesda; he detected a marble sized lump in the right breast. Captain William Fouty, chief of surgery, was asked to corroborate Knab's finding. Fouty determined that the lump was "suspicious." The caution that is a hallmark of VIP medicine was observed; the physicians desired additional consultation. As a result, the patient left the hospital without being informed of her probable diagnosis.

Both physicians contacted the White House physician, William Lukash. Lukash in turn scheduled an examination to be preformed at the White House by Dr. Richard Thistlethwaite, Bethesda's civilian consultant and chief of surgery at the George Washington School of Medicine. Thistlethwaite, the fourth doctor involved, after his examination joined Lukash in informing President and Mrs. Ford that the breast lump required immediate surgery. Betty Ford decided to fulfill her scheduled commitments the following day. The *New York Times* soon broke the story: "Mrs. Betty Ford … entered Bethesda late this afternoon [9/27] for surgery tomorrow to determine whether a nodule in her right breast is benign or malignant."[10]

On Saturday morning, September 28, under general anesthesia, a two centimeter cancer was excised from the outer upper quadrant of Betty Ford's right breast. After a malignant diagnosis was established, by advance consent surgeon Fouty performed a standard radical mastectomy. Bill Fouty was a navy specialist in female surgery; previously he had performed hundreds of mastectomies. Two of thirty regional lymph nodes that were removed contained metastatic cancer.[11]

Cancer of the breast was the most feared disease of women. Contemporary 1974 statistics showed 90,000 cases and 33,000 deaths annually from female breast cancer. Mrs. Ford, in good health and not overweight, was judged to have a favorable prognosis with a 75–90 percent ten-year survival.[12] The first lady was released from Bethesda on the thirteenth post-operative day. She soon resumed her social duties as a hostess at the farewell dinner party for retiring White House chief of staff brigadier general Alexander Haig.[13]

Because the cancer had metastasized to lymph nodes, postoperative therapy was required. Chemotherapy in the form of a "little brown bottle of pills" was supplied by White House doctor Lukash. The regimen called for this treatment five days in a row every five weeks for two years. In addition, a bone scan was scheduled for every six months to determine whether the tumor had spread. Mrs. Ford's treatment was a success; there was no recurrence. Her physicians never discussed reconstructive surgery, but she wore a prosthesis.[14]

The public effect of Betty Ford's candor was enormous. During her hospitalization thousands of letters and cards inundated the White House. Many were written by women with mastectomies and many from women who were encouraged to have breast examinations. One year later, there was a six-fold increase in breast screening examinations. Happy Rockefeller, the wife of Ford's vice president, credited the publicity for her own examination, which detected cancer.[15]

Mrs. Ford was personally responsible for increased public awareness of this serious issue. She shrewdly acknowledged the value of a White House podium: "I'd come to recognize more clearly the power of the woman in the White House. Not my power, but the power of the position, a power which could be used to help."[16] Moreover, her openness was critical in changing the discussion of cancer of the breast from a private and stigmatized medical condition to a publicly acknowledged illness. No longer were breast cancer and mastectomy taboo topics for open discourse. Now susceptible women were encouraged to approach these issues without shame or embarrassment.[17] For her efforts, the first lady received an award from the American Cancer Society in November 1975 and was named a "Communicator of Hope" by the American College of Surgeons in December 1976.[18]

Drug and Alcohol Dependency

Betty Ford's medical story has a second chapter. Its subject matter is alcoholism and analgesic drug dependency. These dependencies were long in developing, and were substantially masked during her residency in the White House. However, these problems, long simmering, detonated shortly after the Fords retired to Rancho Mirage, California. Subsequently, the former first lady wrote two autobiographies to tell her story.[19]

Betty Ford's environment predisposed her towards alcohol dependency. Her father and her brother, Bob, were both alcoholics. Her first husband, Bill Warren, an itinerant salesman, also was a heavy drinker.[20] Congressman Gerald Ford and his wife lived in Washington, D.C., for many years prior to his presidency. Betty referenced its social environment: "In Washington there is more alcohol consumed per capita than in any other city in the United States."[21]

A successful politician's wife frequently leads a lonely existence. Mrs. Ford's expected tasks were homemaker and mother of the couple's children—four in the Ford family. Gerald Ford's absences were commonplace. His wife lamented: "Jerry ended up being gone from home two hundred days a year throughout much of the time when our kids were growing up."[22] Mrs. Ford continued: "During the time that Jerry was gone so much I developed a problem, and I quit drinking entirely for a couple of years." She was unable to set a date when she descended from just drinking socially to alcohol addiction, but she thought that her descent was quite gradual.[23]

At some time in 1965 or possibly later, Betty Ford was hospitalized for pancreatitis. Her presenting complaint was "stomach trouble." After her physicians excluded the stomach, gallbladder and kidneys as a source, a specialist diagnosed her illness as pancreatitis. He said, "Young lady, if I were you, I would just stay on the other side of the room from the bar for a while."[24]

Cervical Spine Osteoarthritis and Depression

In August 1964 the congressman's wife was awakened by excruciating neck pain that was referred down her left arm. A diagnosis was made of cervical spine osteoarthritis with impingement of the nerve to the left arm. Betty Ford was hospitalized in the National Orthopedic Hospital, placed in traction, and given gold injections and cortisone shots. The pain continued despite traction at home for several weeks, thrice weekly visits to the hospital for massage, and heat therapy. She consulted doctor after doctor as the pain continued. Subsequently a neurosurgeon admitted her to George Washington Hospital for ten days of testing and manipulative treatment. Unfortunately, Mrs. Ford was informed that an operation was not indicated since an operable lesion could not be located. Instead, she was prescribed increasing doses of pain-killing drugs.[25]

The future first lady was depressed; loneliness and physical pain had exacted a price. Depression has a familial component. Many years earlier her alcoholic father probably committed suicide by carbon monoxide poisoning.[26] A crisis in 1965 dramatized her depression. She lost control and cried uncontrollably on her bed. Clara, her close friend and longtime housekeeper, summoned Representative Ford home from a meeting with President Lyndon Johnson. A physician was called and Mrs. Ford said she "started seeing a psychiatrist twice a week."[27] At some time thereafter, a psychiatrist prescribed valium, which she continued to use in the White House.[28]

As First Lady

Mrs. Ford wrote that her addictions were "better in the White House," since her husband was around and she was an important person as the First Lady of the Land. Her family and friends were concerned about her dependencies but acted as her enablers since they were allied in suppressing any news of her problem. Her drinking continued after she returned from her breast surgery. She and her close friend Nancy Howe would drink: "The two would sit for a cocktail hour that was viewed with displeasure by the president."[29] A link between the first lady's medical and dependency afflictions and Ford's performance as chief executive has not been found.

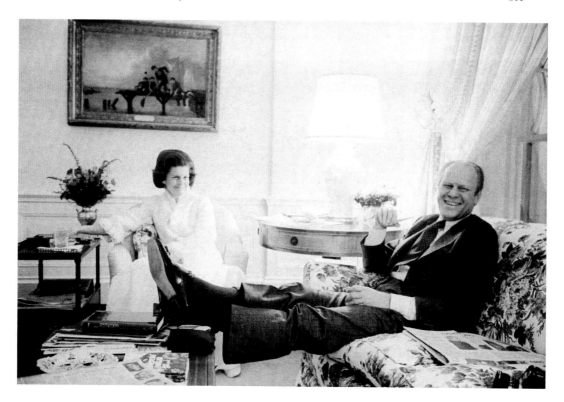

Betty Ford, the wife of Gerald Ford. She survived breast cancer, alcoholism and prescription drug addiction (Library of Congress).

After the White House

When Betty departed the White House for the Ford retirement home in Rancho Mirage, her psychological support vanished. Her husband, as ex-president, was much in demand and he resumed his frequent political travels. Her children were grown and gone; she was no longer prominent and in the public spotlight. She reacted by drinking more and consuming more pills than when she was in the White House. Betty visited her physician twice a week for her arthritis but the doctor "was unaware or didn't want to recognize my dependency on the drugs. I don't think that he knew anything about my use of alcohol." Her family could no longer ignore the slurring of speech, frequent appearances at cocktail parties, and absences at previously scheduled appointments.[30]

Daughter Susan Ford and her gynecologist, Dr. Joseph Cruise, a recovering alcoholic, organized an intervention. The initial attempt failed, but a second, attended by the entire Ford family, was successful. Mrs. Ford checked into the Long Beach Naval Hospital's Alcohol and Drug Rehabilitation Service on April 10, 1978.[31] Mrs. Ford then publicly acknowledged her alcoholism and drug dependency. In July 1979, Jerry Ford stopped drinking in support of his wife.[32] As a result of her prodigious efforts, on October 3, 1982, the Betty Ford Center for the treatment of alcohol and drug dependency was dedicated at Palms Springs, California. Vice President George H. W. Bush was the principal speaker.

Mrs. Ford died on July 8, 2011, at the age of ninety-three. The Betty Ford Center is a direct and lasting result of her victory over alcoholism and drug dependency.[33]

Nancy Reagan

"Perhaps Nancy Reagan's largest and most important work as First Lady, however, was her role as the President's personal protector."[34]

Early Life and Marriage to Ronald Reagan

Nancy Reagan was the only child of the marriage between Edith Luckett and Kenneth Robbins. She was born Anne Francis Robbins in New York City on July 6, 1921. Edith Luckett, an actress, divorced Robbins and bequeathed her daughter, among many other gifts, the new surname of Davis, after remarriage to prominent Chicago neurosurgeon Dr. Loyal Davis. The future first lady also inherited from her mother a strong interest in acting, and more important, longevity. Edith Davis is the longest-lived mother of a first lady; the actress died in Phoenix, Arizona, on October 26, 1987, at the age of 99 years, 3 months.[35]

A Hollywood acting career introduced Nancy Davis to actor Ronald Reagan. The thirty-year-old bride was wed to the forty-one-year-old groom on March 6, 1952. Their marriage of fifty-two years (1952–2004) was an enduring romance and Mrs. Reagan's greatest joy. The Reagans had two children, Patti and Ron. Two miscarriages occurred during the six-year interim between Patti's and Ron's births. Ronald Reagan also had two children from his prior marriage to actress Jane Wyman.[36]

Breast Cancer

Nancy Reagan was the bastion that buttressed President Reagan during three significant medical crises during his eight-year presidency (1981–89). An assassination attempt, a colon resection for cancer of the right colon, and prostate surgery marked his presidential tenure. Mrs. Reagan's sole illness was breast cancer that was detected in October 1987.

Annual mammograms have been recommended by the American Cancer Society for women fifty years of age and older since 1976.[37] Nancy Reagan abided by this schedule and a routine mammogram at Bethesda Naval Hospital on October 5, 1987, detected a tiny malignant tumor in her left breast. She was accompanied to the hospital by the respected White House physician John Hutton. Hutton informed the first lady: "We think we've seen something…. There is an outside chance it isn't malignant, but it probably is."[38] Nancy Reagan became a beneficiary of the escalating advances in medical technology; a single mammographic examination detected a tiny breast cancer while the diagnosis of Betty Ford's much larger malignancy thirteen years earlier required examination by four physicians.

Her initial response to Dr. Hutton was, "Please call Ollie Beahrs. I want him to be involved." Mayo Clinic surgeon Dr. Oliver Beahrs flew to Washington almost immediately, met the patient in the White House physician's office on the mansion's first floor, reviewed the breast X-rays, and examined the patient. He discussed treatment options with Mrs. Reagan and a decision was made to enter Bethesda ten days later with surgery the next day, October 17.[39]

The first lady immediately reached out to Beahrs out of respect for his skill as a physician and for his comfort and support as a dear friend. The doctor previously had consulted with and supported the Reagans during the president's colon surgery. Beahrs was an internationally renowned surgeon, and a leader both at the Mayo Clinic and the American College of Surgeons. He had been a student of Loyal Davis, Nancy's stepfather, at Northwestern University School of Medicine. Another bond was a result of the doctor's skill as a magician, which he practiced for fun and sometimes for profit—to pay his medical school bills: "Throughout medical school, he continued to hone his skills as a magician and became so in demand that he actually had a booking agent, Mrs. Edith Luckett Davis," Nancy's mother.[40]

During the Reagans' final years in the White House, significant elements of their medical diagnoses and treatment were delegated to teams of physicians from the Mayo Clinic of Rochester, Minnesota. Dr. Hutton apparently acted as liaison with the Mayo physicians, and the Washington military/civilian medical establishment thereby was bypassed. One reason, among others, for this strategy may have been Mrs. Reagan's desire to control the flow of medical

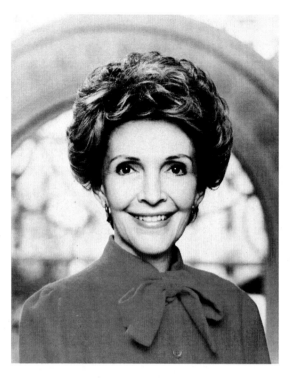

Nancy Reagan, the wife of Ronald Reagan. Her transparency about her choice of treatment for breast cancer was met with much disapproval (Library of Congress).

information. Mayo doctors flew to Washington on at least four occasions to perform a colonoscopy, a cystoscopy, and a major prostate surgery on the president, and a (modified) radical mastectomy on the first lady.[41]

Nancy Reagan determined that she would hold to her public schedule during the ten days between her diagnosis and hospitalization. Only the day prior to entering the hospital did she inform the press secretary and discuss and approve the statement to be released when she entered Bethesda. In two ways, chronicled above, the narrative did not depart from the norm for first ladies' medical treatment. First was the principal-practiced secrecy which revealed only the minimum information when necessary. Secondly, the wife of an American president is able to select the most renowned and expert medical consultants to participate in her care, a privilege attainable by only a minuscule minority of her constituents.[42]

Mrs. Reagan preoperatively directed her physicians to perform a modified radical mastectomy under general anesthesia with no interval wake-up between biopsy and definitive therapy. Dr. McIlrath from the Mayo Clinic was the lead surgeon. The cancer measured 7 millimeters and was defined as "non-invasive," that is, it was confined to the breast ducts and had not invaded into the breast tissue itself. John Hutton reported that the lymph nodes were free of cancer as expected. He further announced that no further treatment was necessary beyond regular follow-up. The cure rate for this type of breast malignancy is close to, if not at, 100 percent.[43]

The publicity surrounding this news event initiated a rush by women towards doctors' offices and mammography clinics for breast exams, as did news of Betty Ford's cancer thirteen years previously. Immediately after the news reports, there was a 30–50 percent increase in mammography screening. A retrospective analysis published two years later noted a lower twelve percent increase. This surely cheered the first lady, who, while still in the hospital, released he following statement through a spokesperson: "I can only hope and pray that women everywhere are calling their doctors for appointments."[44]

The first lady returned to the White House after six days in the hospital. Advances in medical care had significantly reduced hospital stays; Mrs. Ford's hospitalization for breast cancer surgery lasted two weeks. A one-year follow-up examination on Mrs. Reagan was negative for tumor, and there has been no recurrence twenty-six years later.[45] The thirteen-year interval between the surgeries of these two first ladies saw dramatic changes in the surgical approach towards this cancer. The destructive and excessive radical mastectomy had been replaced by the modified radical mastectomy for most tumors. In this procedure only a small amount of chest muscle is removed. A further advance was the substitution of a lumpectomy for small cancers similar to Mrs. Reagan's. A lumpectomy excises the tumor with an adequate margin of uninvolved breast tissue; this surgery is usually supplemented with radiation or chemotherapy.

The first lady's treatment option was widely criticized by the press and medical "experts" on two counts: First, her choice of a more extensive operation than was necessary, and second, her avoidance of an interval between biopsy and definitive surgery to allow an opportunity for the patient to carefully review treatment options. The headline in the *New York Times* the day after the surgery shouted, "Mastectomy Seen as Extreme for Small Tumor." A lay expert was quoted that Nancy Reagan's decision "set us back years." Contemporary articles in both the *Washington Post* and the *Chicago Tribune* also second-guessed Nancy Reagan. The furor came close to negating the beneficial publicity that her surgery had evoked.[46]

This controversy deeply troubled and frustrated the patient involved. Five months later in a television interview Nancy Reagan responded that a lumpectomy probably would have required radiation or chemotherapy, and both would have interfered with her schedule as first lady. She elaborated: "I couldn't possibly lead the kind of life I lead and keep the schedule I do." She added that doctors who were not involved in her case had no business criticizing the treatment choices she made. She stressed "it was she, and not her husband or her doctors, who had made the decisions about which treatment to follow. It was my choice to make, so don't criticize me for making what I thought was the right choice for me."[47]

The carping may have had a small element of merit. In the six months after Mrs. Reagan's surgery there was a documented 25 percent reduction in the use of breast conserving surgery (lumpectomy) as opposed to mastectomy among women with local or regional breast cancer. The effect was greatest among women who were demographically related to her. But this reduction was transient and disappeared after about six months.[48]

Nancy Reagan has been healthy but increasingly frail in the quarter-century after leaving the White House. A basal cell carcinoma was removed from beneath her left nostril during a 1990 physical examination at the Mayo Clinic. Her sense of balance has deteriorated; she experiences frequent falls, and she has been hospitalized for a fractured pelvis and fractured ribs. A recent visit to a favorite Beverly Hills restaurant shocked customers with her frailty and noticeable leg bruises due to her falls.[49]

Rosalynn Carter

Rosalynn Carter, first lady to President Jimmy Carter (1977–1981), was the second of three successive first ladies to undergo a biopsy for a breast lesion. A lump was detected in her breast during a routine six-month physical examination at Bethesda Naval Hospital in April 1977. Navy captain Dr. William Fouty removed the lesion. Pathological examination confirmed its benign nature. Mrs. Carter remains free of breast tumors thirty-seven years later.[50] The first lady again had minor surgery at Bethesda Naval Hospital in August 1977. Navy captain Dr. Douglas Knab performed a dilatation and curettage (D&C) of the uterus. Mrs. Carter's press secretary gave a succinct and unrevealing report to the press: "It is a routine procedure and a private matter."[51]

Chapter Sixteen

Modern-Day First Ladies

*Barbara Bush, Hillary Clinton,
Laura Bush and Michelle Obama*

Introduction

This quartet of first ladies served in the White House from 1989 to the present. All four were relatively healthy; their illnesses were either underemphasized in the press or concealed from the public: Their diseases were neither nettlesome to their presidential husbands nor disruptive of the presidential routine. All were under the constant medical care of a modernized and upgraded White House Medical Unit (WHMU), the military organization responsible for the wellness and medical treatment of the first family.

Barbara Bush (1989–1993)

"George is very healthy, and I always questioned the press' right to know things about his body that had nothing to do with his ability to govern."[1]

Barbara Pierce Bush remains an outspoken and universally admired mother and grandmother. She is the wife to a two-term vice president (1981–1989) and one-term president (1989–1993). Barbara Pierce married navy pilot George H. W. Bush on January 6, 1945.[2] Their marriage has lasted for 68 years and counting. Barbara Bush had six successful pregnancies between 1946 and 1959, giving birth to four sons and two daughters.[3] However, the Bush's oldest daughter, Robin, died from leukemia seven months after the diagnosis. The child was one month shy of her fourth birthday.[4]

Mrs. Bush's health had always been robust. In the 18 months leading up to her husband's presidential inauguration in 1989, she never had felt better and was very pleased that she was losing weight, a reduction of eighteen pounds. However, during the week before George Bush's January 1989 inauguration, her eyes began to bother her.[5] The new first lady described her symptoms in a March 20 diary entry: "They started acting up the week before the inauguration. I thought it was a makeup problem, allergy to makeup, etc. But it didn't stop. They are red, sort of tearing all the time, itch, are puffy and I see double.... Frankly, it is a little scary."[6]

The innately voluble Barbara Bush was the first to inform the public about her illness. She broke the news at an informal March 29 news conference in the White House: "I wouldn't have told you this, but I'm so bored reading about my weight; people keep saying: 'She's dieting.'" She revealed that Dr. Burton Lee III, the Bush family's personal physician in the White House, insisted on diagnostic tests after he was informed of her symptoms. She added that her eyes looked like "horrible-big puffy, horrible eyes." "Pop eyes," she described their appearance.[7]

The tests were performed at Walter Reed Army Medical Center, where the diagnosis of Graves' disease (hyperthyroidism) was established. Mrs. Bush colorfully described her problem as "an overactive thyroid—it just went wacko." Her diary entry, dated March 20, 1989, reads colloquially: "they think I have a thyroid gone berserk."[8] The first lady determined that the public should be informed immediately since Graves' disease was not a life-threatening condition if treated. Later in the day of her news conference, her press office belatedly caught up with the story. It formally announced that Barbara Bush had Graves' disease. In addition, its official statement disclosed that treatment with methimazole had commenced and that marked improvement of her eye symptoms had occurred. Methimazole is a drug that inhibits the synthesis of the thyroid gland's hormones.[9] The following month Mrs. Bush was again an outpatient at Walter Reed. She sipped a solution of a radioactive form of iodine to further suppress the hyperactivity of her thyroid gland.[10]

Graves' disease is the most common cause of hyperthyroidism, i.e., increased activity of the thyroid gland. For reasons still unknown, antibodies to the patient's own thyroid are produced which lead to an uncontrolled production of thyroid hormone. The hormone controls the body's metabolism and is critical for regulating mood, weight, and mental and physical energy levels. Surprisingly, thyroid hormone receptors are also present elsewhere in the body other than the thyroid. The adipose (fat) and muscle cells of the eye orbit contain such receptors. In Graves' disease, these orbital constituents expand and crowd out the eyeball; protrusion of the eyes is a result. Eye protrusion, also known as exophthalmos, is a diagnostic sign of Graves' disease and in Mrs. Bush's case it produced weight loss and eye problems. At sixty-two years of age, she was older than the usual patient—a woman closer to the age of twenty.[11]

Graves' disease was named for an astute nineteenth-century Irish physician, Robert Graves, who at age thirty-nine described four young women with the condition. Three presented symptoms of an enlarged thyroid gland and tachycardia (an abnormally increased heart rate). The fourth exhibited severe exophthalmos. Graves' insight was to connect the symptoms of the four women into a single clinical entity. However, as frequently is the case with eponyms, the namesake was mistaken regarding its essential features. Graves erroneously concluded that the diseased organ was the heart, not the thyroid gland.[12]

Mrs. Bush's ocular symptoms continued. Despite initial optimism, the double vision, tearing, and irritation did not improve. An August return visit to Walter Reed concluded that although her thyroid function was under control the uncomfortable eye complaints persisted. Consequently, another treatment was instituted: Oral steroids in the form of prednisone.[13] Despite prednisone therapy, the symptoms still persisted three months later. Therefore, the first lady sought a second opinion apart from Doctor Lee and the specialists attached to the military hospitals in the Washington, D.C., area. She flew to the Mayo Clinic in Rochester, Minnesota, for a series of tests and recommendations for alternative treatment.

Perhaps her choice of an external consultant was influenced by the Reagans' past successful treatments by physicians from this esteemed institution. The Mayo Clinic reduced the daily prednisone dosage and recommended a course of radiation to her eye orbits.[14] Prednisone is not without side effects, which Mrs. Bush acknowledged: "I was weaning myself off the prednisone ... and it was very painful. I was taking therapy to strengthen my muscles.... [P]rednisone ... killed something in my right hip and caused muscles to weaken, especially around my knee and hips. I confess that I was in a lot of pain that would last through the fall."[15]

A ten-day course of low-level X-rays at Walter Reed Army Medical Center followed in January 1990. The objective of the irradiation was shrinkage of the muscles and fat of the eye orbits in order to reduce swelling and inflammation. The hope was to provide more room for the eye muscles to adjust, limit double vision, and reduce the exophthalmos.[16]

There is no indication that the first lady's disease affected the functioning of the president. Mrs. Bush's account of the first hundred days of the Bush administration showed no let-up in the 41st president's hectic executive, travel, and social schedule.[17]

Two decades later, in March 2010, the eighty-four-year-old Mrs. Bush was briefly hospitalized in Houston with undisclosed, but baffling, symptoms. After several days of testing the diagnostic conclusion was a mild relapse of Graves' disease. The Bush family spokesman "described her symptoms as not life-threatening but would not go into further detail at the time." A slight adjustment was made to her medications that she had been taking for twenty years. Since 1990, there has been no reference to exophthalmos.[18]

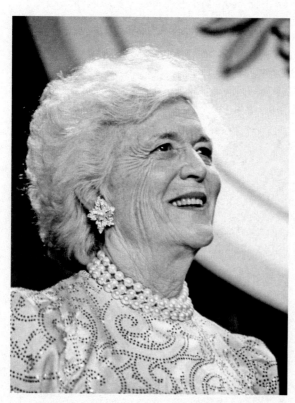

Two years after her diagnosis of Graves' disease, her husband, President George Bush, became symptomatic with the same condition in a dramatic fashion. Bush collapsed while jogging; the cause was atrial fibrillation, a significant abnormality of the heart rhythm (cardiac arrhythmia). Hospital tests disclosed Graves' disease, for which he was then treated successfully. Fortunately for the president, his symptoms did not include eye problems, the symptoms that were most bothersome for his wife.[19] Doctor Burton Lee III, the civilian who served as the first family's personal physician in the White House and who astutely directed Mrs. Bush for medical testing when her symptoms appeared in 1989, failed to diagnose the President's illness. Lee inserted his academic philosophy into his practice of medicine. In an interview for the *Journal of the American*

Barbara Bush, the wife of George H. W. Bush. Both Bushes developed Graves' disease (Library of Congress).

Medical Association, the White House physician criticized physicians for ordering too many unnecessary blood tests, including screening tests for thyroid disease. Lee did not order these for President Bush's annual physicals, and as a result, an early diagnosis of Graves' disease was missed.[20]

Barbara Bush mused about the rarity of a husband and wife contracting an uncommon disease: "What a peculiar illness—it attacked my eyes and George's heart. It is unusual for a husband and wife to both have this problem, but not unheard of. I received several letters telling me of other couples who shared our same disease." The Bushes' dog, Millie, contracted lupus, another autoimmune disease, which led to all sorts of crazy speculation, including an investigation of the water supply at the vice president's house. The search for answers continued, and in response "in December 1993, George, Millie and I [Barbara] gave blood to Dr. Jonathan Jaspan at Tulane University to be tested for a common virus that might be responsible for our autoimmune diseases."[21]

Barbara Bush's public advocacy for thyroid disease awareness, detection, treatment, and research barely outlasted her years in the White House. In 1992 she gave an address in Boston for Dr. Lawrence C. Wood and the Thyroid Foundation of America, which he started and headed at the Massachusetts General Hospital.[22] In addition, the Bushes made public service announcements for the Thyroid Foundation in Houston and were made honorary members of the Graves' Disease Foundation, an organization founded in 1990, a year after the first lady's diagnosis.[23]

However, publicity was fleeting regarding the extremely unusual occurrence of an uncommon malady in both a president and his first lady. Perhaps this resulted from the treatability of Graves' disease and very good prognosis. Mrs. Bush's name now has become unassociated with her malady, outside of biographies and history books. The Graves' Foundation has received little feedback and minimal support from the White House connection. The Foundation's director speculated that Mrs. Bush's inattention and reluctance to speak out was due to a desire to keep her disease a private matter.[24]

At the time of this writing, it has been twenty years since George and Barbara Bush were tenants of the White House. For most of the time, the genial couple have enjoyed a peripatetic existence. Barbara Bush, like Betty Ford before her, chronicled her post–White House experiences in two autobiographies.[25]

The medical care of an ex–first lady is her responsibility; no longer would her health be under the close scrutiny of the physicians of the White House Medical Unit. Barbara Bush, pleased with her previous experience in Rochester, Minnesota, like her predecessor Nancy Reagan, selected the Mayo Clinic facilities in Minnesota and Scottsdale, Arizona, to monitor her care. The bond was fortified by the appointment of Mrs. Bush to the Mayo Clinic Foundation Board, an honor that "happened because I married well."[26]

The Mayo Clinic was the site for most of the operations Mrs. Bush underwent during her first decade as a private citizen. Osteoarthritis necessitated nine surgeries: replacements of both hips, five foot operations, and two back surgeries.[27] The Bushes selected a Houston physician, Dr. Ben Orman, to be their primary care doctor. The former first lady has since been hospitalized several times at Houston's Methodist Hospital. The most recent admission was for pneumonia on December 30, 2013.[28]

Hillary Clinton (1993–2001)

"She did have pain in her calf, but her staff thought she had pulled a muscle exercising."[29]

Hillary Clinton was America's first lady during the two-term presidency of Bill Clinton (1993–2001). Hers was not the traditional narrative of a president's wife. Her activities, both during and subsequent to her White House residency, were remarkably political in nature, even exceeding those of her cherished predecessor Eleanor Roosevelt.[30]

Early in 1993 President Clinton announced that his wife would chair the President's Task Force on National Health Care Reform, which included seven cabinet secretaries and numerous White House staff members.[31] A few months later a federal appeals court ruled that her open advocacy as chair of the task force made her a "de facto" fulltime government official.[32]

In her last year as first lady, Mrs. Clinton campaigned for and won a seat as United States senator from New York. She was reelected in 2006 and served as secretary of state between 2009 and 2013. She sought the 2008 Democratic nomination for president and is rumored to be very interested in its 2016 nomination.

Little is known about Hillary Clinton's past or present medical history. She is the mother of one child. "Chelsea Victoria Clinton arrived three weeks early on February 27, 1980."[33] Hillary was healthy as first lady, as noted by the Clintons' personal physician in the White House: "Hillary rarely had a sick day nor did she complain of feeling ill unless her illness risked compromising her scheduled activities."[34]

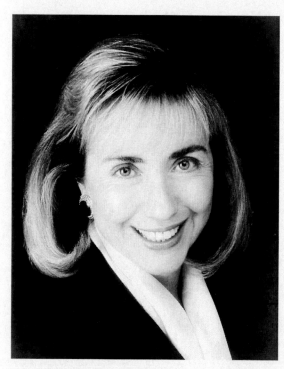

Hillary Clinton, the wife of Bill Clinton. She concealed a dangerous deep vein thrombosis while first lady (Library of Congress).

Transparency regarding her health was absent from this first lady's credo, in contrast to Barbara Bush, who, although she had some misgivings about the release of intimate medical information, was forthcoming with information about her non–life threatening Graves' disease. Hillary Clinton, however, was silent about a more threatening condition, a deep vein thrombosis within the major vein of her right leg. This event became public knowledge only after a brief mention in her biography, *Living History*, five years after the fact.[35] Her physician, navy captain Connie Mariano, was prohibited by professional ethics from releasing the information. It was only in Mariano's 2010 memoir, *The White House Doctor*, that a comprehensive report of the incident became available.[36]

The first lady was a very active campaigner during the 1998 mid-term elections. While in New York City to attend a fund-raiser for her future New York State senatorial colleague, Charles Schumer, she realized her "right foot was so swollen that I could barely put my shoe on." White House physicians are always at the beck and call of a first lady. Dr. Mariano was summoned to the White House upon Hillary Clinton's return. An initial cursory examination diagnosed a deep vein thrombosis (DVT) behind the right knee. This was confirmed at Bethesda Naval Hospital by an ultrasound and consultation with Captain Frank Maguire of the hospital's pulmonary medicine and critical care service.[37]

A DVT is a blood clot that forms in one or more deep veins of the body, usually in the legs. A deep vein thrombosis is a serious condition because a blood clot may break loose, travel through the bloodstream and lodge in the lungs. The result, a pulmonary embolism, may be fatal. In the United States, 600,000 cases of DVT occur each year. One of every 100 patients dies.[38] Mrs. Clinton accurately identified the cause of the clot, her nonstop flying

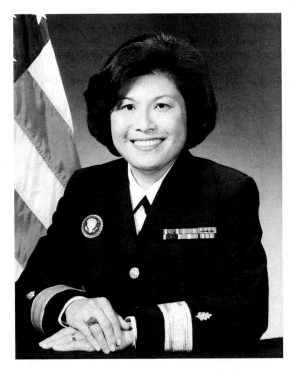

Navy physician Connie Mariano was the personal physician to Bill and Hillary Clinton during their two terms in the White House (courtesy Bureau of Medicine and Surgery Archives).

around the country. Sitting for long periods of time in a car or on an airplane is its most common risk factor. Other risk factors include prolonged bed rest, leg injury, pregnancy, and anovulants.[39]

Drs. Mariano and Maguire recommended hospitalization and anticoagulation. However, the first lady balked and forced the physicians to compromise. She was treated as an outpatient with a newly released blood thinner (anticoagulant). The first lady returned shortly to the campaign trail, repeating the long episodes of sitting that placed her at risk in the first place. Mariano assigned a White House nurse in civilian attire to accompany Mrs. Clinton on the campaign trail. As an added precaution the doctor informed the Secret Service that the first lady was on anticoagulant medication, to warn them: "In the event she was injured, excessive bleeding would be a dangerous complication."[40]

The reasons for this first lady's clandestine handling of a serious disease are best known only to her. Was it bravado, the belief that as a private citizen it was no one's business, or a strictly political motive? "Very few people knew of Hillary's blood clot at the time…. [S]he did have pain in her calf, but her staff thought that she had pulled a muscle exercising."[41] One result of this incident was medical coverage of a first lady on a domestic air flight. In the future, first ladies would be accompanied by a nurse from the WHMU. A physician and a nurse or physician assistant continues to escort a president's wife on all international trips. At least one member of the WHMU contingent is a woman.[42]

During the Clinton presidency, the White House Medical Unit consisted of six military physicians, five physician assistants, five nurses, three hospital corpsmen, and three administrative personnel. All are military except for a few administrative members.[43] During the Bush presidency, his personal physician and chief of the WHMU, Colonel Richard Tubb, tasked a physician to accompany Mrs. Bush on all her trips, both domestic and international. The responsibilities of the WHMU increased and its corresponding personnel expanded to more than thirty. Its members now include eight or nine physicians, six nurses, and six physician assistants.[44]

Recent first ladies have undergone annual physicals during their tenure. Moreover, personalized physician examinations are available at their convenience. For gynecologic examinations, the president's wife would visit a private gynecologist's office, or the gynecologist would visit the White House. The annual physicals and other medical examinations are conducted without publicity or public comment.[45]

Mrs. Clinton's past silence about her health, as well as her political and personal behavior during two decades on the national stage, produced significant cynicism over the initial silence and the subsequent explanation of a subdural hematoma suffered at the conclusion of her tenure as secretary of state in December 2012. The secretary of state contracted a viral infection which enervated her; the consequence was a fall and a head injury. Hemorrhage between the coverings of the brain resulted (subdural hematoma). The condition was diagnosed; it was treated appropriately; and the patient recovered completely.[46]

This chapter on Mrs. Hillary Clinton's eventful career remains unfinished. An addendum may be required in the future.

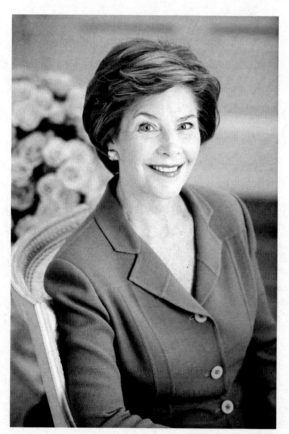

Laura Bush, the wife of George W. Bush. Her small skin cancer caused a controversy with the White House press corps (Library of Congress).

Laura Bush

"She's got the same right to medical privacy that you do."[47]

Laura Welch married George W. Bush, the oldest child of George H.W. and Barbara Bush, when they were both thirty years old. Laura was an only child; her mother's three other pregnancies ended in failure. Laura taught elementary school and, after attaining a graduate degree in library science, she worked as a school librarian.[48]

Despite the couple's desire for children, Mrs. Bush's one and only pregnancy was delayed until the age of thirty-four years. "I was anxious the entire time that I was pregnant. The memories of Mother's late miscarriages hung over me." The prospective parents flew to Houston, Texas, to undergo suturing of the expectant mother's uterine cervix, a maneuver to prevent an aborted pregnancy. A subsequent sonogram diagnosed a twin pregnancy.[49]

The future first lady's obstetrician, Dr. Charles Stephens of Odessa, Texas, diagnosed preeclampsia at seven months of pregnancy; he referred her to Baylor Hospital in Dallas, noted for its excellent obstetrical and prenatal care. Mrs. Bush was placed on bed rest, but toxemia-related hypertension increased to a degree that a caesarean-section was mandated. Healthy twin girls were born five weeks early.[50] Laura Bush certainly was not the only first lady to undergo a difficult pregnancy, though she was more fortunate than her predecessors due to the progress and advances in medical care.

Mrs. Bush was healthy during six years as the wife of the governor of Texas and eight years as first lady of the United States. She experienced two medical problems in the White House, one more consequential politically than medically. The second required surgery.

An observant reporter noted a bandage on Mrs. Bush's right pretibial region (shin) at a Hanukkah ceremony and asked if she had been bitten by Barney, her pet dog. Press speculation boiled over, leading to heated inquiries that evening to Susan Whitson, her press secretary, and the following day to Tony Snow, President Bush's press secretary. In high dudgeon and in anticipation of a nefarious motive during a slow news day, the denizens of the White House press corps demanded answers. They were informed that five weeks previously, a biopsy was taken from a non-healing irritation on the skin of the leg. The pathologist reported a diagnosis of a skin squamous cell carcinoma. The lesion, the size of a nickel, was widely excised.[51]

Squamous cell carcinoma is the second most frequent "cancer" of the skin, but is much less common than its cousin, basal cell carcinoma. ("Cancer" is in quotation marks since this disease almost never spreads or causes death.) Press secretary Snow defensively asserted to the hectoring reporters that Mrs. Bush was not an elected official and that the problem was trivial. He added, "Perhaps if there's something major, this would be discussed."[52] Snow added to the questioners: "She's got the same right to medical privacy that you do."[53]

Some constituents criticized Laura Bush on the grounds that she had missed an opportunity to educate the public about the various kinds of skin cancer and the importance of regular dermatologic examinations.[54] The first lady summed up the issue during a December 24, 2006, interview on CBS's *Face the Nation*: "It just didn't occur to me. Also of course, I am a private citizen. I mean, I have to say that as well. I don't release the results of my regular physicals, like the president does, of course. And so it never really occurred to me. But I'm glad it's out, because I'm glad that people will pay attention. If they have spots, if they don't know what they are, certainly, people like me who are very fair-complected and who grew up in the southern part of the United States and in west Texas where I grew up, where the sun is pretty intense."[55]

The second medical incident was more significant. The first lady developed a seasonal affliction over several Decembers, a pain in her left forearm. Since the problem resolved with the New Year, she discounted it and reasoned that the pain was a result of many hours spent standing and holding the left arm by her side during the numerous White House Christmas social events. However, in 2007, the pain continued into the spring; it worsened after a hiking trip to Zion National Park.[56] Her physical impediment became public in an

August 27 *Los Angeles Times* article. The newspaper reported that the first lady cancelled a trip to Australia due to commence on September 4, 2007. The reason was identified as a pinched nerve in her neck and shoulder. She had received physical therapy for several months; nevertheless her symptoms persisted.[57]

Laura underwent a two-and-a-half-hour operation on September 8, 2007, at the District's George Washington University Hospital. The surgical team was led by Dr. Anthony Caputy, chairman of its Department of Neurosurgery and codirector of its neurological institute. Colonel Richard Tubb, the Bush White House personal physician, was responsible for the first lady's care. When physical therapy was not successful in eliminating the pain, Dr. Tubb recommended several surgeons to his patient. Mrs. Bush had the final say in the selection of the surgeon.[58]

The diagnosis was osteoarthritis of the cervical (neck) vertebral column. Bone spurs and calcifications impinged upon the opening of the nerve to the left arm. These were removed, thus opening up the course of the nerve. Since the procedure was performed on an outpatient basis, Mrs. Bush returned to the White House that afternoon. The arm pain disappeared and she resumed full activity. "The calcifications and bone spurs don't necessarily occur with repetitive motion, so Mrs. Bush's First Ladies duties could ... not explain the pain."[59]

Forty years previously Betty Ford suffered greatly from the same disease. Osteoarthritis of the neck produced excruciating neck and arm pain that were responsible for her prescription drug addiction. Precise radiological instrumentation, e.g., the MRI employed in Mrs. Bush's case, was unavailable at the time. Laura Bush was the fortunate recipient of continuous medical observation and had her choice of many very talented neurosurgeons. She remains well five years after the Bushes departed from the White House. There is no evidence that this incident affected the president's performance of his responsibilities.[60]

The White House revealed Laura's medical malady only after months of physical therapy because her absence on a planned international trip required an explanation. The pending surgery was announced the day before by her press secretary. In a curious fashion, "[Sally] McDonough would not reveal where the surgery would be performed, saying that Mrs. Bush is a private citizen and not an elected official."[61]

Michelle Obama

Michelle Obama was forty-five years of age when Barack Obama, her husband, took the oath of office as the 44th president of the United States. The Obamas are the parents of two daughters. Mrs. Obama has been healthy both before and during her days in the White House. There is no public record of any significant disease. The record of this first lady's health remains to be written.

Chapter Seventeen

The Diseases, Burdens and Confidentiality of First Ladies

It is not possible to summarize the illnesses and the resultant consequences of America's forty first ladies in a concise and comprehensive fashion. However, a few conclusions are appropriate.

The Incidence of Diseases Changes with Time

In general, America's first ladies were affected by the same categories of diseases that afflicted their peers in American society. In the early republic and for most of the nineteenth century infectious and contagious diseases were dominant.

Yellow Fever epidemics in Philadelphia during the 1790s disrupted the operations of the infant United States government and influenced the travel plans of Martha Washington and Abigail Adams. The disease felled the first husband of Dolley Payne Madison and one of her two sons. The new widow also may have been infected. Malaria became almost a first lady's occupational hazard. Sarah Polk, Lucretia Garfield, and possibly Elizabeth Monroe were infected while their husbands toiled amidst the fever swamps of Washington, D.C. Abigail Adams likely was infected when John Adams was vice president, in New York City. Margaret Taylor almost died from the disease when she lived in subtropical Louisiana. Public health measures subsequently eliminated this disease, which is no longer endemic in the United States.

Tuberculosis was the "White Plague" of urban America during the latter part of the nineteenth century. It caused the death of first lady Caroline Harrison in 1892 during her husband's presidency. It persisted as a chronic illness for both Eliza Johnson and Jane Pierce and killed the latter. Tuberculosis remained dormant for decades within the lung of Eleanor Roosevelt, was reactivated possibly by steroid treatment, and contributed to her death in 1962.

Nondescript bacterial infections targeted the urinary tracts of Florence Harding and Grace Coolidge when they resided in the White House. Abigail Fillmore became ill when she attended the inauguration of Franklin Pierce on a cold March morning; pneumonia and death soon followed. A childhood streptococcal infection sickened Mamie Eisenhower; its immediate symptom was Saint Vitus' dance (rapid, irregular, aimless, involuntary movements of the limbs, neck, and trunk that resemble continuous restlessness), and its long-term consequence was rheumatic damage of her cardiac valve. Over the past sixty years antibiotics have controlled and often eliminated the consequences of bacterial infections.

Morbidity related to pregnancy was prevalent until the introduction of modern obstetrics at the beginning of the twentieth century. Toxemia of pregnancy struck Ellen Wilson, Lucy Hayes, Ida McKinley and possibly Letitia Tyler. Mrs. Wilson developed chronic renal failure, Ida McKinley epilepsy, and Lucy Hayes probable hypertension. Although toxemia cannot be documented for Mrs. Tyler, it is likely that pregnancy-induced hypertension was a factor in her debilitating and deadly strokes. Alice, the first Mrs. Theodore Roosevelt, died from acute toxemia of pregnancy. Caroline Harrison underwent surgical correction of a likely vesico-vaginal fistula, a consequence of a difficult vaginal delivery. Postpartum depression became a problem for several of the women, usually prior to living in the White House, but it was most pronounced in Jackie Kennedy. Her malaise and depressed mood after John Jr.'s birth in late 1960 were the circumstances for receiving Dr. Feelgood's amphetamine injections during 1961 and later.

Hypertension and stroke afflicted several first ladies. Although hypertension now is recognized as a leading cause of cerebrovascular accidents, the sphygmomanometer, the device employed to measure a patient's blood pressure, was not widely used until the early 1900s.[1] Therefore it may be reasonable to theorize that the strokes suffered in retirement by Dolley Madison, Louisa Catherine Adams, Lucy Hayes, and in the White House by Nellie Taft, were hypertension-related. Pat Nixon's blood pressure was elevated significantly at 175/100 when she was admitted to the hospital with a hemorrhagic cerebrovascular accident. Both Bess Truman and Lady Bird Johnson were afflicted by strokes in their old age; in neither case were their blood pressure readings released to the press.

Two classes of disease appear, at first glance, to be less frequent than expected: coronary artery disease and cancer, the former, perhaps, because the recognition of coronary artery disease and its relationship to heart attacks were not acknowledged until the early years of the twentieth century.[2] Edith Wilson died from the complications of unspecified heart disease. Grace Coolidge had heart trouble during the last five years of her life; it was listed on her death certificate as kyphoscoliotic heart disuse. Her markedly twisted and curved spinal column allegedly restricted the normal pumping of her heart.

The near absence of cancer is less explicable. It cannot be due entirely to better preventative medicine and screening. This diagnosis has been surprisingly uncommon before and during the subjects' White House years. First ladies Ford and Reagan had well-publicized breast cancers and Nancy Reagan and Laura Bush innocuous skin cancers. Jackie Kennedy and Pat Nixon died from cancer years after living in the White House. In contrast, the American Cancer Society recently reported that one in three American women will develop invasive cancer during their lifetime.[3]

Conversely, the medical histories of presidential wives may include rare disorders. Mamie Eisenhower suffered from Menière's disease, which affects only two per thousand American citizens.[4] Graves' disease is even less common: Only 0.3 persons per year are diagnosed with that disease.[5]

Problems and Prestige. The Burdens of a Public Life

Although the status of first lady may bring prestige, praise, and political power, it also brings problems, some of them physical. Nellie Taft coveted the White House but was unable to savor it. Both Eleanor Roosevelt and Hillary Clinton delighted in a first lady's prestige and podium. The former used these for social and international causes both during and after her husband's presidency; the latter employed her eight years of White House residency to construct her own political career.

Profound grief assailed several first ladies. The office of the president triggered the assassinations of four of its occupants, Lincoln, Garfield, McKinley, and Kennedy. Mary Lincoln and Jacqueline Kennedy were first-person witnesses to their husbands' murders. Nancy Reagan was permanently rattled by John Hinckley's near-fatal attempt on President Reagan's life.

Some first ladies experienced the loneliness of a spouse of an ambitious public figure. John Quincy Adams' personality and political ambition took precedence over any intellectual or emotional intimacy with Louisa Catherine Adams. However, physical intimacy was not eschewed; Louisa's twelve pregnancies were the proof, but loneliness and depression were her rewards. Mrs. Betty Ford acknowledged marital isolation from Gerald Ford both before and after the White House. Paradoxically, her abbreviated White House residence was somewhat beneficial. However, the cumulative years of loneliness resulted in depression and alcoholism. Barbara Bush, the epitome of assurance and composure while a president's spouse, became lonely and depressed when George Bush previously was director of the CIA.[6]

A president's career can sometimes place the first lady in a place or a situation disadvantageous to her health. Geography may have been instrumental in the malaria of Abigail Adams (New York City swamps), Sarah Polk and Lucretia Garfield (the District's stagnant waterways), and possibly for Caroline Harrison's tuberculosis (long hours in the dank basement of the executive mansion as she catalogued its furniture and furnishings). Last, why would Abigail Fillmore attend Franklin Pierce's inauguration in Washington's dismal March weather other than as the departing first lady? Pneumonia and death were her compensation.

As a public figure, the privacy of their medical history is subject to challenge. Only Florence Harding, Betty Ford, and to a lesser extent, Nancy Reagan, were transparent. Many, like Laura Bush, resented the intrusion.

Is the First Lady Merely a Private Individual or Should Her Health Be Transparent?

Both tradition and contemporary medical ethics believe that confidentiality is the best way to protect the well-being of a patient. The principle that the physician-patient relationship is sacrosanct, requiring that all patient medical information must remain private, is both respected and followed. Medical confidentiality has its basis in the Hippocratic oath, which states, "What I may see or hear in the course of the treatment or even outside of the treatment in regard to the life of men, which on no account one must spread abroad, I will keep to myself holding such things shameful to be spoken of."[7]

White House physicians have adhered strictly to complete confidentiality of a first lady's medical information. Burt Lee, President George Bush's personal physician, directed Dr. Connie Mariano upon her selection as a White House physician: "The health of the First Lady is off limits completely to the press."[8]

Tony Snow, then President George W. Bush's press secretary, defended first lady Laura Bush's nondisclosure of a skin cancer. He posited that she was not an elected official, and as a result, had the same right to medical privacy as an ordinary citizen.[9] An analyst agreed, admitting that, although the first lady is a public figure, she has no policy role and the removal of the skin lesion had no bearing on the commonweal.[10]

However, modern society acknowledges several exceptions to complete medical privacy. These include a personal waiver by the patient; specific diseases, injuries or treatments; threats of self-harm including suicide; and danger to third parties.[11]

This author proposes that the practice of strict confidentiality afforded to a first lady's health be reexamined. The first lady is usually the president's closest confidante and intimate. History has demonstrated that her illness may affect the performance of her husband. Examples include the following: (1) the depression of Jane Pierce damaged the effectiveness of antebellum president Franklin Pierce during the country's drift to civil war; (2) Caroline Harrison's fatal disease severely limited Benjamin Harrison's campaign for reelection, which he lost; (3) Ellen Wilson's terminal disease, her death, and its aftermath led to President Wilson's apathy and delayed decision-making during early World War I. Is it not possible that a wife's illness may present a danger to a third party, i.e., the citizens of the United States?

Moreover, a first lady cannot candidly be considered a "private citizen," as claimed.[12] She is housed, fed, transported, and protected at public expense. Moreover, she is provided constant and continuous medical care by the many members of the White House Medical Unit. A president's wife occasionally intrudes into policy-making. The most striking example was Hillary Clinton's attempt in the early 1990s to rearrange America's health care system. As a result, on June 22, 1993, the United States Court of Appeals for the District of Columbia ruled that Hillary Rodham Clinton was a full-time government official.[13]

In addition, the revelation of a first lady's illness may benefit the public. The publicity attached to Mrs. Ford's and Mrs. Reagan's breast cancers encouraged their peers in the public to arrange for early breast screenings.[14]

Unfortunately twenty-first century practices by the United States government,[15] as well as widespread abuse and mishandling of Internet-obtained personal information,[16] have made the confidentiality of personal information, including medical, nearly obsolete.

In this atmosphere there is little reason why the spouse of the leader of the American government should be exempt from such scrutiny. Such specialized treatment is unfair while at the same time average citizens going about their daily business are subjected to all sorts of intrusive surveillance against their will. After all, the decision to strive for the position of first lady was voluntary.

In my opinion, the first lady should waive the confidentiality of her medical record. It would be an affirmative gesture on her part, since in almost any case the public will find out about any medical problems sooner or later—probably sooner than later, given the vastly expanded and intrusive media outlets.

Chapter Notes

Preface

1. John B. Roberts II, *Rating the First Ladies* (New York: Citadel, 2003).

2. Jonah Goldberg, "The Irony of Michelle Obama's Water Campaign," *Los Angeles Times*, October 1, 2013.

3. Carl Sferrazza Anthony, ed., *This Elevated Position: A Catalogue and Guide to the National First Ladies' Library* (Canton, OH: National First Ladies' Library, 2003).

4. Hillary Clinton, *Living History* (New York: Scribner, 2003). The former first lady's autobiography sat near the top of nonfiction sales charts for many months in 2003; Sylvia Jukes Morris, *Edith Kermit Roosevelt: Portrait of a First Lady* (New York: Coward, McCann and Geoghegan, 1980). This biography of Theodore Roosevelt's second wife, Edith Carow, was very favorably reviewed when published.

5. Laura C. Holloway, *The Ladies of the White House; or, In the Home of the Presidents; Being a Complete History of the Social and Domestic Lives of the Presidents from Washington to the Present Time, 1789–1881* (Philadelphia: Bradley, 1881).

6. Betty Boyd Caroli, *First Ladies* (New York: Oxford University Press, 1987), xxii.

7. Carl Sferrazza Anthony, *First Ladies: The Saga of the Presidents' Wives and Their Power, 1789–1961*, vols. 1 and 2 (New York: William Morrow, 1990).

8. Margaret Truman, *First Ladies* (New York: Random House, 1995).

9. Robert P. Watson, *The Presidents' Wives: Reassessing the Office of the First Lady* (Boulder, CO: Lynne Rienner, 2000).

10. Lewis L. Gould, *American First Ladies: Their Lives and Legacy*, 2d ed. (New York: Routledge, 2001).

11. Cynthia D. Bittinger, *Grace Coolidge: Sudden Star* (New York: Nova History, 2005), viii.

12. Robert H. Ferrell, *Grace Coolidge: The People's Lady in Silent Cal's White House* (Lawrence: University Press of Kansas, 2008), viii.

Introduction

1. Robert P. Watson, *The Presidents' Wives: Reassessing the Office of the First Lady* (Boulder, CO: Lynne Rienner, 2000), 16n.

2. Margaret Truman, *First Ladies* (New York: Random House, 1995), 17–18; Betty Boyd Caroli, *First Ladies* (New York: Oxford University Press, 1987), xv.

3. Watson, *The Presidents' Wives*, 10–11.

4. Ibid.; Caroli, xv.

5. Caroli, xv; Watson: *The Presidents' Wives*, 10.

6. Harriet Lane, Biography, National First Ladies' Library, http://www.firstladies.org/biographies/firstladies.aspx?biography=16 (accessed February 3, 2014).

Chapter One

1. Jim Murphy, *An American Plague: The True and Terrifying Story of the Yellow Fever Epidemic of 1793* (New York: Clarion, 2003), 43.

2. Abigail Adams, Biography, National First Ladies' Library, http://www.firstladies.org/biographies/firstladies.aspx?biography=2 (accessed October 10, 2013).

3. Robert P. Watson, *First Ladies of the United States: A Biographical Dictionary* (Boulder, CO: Lynne Rienner, 2001), 16–7.

4. Catherine Allgor, *A Perfect Union: Dolley Madison and the Creation of the American Nation* (New York: Henry Holt, 2006), 6, 247; Watson, 33; Dolley Madison, Biography, National First Ladies' Library, http://www.firstladies.apx?biography=4 (accessed February 8, 2010; Allen C. Clark, *Life and Letters of Dolly Madison* (Washington: W.F. Roberts, 1914), 93, 190.

5. Murphy, 3.

6. http://millercenter.org/president/events/12_06.

7. Murphy, 9.

8. Ibid., 12–14.

9. Ibid., 15–16, 57, 85.

10. Douglas Southall Freeman, *Washington* (New York: Simon & Schuster, 1992), 638–9.

11. Helen Bryan, *Martha Washington: First Lady of Liberty* (New York: John Wiley, 2002), 325; Stephen Decatur and Tobias Lear, *Private Affairs of George Washington, from the Records and Accounts of Tobias Lear, Es-*

quire, His Secretary (New York: Da Capo, 1969 [1933]), 181, 194, 205.

12. Murphy, 42.

13. Anne Hollingsworth Wharton, *Martha Washington* (New York: Scribner's, 1899), 245; Bryan, 327; Joseph E. Fields, ed., *"Worthy Partner": The Papers of Martha Washington* (Westport, CT: Greenwood, 1994), 252n; Murphy, 42; Freeman, 638–9.

14. Allgor, 22–3.

15. Paul Zall, *Dolley Madison* (Huntington, NY: Nova History, 2001), 9–10; Allgor, 25; Catharine Anthony, *Dolly Madison: Her Life and Times* (Garden City, NY: Doubleday, 1949), 49–50; Lewis L. Gould, *American First Ladies: Their Lives and Legacy*, 2d ed. (New York: Routledge, 2001), 22.

16. Gould, 22; Clark, 18–9.

17. Anthony, 49–50, the author's definite diagnosis of yellow fever; Allgor, 25: "whether she contacted yellow fever is unclear."

18. Murphy, 104; Allgor, 25.

19. Murphy, 108, removal of government to Germantown; David McCullough, *John Adams* (New York: Simon & Schuster, 2001), 491–2, Adams to Eastchester in 1797; Gould, Trenton in 1799.

20. Murphy, 131

21. Ibid., 132.

22. "Yellow Fever Epidemic of 1793," Wikipedia, http://en.wikipedia.org/wiki/Yellow_Fever_Epidemic_of_1793 (accessed October 9, 2011).

23. Ibid.

24. Ibid.; Mary T. Busowki, Burke A. Cunha, et al.: "Yellow Fever," http://emedicine.medscape.com/article/232244 (accessed October 20, 2011).

25. Ludwig M. Deppisch, M.D.: *The White House Physician: A History from Washington to George W. Bush* (Jefferson, NC: McFarland, 2007), 9.

26. Ibid., 11; Wharton, 105–6; Bryan, 205–6.

27. Fields, 168–9.

28. Martha Washington Biography, National First Ladies' Museum.

29. Freeman, 710; Wharton, 148–9; Bryan, 139–141; Fields, 186.

30. Deppisch, 7–9, 14–17.

31. Fields, 186.

32. Ibid., 237.

33. Ibid., 23.

34. Patricia Brady, *Martha Washington: An American Life*, Google Books, http://books.google.com/books?id=vqCIBnJOwsC&pg=PT170&lpg (accessed October 11, 2011).

35. Bryan, 72–4.

36. Fields, 15–16, 123–4.

37. Bryan, 139–40.

38. Deppisch, 7–10, 12.

39. Freeman, 740; Bryan, 365–6.

40. Bryan, 377, 379.

41. Gould, 23; Anthony, 165–7; Allgor, 108–110; Zall, 39–40: various names applied to Mrs. Madison's knee abnormality; Clark, 72–3: attempts to cure malady at Montpelier; Ralph Ketcham, *James Madison* (Charlottesville: University Press of Virginia, 1990), 442–5: "a complaint near her knee, which from a very slight tumor had ulcerated into a very obstinate sore."

42. Anthony, 165–7; Allgor, 108–110; Zall, 39–40.

43. Deppisch, 12.

44. Ira M. Rutkow, "Philip Syng Physick," *Archives of Surgery* 136, no. 8 (August 2001), 968.

45. J. Randolph, *Life and Character of Philip Syng Physick* (Philadelphia: T.K. and P.G. Collins, 1839), 33.

46. Ibid., 37.

47. Ibid., 51–2.

48. Ibid., 11.

49. Zall, 39–40; Gould, 23; Ketcham, 442–5; David B. Mattern and Holly C. Shulman, eds., *The Selected Letters of Dolley Payne Madison* (Charlottesville: University of Virginia Press, 2003), 49; Allgor, 113; Clark, 83: "I may hopefully leave this place in a fortnight."

50. Mattern, 149.

51. Ibid., 86; Ketcham, 459–60; Tiffany Cole, e-mail.

52. Allgor, 251.

53. Ketcham, 481.

54. Mattern, 103; Anthony, 208.

55. Mattern, 141, 144, 169; Clark, 193.

56. Mattern, 153; Robert Honyman, Virginia Center for Digital Research at the University of

Virginia, http://www2.vcdh.virginia.edu/xslt/servlet/XSLTServlet?xml=/xml_docs/Dolley/Glossary.xml&xsl=/xml_docs/Dolley/glossary.xsl&area=glossaryr (accessed October 2011).

57. Allgor, 357; Zall, 74.

58. Clark, 242 (September 18, 1831), 277 (November 8, 1836).

59. Ibid., 324.

60. Zall, 101; Clark, 450.

Chapter Two

1. Woody Holton, *Abigail Adams* (New York: Free, 2009), 284.

2. World Health Organization, "Malaria," October 2011, http://www.who.int/mediacentre/factsheets/fs094/en/index.html (accessed November 19, 2011); Randall M. Packard, *The Making of a Tropical Disease: A Short History of Malaria* (Baltimore: Johns Hopkins University Press, 2007), xvi; "The World Malaria Report, 2010" (Malaria, WHO). Recent progress has significantly reduced the annual deaths from between 2 million and 3 million (Packard, xvi) to 850,000 (UN News Center) to 781,000 (WHO 2010). The annual case load has declined from 350 million to 500 million (Packard xvi) to 225 million (WHO 2010).

3. Fiammetta Rocco, *The Miraculous Fever Tree* (Great Britain: HarperCollins, 2003), xviii, 253. Pages 170 and 173 describe malaria's seasonality in America.

4. Lynne Withey, *Dearest Friend: A Life of Abigail Adams* (New York: Simon & Schuster, 2002), 208; Holton, 262.

5. Holton, 277.

6. Holton, 277: "seamy and unsanitary"; http://www.irishinnyc.freeservers.com/custom.html (accessed November 20, 2011): "Irish in New York City."

7. Withey, 212; Holton, 277.

8. Withey, 214–5: description of Philadelphia trip in a much weakened state.

9. David McCullough, *John Adams* (New York: Simon & Schuster, 2001), 513; Withey, 220–1; Holton, 217. Plasmodium vivax

is the species of protozoan parasite that was endemic to the United States when Mrs. Adams was infected and was rarely fatal by itself. An African species, plasmodium falciparum, rarely present in North America, may frequently cause fatal disease.

10. Withey, 217.

11. Phyllis Lee Levin, *Abigail Adams* (New York: St. Martin's, 1987), 393: "Physical complaints from rheumatism and malaria increased to the point that she worried how she could manage the journey home when Congress adjourned"; Stewart Mitchell, ed., *New Letters of Abigail Adams, 1788–1901* (Boston: Houghton Mifflin, 1947), 78: Abigail Adams, letter to sister, March 20, 1792, from Philadelphia.

12. Mitchell, 66; Abigail Adams letter to sister, December 12, 1790, from Philadelphia: "a kind friend as well as physician"; McCullough, 433 (Autumn 1791): Dr. Rush's visits; Paul C. Nagel, *The Adams Women: Abigail and Louisa Adams, Their Sisters and Daughters* (New York: Oxford University Press, 1987), 85. In 1798 Abigail consulted Rush about her niece, her "holy trinity" of treatments; Levin, 448–9; Withey, 302, 306, Nabby.

13. Deppisch, 11–12, 18, 21–2.

14. M.L Duran-Reynals: *The Fever Bark Tree: The Pageant of Quinine* (Garden City, NY: Doubleday, 1946), 38–40; Rocco, 52.

15. Withey, 220–1.

16. John Ferling, *John Adams* (New York: Henry Holt, 1992), 368–9; McCullough, 513; Withey, 258; Howard A. Kelly, *A Cyclopedia of American Medical Biography Comprising the Lives of Eminent Deceased Physicians and Surgeons from 1610 to 1910* (New York: W.B. Saunders, 1920), 1164–5.

17. Ferling, 368–9; Withey, 258; Nagel, 137: bilious fever reference.

18. Levin (388–9) described her early arthritic symptoms; Levin, 192, and Holton, 196, described the 1784 trans–Atlantic journey.

19. McCullough, 433.

20. Levin, 293.

21. Mitchell, 78.

22. Ibid., 131. Letter from AA in Philadelphia to sister, February 6, 1798.

23. Levin, 388–9.

24. Levin, 423. In March 1807, AA had barely recovered from a rheumatic attack; Holton, 407. In the 1815–6 winter, she suffered through her usual cold weather ailments, especially rheumatism.

25. Holton, 109–114; Withey, 83–4.

26. Holton, 21.

27. Jennifer Carrell, *The Speckled Monster: A Historical Tale of Battling Smallpox* (New York: Plume/Penguin, 2004), 392–3.

28. Holton, 282, 284, 307; Ellis, 163; Levin, 294; Withey, 217, 220; Joseph J. Ellis, *First Family: Abigail and John Adams* (New York: Alfred A. Knopf, 2010), 163.

29. Levin, 305.

30. Holton, 307.

31. McCullough, 447.

32. Holton, 307–9.

33. Holton, 311, 315.

34. Ferling, 368–9; Holton, 322; Levin, 356, McCullough, 526; Nagel, 12.

35. McCullough, 530–2; Holton, 328.

36. Levin, 388–9.

37. Ellis, 194.

38. Holton, 324–6; Withey, 261.

39. Robert P. Watson, *The Presidents' Wives: Reassessing the Office of the First Lady* (Boulder, CO: Lynne Rienner, 2000), 138.

40. Walter R. Borneman, *Polk: The Man Who Transformed the Presidency and America* (New York: Random House, 2008), 13.

41. John Reed Bumgarner, *Sarah Childress Polk: A Biography of a Remarkable First Lady* (Jefferson, NC: McFarland, 1997), 15, 26.

42. Barbara Bennett Peterson, *Sarah Childress Polk: First Lady of Tennessee and Washington* (New York: Nova History, 2002), 5–8, 19.

43. Borneman, 7–8.

44. Bumgarner, 34; Jimmie Lou Sparkman Claxton, *Eighty-Eight Years with Sarah Polk* (New York: Vantage, 1972), 36.

45. Bumgarner, 94.

46. Milo Milton Quaife, *The Diary of James K. Polk During His Presidency* (Chicago: A.C. McClurg, 1910; Claxton, 87–8.

47. Quaife; Bumgarner, 92–4; Borneman, 282.

48. Deppisch, 20–23, 30.

49. Ibid., 20–31.

50. Quaife, May 4; Claxton, 95–6.

51. Bill Severn, *Frontier President: The Life of James K. Polk* (New York: Ives Washburn, 1965), 67–117.

52. Bumgarner, 150–1.

53. John Shaw, *Lucretia* (New York: Nova History, 2004), 89.

54. Ibid., 71.

55. Ibid., 100–102; Harry James Brown and Frederick D. Williams, eds., *The Diary of James A. Garfield, 1878–1881*, vol. 4 (Lansing: Michigan State University Press, 1981 [May 4, 1881]).

56. Allan Peskin, *Garfield* (Kent, OH: Kent State University Press, 1978), 573.

57. Deppisch, 48, lists Lucretia Garfield's physicians; 18 quotes Thomas Jefferson's observation.

58. Ludwig M. Deppisch, "Homeopathic Medicine and Presidential Health," *PHAROS* 60, no. 4 (Fall 1997), 5–10; James C. Clark, *The Murder of James A. Garfield: The President's Last Days and the Trial and Execution of His Assassin* (Jefferson NC: McFarland, 1993), 42–3; Peskin, 573; Shaw, 100–102.

59. Shaw, 100–102.

60. Clark, 51–115; Shaw, 100–102.

61. Shaw, 100–102.

62. Clark, 42.

63. Peskin, 573.

64. Candice Millard, *Destiny of the Republic: A Tale of Madness, Medicine and the Murder of a President* (New York: Doubleday, 2011), 112.

65. John Duffy, "The Impact of Malaria on the South," in *Disease and Distinctiveness in the American South*, ed. Todd L. Savitt and James Harvey Young, (Knoxville: University of Tennessee Press, 1988), 29–54; Margaret Humphreys, *Malaria, Poverty, Race and Public Health in the United States* (Baltimore:

Johns Hopkins University Press, 2001), 40.

66. Ibid.

67. Randall M. Packard, *The Making of a Tropical Disease: A Short History of Malaria* (Baltimore: Johns Hopkins University Press, 2007), 7.

68. *History of the Medical Society of the District of Columbia* (Washington, D.C.: Medical Society of the District of Columbia, 1909), 143.

69. *New York Times*, July 16, 1879.

70. Shaw, 119.

71. Rocco, 170–2.

72. Deppisch, 23.

73. Peskin, 13.

74. Deppisch, 24.

75. John G. Sotos, *The Physical Lincoln Sourcebook: An Annotated Medical History of Abraham Lincoln and His Family* (Mount Vernon, VA: Mount Vernon Book Systems, 2008), 146.

76. Deppisch, 127.

77. William S. McFeely, *Grant: A Biography* (New York: W.W. Norton, 1982), 63.

78. Edmund Morris, *Colonel Roosevelt* (New York: Random House, 2010), 16.

Chapter Three

1. Lewis L. Gould, *American First Ladies: Their Lives and Legacy*, 2d ed. (New York: Routledge, 2001), 67.

2. The number of children that resulted from the John/Letitia mating remains uncertain. Craig Hart, *A Genealogy of the Wives of American Presidents and Their First Two Generations of Descent* (Jefferson, NC: McFarland, 2004), 228–9, lists eight children. Christopher Leahy, "Torn Between Family and Politics: John Tyler's Struggle for Balance," *Virginia Magazine of History and Biography* 114, no. 3 (2006), 322–355), and Lewis L. Gould, *American First Ladies: Their Lives and Legacy*, 2d ed. (New York: Routledge, 2001, 66) counted nine pregnancies. All agree that seven Tyler children attained adulthood.

3. William Degregorio, *The Complete Book of U.S. Presidents* (New York: Wings, 1993), 153–4.

4. Leahy, 330.

5. Gould, 67: "presided over the governor's mansion with charm"; *Washington Globe*, September 12, 1842: "then in perfect health and adorned with beauty."

6. Leahy, 331, 345.

7. Ibid., 345–6.

8. Lyon G. Tyler, *The Letters and Times of the Tylers*, vol. 1 (Richmond, VA: Whittet & Shepperson, 1884), 562, Letter from John Tyler to Mary Tyler, June 16, 1832.

9. Laura C. Holloway, *The Ladies of the White House, or, In the Home of the Presidents; Being a Complete History of the Social and Domestic Lives of the Presidents from Washington to the Present Time, 1789–1881* (Philadelphia: Bradley, 1881), 375; this part of Virginia seceded in 1863 to become the state of West Virginia.

10. Robert Byrd, "The Greenbrier," Congressional Record, 106th Congress (1999–2000), July 10, 2000, http://thomas.loc.gov/cgi-bin/query/z?r106:S10JY0-0008 (accessed October 19, 2013).

11. *Washington Globe*, obituary (September 13, 1842); *Baltimore Sun*, obituary (September 14, 1842); Holloway, 387; Gould, 67; Carl Sferrazza Anthony, *First Ladies: The Saga of the Presidents' Wives and Their Power, 1789–1961*, vols. 1 and 2 (New York: William Morrow, 1990) on 127 states: "Although Mrs. Tyler's stroke evidently took her powers of speech in its first stage, she regained it"; The *Baltimore Sun* (above) suggests otherwise: "The loss of speech, to an extent, was one of the unhappy effects of the attack"; The description of Letitia's silent joy over her son's marriage is from Elizabeth Tyler Coleman, *Priscilla Cooper Tyler and the American Scene, 1816–1889* (Birmingham: University of Alabama Press, 1955), 69.

12. Leahy, 329.

13. Coleman, 73; Chitwood, Oliver Perry: *John Tyler: Champion of the Old South* (New York: Russell and Russell, 1964), 199; Gould, 68: remained in her bedroom.

14. Sally G. McMillen, *Motherhood in the Old South: Pregnancy, Childbirth and Infant Rearing* (Baton Rouge: Louisiana State University Press, 1990), 180, 91.

15. Vivek Dhawan, et al.: "Long-Term Effects of Repeated Pregnancies (Multiparity) on Blood Pressure Regulation." *Cardiovascular Research* 64 (2004), 179–186.

16. Gould, 68.

17. Gould, 68; Anthony, 122; Coleman, 83; Robert II Seager, *And Tyler Too: A Biography of John and Julia Gardiner Tyler* (New York: McGraw-Hill, 1963), 172–3.

18. Coleman, 86–7.

19. Ibid., 87–8.

20. Ibid., 89.

21. Hart, 224–5.

22. Coleman, 99; Dan Monroe, *The Republican Vision of John Tyler* (College Station: Texas A&M University Press, 2003), 136.

23. Holloway, 385–6.

24. *Washington Intelligencer*, September 12–13, 1842; *Washington Globe*, September 12, 1842; Holloway, 395.

25. Edward Crapol, *John Tyler: The Accidental President* (Chapel Hill: University of North Carolina Press, 2006), 268: a comprehensive review of Tyler's difficult presidency.

26. Virginia Miller, "Dr. Thomas Miller and His Times," *Records of the Columbia Historical Society* 3 (1900): 303–323.

27. *History of the Medical Society of the District of Columbia*, 25, 229, 433.

28. Samuel Busey, *Personal Reminiscences and Recollections of Forty-Six Years' Membership in the Medical Society of the District of Columbia* (Washington, D.C.: 1895), 24.

29. Busey, 205; *American Mercury* (December 21, 1821) details Sewall's appointment; *New Hampshire Gazette* (March 10, 1834) contains a letter to the editor supporting Beaumont's experiments; *Baltimore Sun* (November 6, 1839): The operation was performed at the Washington alms house by Dr. Thomas

Miller, who was assisted by Drs. Sewall, Hall and May.

30. *Madisonian*, May 4, 1841; *Baltimore Sun*, May 13, 1844; *History of the DC Medical Society*, 222, lists many of his civic and professional accomplishments.

31. Mary Roach, *Stiff: The Curious Lives of Human Cadavers* (New York: W.W. Norton, 2004), 14–5.

32. *History of the DC Medical Society*, 148.

33. Roach, 43.

34. "Mind Games: A Look at Phrenology in the 1830s," *Skeptic Report*, http:/www.skepticreport. com/sr/?p=558 (accessed December 15, 2011); van Wyhe, John: "The History of Phrenology on the Web," http://www.historyof phrenology.org.uk/overview.htm (accessed December 15, 2011).

35. Thomas Sewall, *Examination of Phrenology* (Washington City: Honans, 1837); *History of the DC Medical Society*, 148; Catharine Anthony, *Dolly Madison: Her Life and Times* (Garden City, NY: Doubleday, 1949), 336: loan of a book to the widow Madison.

36. *New Hampshire Sentinel*, December 29, 1841.

37. *Amherst* (NH) *Farmer's Cabinet* 39, no. 33 (April 9, 1841): 2.

38. *Connecticut Courant*, February 7, 1835; *Washington National Intelligencer*, February 9, 1835; *Washington Globe*, February 4, 1835.

39. John R. Bumgarner, *The Health of the Presidents: The 41 United States Presidents Through 1993 from a Physician's Point of View* (Jefferson, NC: McFarland, 1994), 81.

40. William Boyd Mushet, *A Practical Treatise on Apoplexy (Cerebral Hemorrhage), Its Pathology, Diagnosis, Therapeutics, and Prophylaxis, with an Essay on So-Called Nervous Apoplexy, on Congestion of the Brain and Serous Effusion* (London: John Churchill and Sons, 1866), 156; George B. Taylor, "The Inaugural Essay on Apoplexia of Apoplexy," submitted to the faculty of the University of Pennsylvania for the degree of doctor of

medicine; Marshall Hall, "The Threatenings of Apoplexy and Paralysis, etc.," the Cronian Lectures delivered at the Royal College of Physicians, March 1851, pp. 1–90.

41. Mushet, 106; Taylor.

42. J.D.B. De Bow, *Mortality Statistics: Life Expectancy by Age, 1850–2004.*

43. Coleman, 99; Monroe, 136.

Chapter Four

1. William Degregorio, *The Complete Book of U.S. Presidents* (New York: Wings, 1993), 75.

2. Elizabeth Monroe, *First Ladies Biography*, http://www. firstladies.org/biographies/first ladies.aspx?biography=5 (accessed October 23, 2013); Degregorio, 75; Robert P. Watson, *The Presidents' Wives: Reassessing the Office of the First Lady* (Boulder, CO: Lynne Rienner, 2000), 36.

3. Degregorio, 75; George Morgan, *The Life of James Monroe* (Boston: Small, Maynard, 1921), 416; Harlow G. Unger, *The Last Founding Father: James Monroe and a Nation's Call to Greatness* (Philadelphia, PA: Da Capo, 2009), 298.

4. Carl Sferrazza Anthony, *First Ladies: The Saga of the Presidents' Wives and Their Power, 1789–1961*, vols. 1 and 2 (New York: William Morrow, 1990), 613n1: absences, 103: "first Queen Elizabeth"; W.P. Cresson, *James Monroe* (Chapel Hill: University of North Carolina Press, 1946), 92: the hauteur of a grande dame.

5. Lewis L. Gould, *American First Ladies: Their Lives and Legacy*, 2d ed. (New York: Routledge, 2001), 40; Monroe, Biography, National First Ladies' Library for Louisa Adams's quote.

6. Cresson, 368, improved acceptance amongst social opinion makers; Harry Ammon, *James Monroe: The Quest for National Identity* (Charlottesville: University of Virginia, 1990) (401) and Unger (324) describe Mrs. Monroe's charm and beauty; Ammon, 542, for Lafayette banquet.

7. Ammon, 64.

8. James Monroe, *The Autobiography of James Monroe*, ed. Stuart Gerry Brown (Syracuse: Syracuse University Press, 1959), 70–1.

9. Ammon, 546; Monroe, *First Ladies' Biography*, records Elizabeth Monroe's post inauguration White House stay.

10. Unger, 65, 142; Craig Hart, *A Genealogy of the Wives of American Presidents and Their First Two Generations of Descent* (Jefferson, NC: McFarland, 2004), 161, for the Monroe children's birthdates.

11. James Monroe, *The Papers of James Monroe, 1776–1794*, ed. Daniel Preston (Westport, CT: Greenwood, 2003).

12. Monroe, *Biography*, First Ladies'; Unger, 153.

13. "Rheumatoid Arthritis: Comparing Rheumatoid Arthritis and Osteoarthritis," http:// www.webmd.com/rheumatoid-arthritis/tc/comparing-rheumatoid-arthritis-and-osteoarthritis-topic-overview (accessed October 24, 2013); Pouya Entezami, et al.: "Historical Perspective on the Etiology of Rheumatoid Arthritis," *Hand Clinics* 27, no. 1 (2011 February): 1–10.

14. Monroe, *Biography*, First Ladies'; Cresson, 205; George Morgan, *The Life of James Monroe* (Boston: Small, Maynard, 1921), 279.

15. Unger, 186–7.

16. James Monroe to Madison, January 10, 1806, *James Monroe Writings* IV, 391–398; Unger, 186–7.

17. James Monroe to Charles Everett, 13 January 1810; James Monroe to Elizabeth Trist, March 6, 1810.

18. Unger, 219: Mrs. Monroe, as the wife of the secretary of state; Ammon, 290: editor's description of Elizabeth; James E. Wootton, *Elizabeth Kortright Monroe*, pamphlet (Charlottes ville VA: Ash Lawn-Highland, 1987).

19. Unger, 279, 323.

20. Gould, 42; Monroe, *Biography*, First Ladies'; Noble E. Cunningham, Jr.: *The Presidency of James Monroe* (Lawrence: Uni-

versity Press of Kansas, 1996), 134.

21. Cunningham, 179.

22. Gould, 41; *Biography,* First Ladies'; Anthony, 102; Unger, 329; Anne Adams, *Elizabeth Monroe: Elegance in the White House; History's Women,* http://www.historyswomen.com/1stWomen/elizabethmonroe.html (accessed November 3, 2012).

23. James Monroe (Washington) to Charles Everett, September 1, 1824.

24. James Monroe to Samuel Gourveneur, December 29, 1826.

25. Anthony, 102–3.

26. Gould 41; *Biography,* First Ladies'; Unger, 329.

27. Anne Adams.

28. Nancy R. Miller, University of Pennsylvania Archives and Records Center, e-mail February 4, 2005.

29. James Monroe (Albemarle County, Virginia) to Charles Everett (Albemarle County, Virginia), July 1, 1820, *Tyler's Historical Quarterly* 5, no. 18 (New York: Kraus Reprint, 1967); James Monroe (Albemarle County, Virginia) to Charles Everett (Albemarle County, Virginia) July 9, 1820, *The Papers of James Monroe;* Wootton.

30. James Monroe (Washington) to Dr. Charles Everett (Richmond, Virginia), December 2, 1822, *Tyler's Historical Quarterly* 5, no. 18 (New York: Kraus Reprint, 1967).

31. Cunningham, 124.

32. James Monroe (Washington) to Charles Everett (Albemarle County, Virginia), November 13, 1823, *Tyler's Historical Quarterly* 5, no. 21 (New York: Kraus Reprint, 1967).

33. Bilious fever, http://www.rootsweb.ancestry.com/~memigrat/diseases.html (accessed October 27, 2013).

34. James Monroe (Oak Hill, Virginia) to Samuel Gourveneur (New York City), February 24, 1826; James Monroe (Oak Hill, Virginia) to James Madison (Montpelier, Virginia), March 20, 1829.

35. James Monroe (Oak Hill, Virginia) to Samuel Gourveneur (New York, NY), September 23,

1930 (James Monroe Papers, Manuscripts and Archives Division, New York Public Library); Hart, 161.

36. Norma Lois Peterson, *The Presidencies of William Henry Harrison and John Tyler* (Lawrence: University Press of Kansas, 1989), 535.

37. Anna Harrison, Biography, National First Ladies' Library, http://www.firstladies.org/biographies/firstladies.aspx?biography=9 (accessed October 27, 2013); Anthony, 120: Anna Harrison's quote.

38. Harrison, Biography, First Ladies' Library.

39. Ibid.; Hart, 114.

40. K. Jack Bauer, *Zachary Taylor* (Baton Rouge: Louisiana State University Press, 1985), 258.

41. John B. Roberts, II: *Rating the First Ladies* (New York: Citadel, 2003), xxiii-xxiv.

42. Bauer, 8, summarized the Taylors' married life; Anthony, 145–6: Margaret Taylor's reluctance to be America's first lady.

43. Anthony, 145–6; Bauer, 258.

44. Anthony, 145: "The Phantom in the White House"; Margaret Taylor, Biography, First Ladies' Library, http://www.firstladies.org/biographies/firstladies.aspx?biography+13 (accessed November 12, 2012); Anthony, 145–6.

45. Anthony, 145–6; Bauer, 258; Taylor, Biography, First Ladies' Library.

46. Taylor, Biography, First Ladies' Library.

47. Ibid., Chapter Two.

48. Hart, 214–5; John S.D. Eisenhower, *Zachary Taylor* (New York: Henry Holt, 2008), 19: "health permanently impaired"; Bauer, 38; Holman Hamilton, *Zachary Taylor: Soldier of the Republic* (Indianapolis: Bobbs-Merrill, 1941), 68–9.

49. Roberts, 80; Degregorio, 176.

50. Bauer, 48, 55, 229.

51. Samuel W. Francis, "Biographical Sketch of General R.C. Wood," *Medical and Surgical Reporter* 20 (April 10, 1869): 275–6; Robert C. Wood, Robert C. Wood's Medical Officer's files, National Archives and Records Administration.

52. Taylor, Biography, First Ladies' Library.

53. Robert J. Scarry, *Millard Fillmore* (Jefferson, NC: McFarland, 2001), 127.

54. Abigail Fillmore, Biography, National First Ladies' Library, http://www.firstladies.org/biographies/firstladies.aspx?biography=14 (accessed October 29, 2013); Degregorio, 192.

55. Watson, 78: quote "Abigail is typical of those"; Fillmore, Biography, First Ladies' Library; Gould, 102–3.

56. Watson, 78; Gould, 102–3.

57. Scarry, 15; Anthony, 152; Gould, 102–3; Degregorio, 188, for information on Abbie' talents.

58. Anthony, 152.

59. Roberts, 82: "What Ms. Fillmore Most Enjoyed," 86: congressional appropriation; Fillmore, Biography, First Ladies' Library; Anthony, 152, 155, for famous authors.

60. Anthony, 153–5, for her influence on President Fillmore; Roberts, 86–7: Abigail Fillmore's opposition to the Fugitive Slave Act, which mandated that escaped slaves be returned to their southern masters even if apprehended in a state that had outlawed slavery.

61. Fillmore, Biography, First Ladies' Library; Anthony, 151.

62. Fillmore, Biography, First Ladies' Library.

63. Ibid.; Gould, 102–3.

64. Scarry, 88–9, 125–7, for Abigail's therapy; Gould, 102–3:Saratoga Springs, New York; Scarry, 126–7 for 1845 letter from Abigail Fillmore to sympathetic correspondent C.F. Perkins.

65. Scarry, 125–7.

66. Ibid.

67. Ibid. for January 1849 letter; Gould, 102–3: Abigail in bed for days; Roberts, 85, concluded that the injured ankle produced the back and hip pain.

68. Gould, 102–3.

69. Millard Fillmore (Buffalo, New York) to Julia, his sister, April 12, 1953 (Buffalo and Erie County Historical Society); Anthony, 155, and Gould, 105, both commented on her illness during the previous winter.

70. Anthony, 105: Mrs. Fill-

more was the first first lady to attend her husband's successor's inauguration; Roy Franklin Nichols, *Franklin Pierce: Young Hickory of the Granite Hills* (Norwalk, CT: Easton, 1931), 234: quote about the weather on inauguration day, 1853.

71. Nichols, for the death of William Henry Harrison.

72. Fillmore, Biography, First Ladies' Library.

73. Millard Fillmore (Buffalo, New York) to Julia, his sister, April 12, 1953 (Buffalo and Erie County Historical Society).

74. Anthony, 155.

75. Ibid.

76. *New York Daily Times*, March 23, 1853.

77. Millard Fillmore (Washington, D.C.) to Franklin Pierce (Washington, D.C.), March 28, 1853 (Special Collections, Penfield Library, SUNY-Oswego).

78. Millard Fillmore: note "Funeral Expenses of Mrs. F at Washington," April 17, 1853 (Special Collections, Penfield Library, SUNY-Oswego).

Chapter Five

1. Alyn Brodsky, *Benjamin Rush: Patriot and Physician* (New York: St. Martin's, 2004), 336; David Barton, *Benjamin Rush* (Aledo, TX: Wallbuilder, 1999), 263.

2. Norman F. Boas, *Jane M. Pierce (1806–1863)*; Pierce-Aiken Papers (Seaport-Aiken Autographs, 1983): "Mrs. Pierce found Benny"; Michael Minor and Larry F. Vrzalik, "A Study in Tragedy: Jane Means Pierce, First Lady," *Manuscripts* 40 no. 3 (Summer 1988): 177–89: "It destroyed her forever."

3. Jane Walter Venzke and Craig Paul Venzke, *The President's Wife: Jane Means Appleton Pierce, a Woman of Her Time*, http://www.nhhistory.org/publications/Revealing_Relationships_Pressidents_wife.pdf (accessed February 27, 2011).

4. Lloyd C. Taylor, Jr.: "A Wife for Mr. Pierce," *New England Quarterly* 28, no. 3 (September 1955), 339–348; Deborah

Kent, *Jane Means Appleton Pierce* (New York: Children's, 1998), 47–9.

5. Minor.

6. Jane Pierce, Biography, First Ladies' Library; http://www.firstladies.org/biographies/firstladies.aspx?biography=15 (accessed February 14, 2011).

7. Robert P. Watson, *The Presidents' Wives: Reassessing the Office of the First Lady* (Boulder, CO: Lynne Rienner, 2000), 59, 64–5; Roy Franklin Nichols, *Franklin Pierce: Young Hickory of the Granite Hills* (Norwalk, CT: Easton, 1931), 230–1.

8. Nichols, 242: She did not appear at table when company was present. She did socialize with friends and accompanied Nathaniel Hawthorne to Mount Vernon. Nichols, 313–4: In February 1854, Mrs. Pierce's customary ill health and melancholy prevented her from giving any attention to society, much less playing the leading part befitting her as mistress of the White House. Accompanied by Daniel Webster and other friends, but never by Mrs. Pierce, the president regularly attended concerts in Washington; Nichols, 360: In August 1854, Mr. and Mrs. Pierce escaped Washington's heat by sailing down the Potomac with a party. Later they spent a week at Capon Springs, Virginia.

9. American President, Reference Resource, Miller Center, University of Virginia, http://millercenter.org/president/events/12_06 (accessed October 19, 2011); Joel Martin and William J. Birnes: *The Haunting of the Presidents: A Paranormal History of the U.S. Presidency* (Old Saybrook, CT: Konecky and Konecky, 2003), 213; "The Fox Sisters: Spiritualism's Unlikely Founders," http://www.histroynet.com/the-fox-sisters-spiritualisms-unlikely-founders.htm. Maggie and Katy Fox were charlatans but had a remarkable career for decades as they duped countless people into "communication" with their beloved deceased.

10. Jane Pierce to (deceased son) Bennie, January 23, 1853

(New Hampshire Historical Society manuscript, Franklin Pierce papers, accession number 1929–001).

11. Nichols, 375, 421, 439.

12. Venzke; Nichols, 76: described as "tubercular."

13. Nichols, 94; Venzke.

14. Nichols, 103–4: "Sewall did his best"; Nichols, chapter three, for Sewall's other patients; Venzke: diagnosis of tuberculosis.

15. Venzke, for Jane Pierce's use of leeches; "Leech," Wikipedia, http:en.wikipedia.org/wiki/Leech (accessed 27 February 2012), for contemporary leech therapy.

16. Nichols, 507–8.

17. Jane Pierce, Biography, First Ladies' Library, for the diagnosis of tuberculosis; Minor for the Pierces' wanderings in search of a cure; Deborah Kent, *Jane Means Appleton Pierce* (New York: Children's, 1998), 78–86: "All during her travels"; Craig Hart, *A Genealogy of the Wives of American Presidents and Their First Two Generations of Descent* (Jefferson, NC: McFarland, 2004), 165, for the date and location of her death.

18. Hart, 165; Kent: 14,16; Venzke.

19. Jane Pierce, Biography, First Ladies' Library; Jonathan R.T. Davidson and Kathryn M. Connor, "The Impairment of Presidents Pierce and Coolidge After Traumatic Bereavement," *Comprehensive Psychiatry* 49 (2008), 413–419.

20. Minor: "Disaster almost from the start. The couple was completely mismatched—she, a shy reclusive sickly introvert"; Nichols, 76: "Her husband presented quite a contrast."

21. Lloyd C. Taylor, Jr.: "A Wife for Mr. Pierce," *New England Quarterly* 28, no. 3 (September 1955), 339–348.

22. Minor; Taylor; Nichols, 140.

23. Nichols, 203, Taylor, Venzke, and Minor all describe Jane Pierce's prayers for her husband's defeat; Davidson for Bennie's comments; Nichols, 204: "the results were too dreadful."

24. Larry Gara: *The Presidency of Franklin Pierce* (Lawrence: University Press of Kansas, 1991), 183–4.

25. C-SPAN: 2009 Historians Presidential Leadership Survey, 2012.

26. Minor

27. Ibid.

28. Davidson.

29. Louisa Adams quote as reported in Paul C. Nagel, *The Adams Women: Abigail and Louisa Adams, Their Sisters and Daughters* (New York: Oxford University Press, 1987).

30. William Degregorio, *The Complete Book of U.S. Presidents* (New York: Wing, 1993), 94; Joan Ridder Challinor, "Louisa Catherine Johnson Adams: The Price of Ambition," PhD diss., American University, Washington, D.C., April 20, 1982; Paul C. Nagel, *Descent from Glory: Four Generations of the John Adams Family* (New York: Oxford University Press, 1983), 63; Michael O'Brien, *Mrs. Adams in Winter* (New York: Farrar, Straus and Giroux, 2010), xv.

31. Alan Levenson, M.D., e-mail, April 15, 2011.

32. Jonathan R.T. Davidson, Kathryn M. Connor and Marvin Swartz: "Mental Illness in U.S. Presidents Between 1776 and 1974: A Review of Biographical Sources," *Journal of Nervous and Mental Disease* 194, no. 1, (January 2006): 47–51.

33. Nagel, *Descent from Glory*, 77–80, 88, 122, 133, 147, 157–9, 171–3, 178.

34. Louisa Adams, *The Adventures of a Nobody: Autobiographical Sketch, Begun 1 July 1840* (Boston: Massachusetts Historical Society, 1956).

35. Challinor, "Mr. Adams has always accustomed me to believe that Women had nothing to do with politics."

36. Nagel, *The Adams Women*, 188–9.

37. Nagel,: *Descent from Glory*, 107–8, 170.

38. Degregorio, 94.

39. Robert Remini, *John Quincy Adams* (New York: Henry Holt, 2002), 30.

40. Paul C. Nagel, *John Quincy Adams: A Public Life, a Private Life* (Cambridge, MA: Harvard University Press, 1997), 253.

41. Presidential Notes: "Louisa Catherine Adams," http://www.essortment.com/presidential-notes-louisa-catherine-adams (accessed January 3, 2012): "reading and writing and spice through story telling"; Louisa Catherine Adams: *Our White House: Looking In, Looking Out*; http://www.ourwhitehouse.org/flpages/ladams.html (accessed January 3, 2012): lists Louisa's musical talents.

42. Presidential Notes: "Louisa Catherine Adams."

43. Adams, *Adventures of a Nobody*. The "old gentleman" is her father- in-law, former president John Adams.

44. Challinor: "At times wished obsessively and overwhelmingly to die"; Hart, 23: The Adams only daughter who was not stillborn was Louisa Catherine, who died September 15, 1812, in Saint Petersburg, Russia.

45. O'Brien.

46. Ibid., 228.

47. Nagel, *Descent from Glory*, 116–7.

48. Jack Shepherd, *Cannibals of the Heart: A Personal Biography of Louisa Catherine and John Quincy Adams* (New York: McGraw-Hill, 1980), 99.

49. Puerperal Fever; *Wikipedia*, http://en.wikipedia.org/wiki/Puerperal_fever#Famous_Victims, (accessed January 23, 2012).

50. Challinor; Shepherd, 190.

51. Challinor.

52. Adams, *Adventures of a Nobody*: "My husband's time was entirely occupied"; Shepherd, 103, and Challinor describe the traumatic birth of George Washington Adams; Shepherd, 111, alludes to John Quincy's absences.

53. Challinor, use of "illness" as a bargaining device; Don Keko, *Louisa Adams: The Reclusive First Lady*, http://www.examibner.com/american-history-in-national/louisa-adams-thr-reclusive-first-lady (accessed January 3, 2012): frequent migraines and fainting spells.

54. Challinor for her use of laudanum both in Massachusetts and in Saint Petersburg.

55. Nagel, *Descent from Glory*, 83.

56. Laudanum: Wikipedia, http://en.wikipedia.org/wiki/Laudanum (accessed March 8, 2012); Laudanum encyclopedia topics: http://www.reference.com/browse/laudanum (accessed March 8, 2012); "What is Laudanum": http://www.laudanumonline.com.drupal/content/what-laudanum (accessed March 8, 2012, for Mary Todd Lincoln and laudanum, see below.

57. Challinor and Shepherd, 329, for the long term recurrences of erysipelas; Nagel, *John Quincy Adams: A Public Life, a Private Life*, 290, and Nagel, *The Adams Women*, 212–3, for Louisa's symptoms and her attempted respite at the Bedford spa; Erysipelas: Pubmed Health National Library of Medicine, http://www.ncbi.nlm.nih.gov/pubmedhealth/PMH0001643/ (accessed January 19, 2012).

58. Shepherd, 220, 221, 223.

59. Ibid., 223, 226–8. 239.

60. Nagel, *Adams Women*, 287–8.

61. Presidential Notes: "Louisa Catherine Adams": "Louisa's Room became a central area"; Keko, First Ladies' History, "Louisa Adams: The Chocoholic Resurfaces," http://firstladyblog.typepad.com/my-year-with-the-first-la/2011/04/first (accessed January 3, 2012): "The Adams residence became a social center"; Catherine Allgor, *Parlor Politics, in Which the Ladies of Washington Help Build a City and a Government* (Charlottesville: University of Virginia Press, 2000), 165, for Louisa's political skills.

62. Allgor, 191, 193, for being sidelined in the White House; Presidential Notes: "Louisa Catherine Adams," http://www.essortment.com/presidential-notes-louisa-catherine-adams (accessed January 3, 2012): description of Louisa's social skills as wife of the secretary of state.

63. Louisa Catherine Johnson Adams: *Our White House: Looking In, Looking Out*, http://www.

ourwhitehouse.org/flpages/ ladams.html (accessed January 3, 2012).

64. Nagel, *Adams Women*, 189, and Challinor record for John Quincy's recommendation of the Rush book; Louisa Catherine Adams, *Diary and Biographical Writings of Louisa Catherine Adams*, Judith Graham, et al., ed. (Cambridge, MA: Belknap Press, 2012), 1812–1814 Diary, 373, records Louisa's reaction.

65. Nagel:, *Adams Women*, 212–13, for the unnamed physician's diagnosis; Hysteria, http:// en.wikipedia.org/wiki/Female_ hysteria (accessed November 5, 2013) for a discussion of hysteria.

66. Shepherd, 256.

67. Nagel, *Adams Women*, 217: opinions on the status of women, and 236: advising niece against marriage; Keko; http://www.ex- amibner.com/american-history- in-national/louisa-adams-thr- reclusive-first-lady (January 3, 2012): chocolate addiction.

68. Shepherd, 260–4; Nagel: *Adams Women*, 220.

69. Nagel, *Adams Women*, 219–20; Shepherd, 256–60.

70. Nagel, *Adams Women*, 214– 5: 1828 recurrence of erysipelas; Shepherd, 307–8, for Huntt's White House treatments; Ludwig M. Deppisch, *The White House Physician: A History from Wash- ington to George W. Bush* (Jeffer- son, NC: McFarland, 2007), 20– 31, for Dr. Huntt's biographical information.

71. Nagel, *Adams Women*, 220–1.

72. Shepherd, 359–60; Hunt, Harriot Kezla (1805–1875), http:// www.jiffynotes.com/a_study_ guides/book_notes_add/amer_ 000 (accessed January 16, 2012).

73. Shepherd, 405, 409–10.

74. Elizabeth Keckley, *Behind the Scenes* (Los Angeles: Indo- European, 2011), 53.

75. Catherine Clinton, *Mrs. Lincoln: A Life* (New York: HarperCollins, 2009): 84, 221; Anne E. Beidler, *The Affliction of Mary Todd Lincoln* (Seattle: Cof- feetown, 2009): 12–13, 32–5: Mary Lincoln's lifelong head- aches; Clinton, 244: Fear of head- ache subservient to desire to ac-

company her husband to Ford's theater.

76. Jason Emerson, *The Mad- ness of Mary Lincoln* (Carbon- dale: Southern Illinois University Press, 2007); W.A. Evans, *Mrs. Abraham Lincoln: A Study of Her Personality and Her Influence on Lincoln* (Carbondale: Southern Illinois University Press, 2010); Mark E. Neely, Jr., and R. Gerald McMurtry: *The Insanity File: The Case of Mary Todd Lincoln* (Car- bondale: Southern Illinois Uni- versity Press, 1986).

77. Evans, 65, 138; Clinton, 88–9.

78. Clinton, 86–7; Emerson, 12; Jerrold Packard, *The Lincolns in the White House: Four Years That Shattered a Family* (New York: St. Martin's Griffin, 2005), 19.

79. Evans, 155: "She kept Mr. Lincoln from making several mistakes"; Carl Sandburg, *Abra- ham Lincoln: The Prairie Years and the War Years* (New York: Harcourt Brace Jovanovich, 1954), 155: Mary provided excel- lent political counsel; David Her- bert Donald, *Lincoln* (New York: Simon & Schuster, 1995),158, summarized Mrs. Lincoln's un- predictable behavior.

80. Packard, 1.

81. Clinton, 127: describes her social and ceremonial activities; Packard, 71, and Robert P. Wat- son, *The Presidents' Wives: Re- assessing the Office of the First Lady* (Boulder, CO: Lynne Rien- ner, 2000), 77: Prince Bonaparte's reception; Donald, 311, for more on her social success; Evans, 165– 6, and Watson, 95–6: Mrs. Lin- coln as political partner.

82. Watson, 36: "brutalized by her husband's critics"; Evans, 178, for Mrs. Lincoln's reaction.

83. Keckley, 45, for Mary's judgment on Seward; Sandburg, 393; Evans, 172; Donald, 427–8.

84. Donald, 271; Evans, 169– 70, for New York City shopping spree; Keckley, 29.

85. Clinton, 219, Evans, 169– 70, and Keckley, 53: Mrs. Lin- coln's continued extravagance; Packard, 210: purchases from Galt Brothers.

86. Emerson, 13; Clinton, 169– 70.

87. Clinton, 165–7; Keckley 34–5; Packard, 119.

88. Clinton, 165–7, 169–70; Packard, 114–6, for typhoid fever diagnosis.

89. Clinton, 212.

90. Evans, 185–6.

91. Emerson, 17.

92. Clinton, 182–89; Donald, 427; Emerson, 36–7; Sandburg, 394. For more on spiritualism, the reader is referred to the fol- lowing: "The Fox Sisters: Spiritu- alism's Unlikely Founders," http://www.histroynet.com/the- fox-sisters-spiritualisms-un- likely-founders.htm. Maggie and Katy Fox were charlatans but had a remarkable career for decades as they duped countless people into communication with their beloved deceased; "Charles J. Colchester," http://www.mrlin colnswhitehouse.org/content_ inside.asp?ID=179&sub.htm. Colchester was a medium who was a fake. He conducted séances for Mrs. Lincoln, including one at the Soldier's Home. Journalist Noah Brooks, a friend of the First Lady, exposed Colchester and de- stroyed Colchester's attempt to blackmail Mrs. Lincoln; Nettie Colburn Maynard, *Séances in Washington: Abraham Lincoln and Spiritualism During the Civil War* (Toronto: Ancient Wisdom, 2011) (originally published as *Was Abraham Lincoln a Spiritu- alist?* in 1891). Nettie Colburn de- scribed séances with Abraham Lincoln and Mary Lincoln in the White House from 1863 to 1865. William Mumler: Louis Kaplan, *The Strange Case of William Mumler, Spirit Photographer* (Minneapolis: University of Min- nesota Press, 2008). Mumler was also a fake. He produced a pho- tograph of Abraham Lincoln su- perimposed upon a photo of Mary Lincoln.

93. Donald, 427; Beidler, 20.

94. Donald, 572–3; Beidler, 23–4; Packard, 229–30; Keckley, 59–60.

95. Emerson, 16.

96. Emerson, 16; Packard, 162.

97. Emerson, 16; Packard, 162; Clinton, 221: Robert Lincoln's conclusion.

98. Packard, 162; Clinton, 121;

255 for Mary Lincoln's state after the funeral events were over.

99. Jonathan R.T. Davidson, Kathryn M. Connor and Marvin Swartz: "Mental Illness in U.S. Presidents Between 1776 and 1974: A Review of Biographical Sources," *Journal of Nervous and Mental Disease* 194, no. 1 (January 2006), 47–51.

100. Robert P. Watson, *The Presidents' Wives*, 143.

101. Ibid., 195; John B. Roberts, II, *Rating the First Ladies* (New York: Citadel, 2003), xxiv.

102. The reader is directed to the following excellent references: W.A. Evans, *Mrs. Abraham Lincoln: A Study of Her Personality and Her Influence on Lincoln*; Mark E. Neely, Jr., and R. Gerald McMurtry, *The Insanity File*; Jason Emerson, *The Madness of Mary Lincoln*; Clinton, *Mrs. Lincoln*.

103. Neely and McMurtry, *The Insanity File*.

104. Evans, 217: account of money; Emerson, 114: her accusation against Robert Lincoln.

105. Emerson, 40, and Evans, 215: "An Indian spirit was removing her scalp"; Evans, 222–3, lists her delusions; Evans, 222–3, and Emerson, 67–70, for discussions of suicide with Keckley; Emerson, 185–90: 1875 suicide attempt.

106. Emerson, 185–190.

107. Evans, 318: as early as 1860; Clinton, 221: began with carriage accident; Emerson, 16: signs of mental illness preceded Lincoln's assassination; Evans, 186, 305:illness a result of Willie's and Abraham's deaths.

108. Roberts, 114.

Chapter Six

1. Ishbel Ross, *The General's Wife: The Life of Mrs. Ulysses S. Grant* (New York: Dodd, Mead, 1959), 220–1.

2. Russell L. Mahan, *Lucy Webb Hayes: A First Lady by Example* (New York: Nova Science, 2011), 72.

3. Ross, 8.

4. Emily Geer, *First Lady: The Life of Lucy Webb Hayes* (Kent, OH: Kent State University Press, 1984), 8, 10, 16; Mahan, 17. Wesleyan Female College was founded in Cincinnati in 1812 but was established as a woman's college only in 1846. At the time of Lucy's matriculation, the school had an enrollment of 340 women. She graduated after three years in 1859 with a well-rounded education that probably included rhetoric, mathematics, geology, painting, French, German and English. The college's notable contribution was the introduction of the terms *alumna* and *alumnae*. Lack of funds forced the school's closure in 1892.

5. Ross, 198.

6. Geer, 93. Rutherford Hayes was governor of Ohio, 1868–1872 and 1876–1877.

7. Julia Grant; National First Ladies' Library, http://www.firstladies.org/biographies/firstladies.aspx?biography=19 (accessed 19 February 2013).

8. Jean Edward Smith, *Grant* (New York: Simon & Schuster, 2001), 473.

9. Julia Grant, National First Ladies' Library.

10. Ross, 207–9.

11. Geer, 138; Mahan, 8.

12. Carl Sferrazza Anthony, *First Ladies: The Saga of the Presidents' Wives and Their Power, 1789–1961*, vols. 1 and 2 (New York: William Morrow, 1990), 227; Geer, 233.

13. Geer, 144: "Washington reporters began to praise Lucy's competence as a hostess and appreciate her"; 188: On June 19, 1878, in the Blue Room of the White House, Emily Platt, Lucy Hayes' niece, companion and efficient secretary married General Russell Hayes, a military colleague of the president.

14. Lucy Hayes, National First Ladies' Library, http://www.firstladies.org/biographies/firstladies.aspx?biography=20 (accessed 19 February 2013).

15. Julia Grant, National First Ladies' Library.

16. Ross, 37: "troubled her considerably"; 329; refusal to wear glasses.

17. Ibid., 37.

18. Ibid., 221–2. Ulysses Grant stopped his wife from surgery at the last minute, saying, "My dear, I know that I am very selfish and ought not to say what I am going to; but I don't want to have your eyes fooled with. They are all right as they are. They look just as they looked the first time I ever saw them—the same eyes I looked into when I fell in love with you."

19. *Surgical Management of Strabismus*, Chapter 1, "History of Strabismus Surgery, http://www.cybersight.org/bins/volume_oage.asp?cid=1-2161-2252 (20 February 2013). In 1839 Diefenbach performed the first successful surgery to correct strabismus. He removed part of the medial rectus extraocular muscle to correct an internal squint. It took some years before modern anesthetic and surgical techniques permitted such surgery to become routine in America.

20. Ross, 234.

21. Mahan, 2–3.

22. Geer, 36–7.

23. Ibid., 106–7.

24. Mahan, 29.

25. Geer, 109.

26. Mahan, 1: "on election day"; 72: "the only drawback."

27. Ibid., 103; Lucy Hayes, National First Ladies' Library.

28. Geer, 109, 210.

29. Mahan, 72: "She is large but not unwieldy."

30. Ibid., 101.

31. Geer, 255.

32. Ibid., 36–7: instances of arthritic attacks; Mahan, 29–30: "For ten days has had her rheumatism creeping over her from one place to another, giving her great pain. It began in her left shoulder and arm and in her neck."

33. Deppisch, *The White House Physician*, 46–7.

Chapter Seven

1. Mary Lord Dimmick diary entry, May 20, 1892: Benjamin Harrison Home, "The medical conclusion of Dr. Franklin Gardiner."

2. Please refer to Chapter One (yellow fever) and Chapter Two (malaria) of this book; J.

Arthur Myers, *Tuberculosis: A Half Century of Study and Conquest* (St. Louis: Warren H. Green, 1970), 305; David L. Ellison, *Healing Tuberculosis in the Woods: Medicine and Science at the End of the Nineteenth Century* (Westport, CT: Greenwood, 1994), 11.

3. Robert P. Watson, *First Ladies of the United States: A Biographical Dictionary* (Boulder, CO: Lynne Rienner, 2001), 56.

4. http://ask.yahoo.com/20020417.html (accessed 26 January 2012. "Consumption" is an old name for tuberculosis (TB) that describes how the illness wastes away, or consumes, its victims. TB is "an ancient enemy" that has plagued humankind for more than five thousand years. The Greeks called it phthisis, and Hippocrates advised his medical students against treating it because it was almost always deadly, and a dead patient was bad for business; *Indianapolis News*, October 24 and 25, 1892.

5. Harry J. Sievers, S.J.: *Benjamin Harrison: Hoosier Warrior* (Chicago: Henry Regnery, 1952): 72–3, 75, 78.

6. Ibid.; Sievers, 194, 224–6, 237, 292.

7. Sievers, *Benjamin Harrison: Hoosier Warrior*, 207; Charles W. Calhoun, *Benjamin Harrison* (New York: Henry Holt, 2005): 143; Dimmick diary entry, January 24, 1891: "Mrs. Harrison's reception, but she was too ill to receive"; Dimmick letter to Mrs. Putzi, September 23, 1891: Mrs. Harrison has been "ill for the past few days"; *Indianapolis News*, October 24 and 25, 1892; Mary Lord Dimmick diary entry, December 29, 1891.

8. Library of Congress, Benjamin Harrison archives: presence at February 16 dinner; Anne Chieko Moore, *Caroline Lavinia Scott Harrison* (New York: Nova History, 2005), 51–2: presence at April 6, 1892, dinner, "catarrhal pneumonia," pallor and cough at April 6 dinner.

9. Dimmick diary entry, April 7, 1892, records the onset of her continuous nursing of her aunt; diary entry, April 23, 1892: "suf-

fers much from depression." The diagnosis of malaria was a diagnostic construct by the uninformed Dimmick. Caroline Harrison never had malaria; diary entry, May 14, 1892: "still very depressed and nervous"; diary entry, May 21, 1892: "very nervous and ill all day"; Mary Lord Dimmick letter to May Saunders Harrison, July 28, 1892: "state of melancholia."

10. *New York Tribune*, October 25, 1892; Medical and Surgical Register of the United States and Canada, 1898.

11. Dimmick diary entries, May 14 and 19, 1892; Dimmick diary, May 20, 1892: Dr. Doughy's erroneous diagnosis.

12. Dimmick diary, several entries, May 22–29, 1892; Calhoun, 143: for initial experience at Loon Lake.

13. *New York Tribune*, October 25, 1892, and Moore, 51, for the diagnosis and treatment of Mrs. Harrison's pleurisy; *New York Tribune*, October 25, 1892, and Dimmick diary, September 14 or 15, 1892, for Edmund Trudeau; Moore, 52, for press release.

14. Harry J. Sievers, S.J., *Benjamin Harrison: Hoosier President* (Newtown, CT: American Political Biography, 1996), 242.

15. *New York Tribune*, October 25, 1892; Dimmick diaries, several entries.

16. Ellison, *Healing Tuberculosis in the Woods*, 1; William G. Rothstein, *American Physicians in the 19th Century: From Sects to Science* (Baltimore: Johns Hopkins University Press, 1985), 267–272.

17. Robert Taylor, *Saranac: America's Magic Mountain* (Boston: Houghton Mifflin, 1986), 75; Thomas M. Daniel, *Captain of Death: The Story of Tuberculosis* (Rochester: University of Rochester Press, 1997), 108–9; Thomas Dormandy, *The White Death: A History of Tuberculosis* (London: Hambledon, 1999), 177–182.

18. Edward Livingston Trudeau, *An Autobiography* (New York: Lea and Febiger, 1915), 243.

19. Benjamin Harrison (Indi-

anapolis) to Dr. E.L. Trudeau (Saranac Lake, New York), March 22, 1899 (Library of Congress Benjamin Harrison Collection).

20. Deppisch, *The White House Physician*, 54, 60.

21. Obituary of Dr. Franklin A. Gardner, *New York Times*, February 13, 1903; Mrs. Franklin Gardner, notes to Benjamin Harrison, March 18, 1892, April 1, 1892.

22. W.H. Crook, *Memories of the White House: The Home Life of Our Presidents from Lincoln to Roosevelt, Being Personal Recollections of Colonel W.H. Crook* (Boston: Little, Brown, 1911), 229–30; Carl Sferrazza Anthony, *America's First Families: An Inside View of 200 Years of Private Life in the White House* (New York: Simon & Schuster, 2000), 211; Franklin A. Gardner, letters to Benjamin Harrison, September 5, 1898, January 15, 1899, and January 22, 1899; Benjamin Harrison, letters to F.E. Doughty, November 10, 1897, and June 3, 1898; Degregorio, 332, 334.

23. The allopathic-homeopathic conflict will be discussed at length in a later chapter; *New York Tribune*, October 25, 1892; *Medical Mirror* 3 (1892), 471–2, 514.

24. John Scott, letter to Henry Scott, May 3, 1858. John Scott was Caroline Harrison's father and Henry was her brother (courtesy of President Benjamin Harrison Home, Indianapolis); Moore, 11; Robert P. Watson, *First Ladies of the United States: A Biographical Dictionary* (Boulder, CO: Lynne Rienner, 2001), 153.

25. Moore, 21–2: In January 1883, "she began a three month convalescence at a New York hospital following surgery"; Sievers, *Benjamin Harrison: Hoosier Statesman*, 227–9: Health "sunk to a new low in January, 1883 and she stayed under doctor's care in New York until the middle of March. Surgery kept her hospitalized"; Valerie J. Riley and John Spurlock: "Vesicovaginal Fistula," http://emedicine.medscape.com/article/267943-overview (July 28, 2009).

26. L. Lewis Wall and Thomas

Addis Emmet, "The Vesicovaginal Fistula and the Origins of Reconstructive Gynecologic Surgery," *International Urogynecology Journal* 13 (2002), 145–155.

27. Wall; Three years before Emmet operated on Caroline Harrison, in 1880, the second edition of his book, *The Principles and Practice of Gynecology*, was published. On page 90, he wrote the following: "Sloughing from continued pressure of the child's head on the vaginal walls during labor, resulting in fistulae, or loss of tissue with subsequent contraction, will often displace the uterus, interfere with the circulation, and cause much irritation to the bladder and rectum. The same cause and injury to the uterus often result in atrophy to the organ and permanent cessation of menstruation, even in early womanhood." Earlier, in 1868, Emmet had elucidated this condition in book-length form (*Parturition and Other Causes with Cases of Recto-Vaginal Fistula* (New York: William Wood).

28. Benjamin Harrison (U.S. Senate), letter to Dr. Thomas A. Emmet (New York), June 13, 1883.

29. Watson, *The Presidents' Wives*, 53.

30. Moore, 39–44.

31. Ibid., 34–8, 83.

32. Ibid., 34–8, for a discussion of her refurbishing efforts; Calhoun, 78: "During her years in the White House"; Craig Schermer letter to the author, September 6, 2008, and Jennifer Capps letter to the author, March 30, 2012, describe her use of solvents.

33. Degregorio, 334–7.

34. Sievers, *Benjamin Harrison: Hoosier President*, 227–21, 236.

35. Degregorio, 346; Sievers: *Hoosier President*, 241; Calhoun, 143, 149; Paul F. Boller, Jr.: *Presidential Campaigns* (New York: Oxford University Press, 1985), 162.

36. Sievers, *Benjamin Harrison: Hoosier President*, 248–250; Boller, 165. Charles Calhoun holds a contrary opinion that Caroline's illness and death contributed to Harrison's defeat. The president was unable to leave her side to engage in the sort of effective campaign speaking that had sealed his victory in 1888; personal correspondence with the author; Homer E. Socolofsky and Allan B. Spetter, *The Presidency of Benjamin Harrison* (Lawrence: University Press of Kansas, 1987), 199; Sievers, *Benjamin Harrison: Hoosier President*, 238–9, 248–9; Boller, 165; Calhoun, 145–6. The steelworkers' strike at Carnegie Steel's Homestead, Pennsylvania, plant in June and July 1892 was one of the most violent labor battles in U.S. history. Twelve people were killed and sixty wounded. Andrew Carnegie, the owner, was widely viewed as being close to President Harrison.

37. Watson, *The Presidents' Wives*, 139–143.

38. See Chapter Five.

39. Jean Choate, *Eliza Johnson in Perspective* (New York: Nova History, 2006), 36, 47. A cough is mentioned in Choate, 50–51, 58, 63, 66–7, 69, 79–80.

40. Ibid., 101; Eliza Johnson, National First Ladies' Library, http://www.firstladies.org/biographies/firstladies.aspx?biography=18 (accessed 27 March 2012); Choate, 154.

41. Barron Lerner, "Charting the Death of Eleanor Roosevelt," http://www.fathom.com/feature/35672/index.html (20 March 2012); B.H. Lerner, "Revisiting the Death of Eleanor Roosevelt: Was the Diagnosis of Tuberculosis Missed?" *International Journal of Tuberculosis and Lung Disease* 5, no. 12 (December 2001): 1080–5.

Chapter Eight

1. Nancy L. Herron, *Ida Saxton McKinley: Indomitable Spirit or Autocrat of the Sickbed in Inventing a Voice; The Rhetoric of American First Ladies of the Twentieth Century*, ed. Molly Meijer Wertheimer, (Lanham, MD: Rowman and Littlefield, 2004), 31.

2. William C. Braisted and William H. Bell, *The Life Story of Presley Marion Rixey* (Strasburg, VA: Shenandoah, 1930), 30.

3. Ibid., 30–31.

4. Ross T. McIntire, *White House Physician* (New York: G.P. Putnam's Sons, 1946), 58–9: McIntire, Franklin Roosevelt's personal and White House physician, wrote: "Dr. Jonathan M. Foltz, the first regular White House physician, was a family friend of James Buchanan and had his own room in the White House. Colonel Robert M. O'Reilly came to Grover Cleveland's attention through their common love of fishing."

5. Braisted and Bell, 240–1.

6. Presley Marion Rixey, "Guarding the Health of Our Presidents," *Better Health*, June 1925.

7. Braisted and Bell, 239.

8. Margaret Leech, *In the Days of McKinley* (New York: Harper, 1959), 567.

9. Leech, 17; John C. DeToledo, Bruno B. Toledo and Meredith Lowe: "The Epilepsy of First Lady Ida Saxton McKinley," *Southern Medical Journal* 93, no. 3 (March 2000), 267–271.

10. DeToledo; Leech, 17; Herron, 32.

11. Craig Hart, *A Genealogy of the Wives of American Presidents and Their First Two Generations of Descent* (Jefferson, NC: McFarland, 2004), 158.

12. Leech, 17; DeToledo offered the description of Mrs. McKinley's attacks.

13. Absence seizure (petit mal seizure): Mayo Clinic, http://www.mayoclinic.com/health/petit-mal-seizure/DS00216/DSEC (accessed April 5, 2012).

14. Leech, 17: "big," "prolonged and violent"; Rixey: "other ailments"; DeToledo.

15. DeToledo; Steven J. Kittner, et al., "Pregnancy and the Risk of Stroke," *New England Journal of Medicine* 335 (September 12, 1996), 768–774; C.A. Davis and P. O'Brien, "Stroke and Pregnancy," *Journal of Neurology Neurosurgery and Psychiatry* 79 (2008), 240–245; James N. Martin, Jr., Brad D. Thigpen, et al.: "Stroke and Severe Preeclampsia

and Eclampsia: A Paradigm Shift Focusing on Systolic Blood Pressure," *Obstetrics and Gynecology* 105, no. 2 (February 2005), 246–253.

16. Leech, 19–20; Ida McKinley, National First Ladies' Library, http:www.firstladies.org/biographies/firstladies.aspx?biography=25 (accessed June 25, 2010).

17. Herron, 35; William Degregorio, *The Complete Book of U.S. Presidents* (New York: Wings, 1993), 358–9, provided the dates of McKinley's political career.

18. "Locock, Sir Charles, Obituary," *British Medical Journal*, July 31, 1875, 151; "Potassium bromide," Wikipedia, http://en.wikipedia.org/wiki/Potassium_bromide (accessed July 1, 2010).

19. Herron, 35.

20. "Potassium bromide," Wikipedia; Walter J. Friedlander, "The Rise and Fall of Bromide Therapy in Epilepsy," *Archives of Neurology* 57 (December 2000), 1782–5.

21. "Mrs. McKinley's Life and Character," *Los Angeles Times*, June 14, 1901.

22. Leech, 199, 432, for McKinley's euphemisms; Braisted and Bell; Presley Marion Rixey, "Guarding the Health of Our Presidents," *Better Health* (June 1925).

23. Braisted and Bell, 35, 43, and Leech, 123, 433, 434, with the euphemisms; Leech, 432, 433: Kate's reaction.

24. "Epilepsy Across the Spectrum: Promoting Health and Understanding," Consensus Report, Institute of Medicine, March 30, 2012.

25. Ibid., 274; "The History and Stigma of Epilepsy," Introduction, *Epilepsia* 44, no. suppl. 6 (2003): 12–14; Ann Jacoby and Joan K. Austin, "Social Stigma for Adults and Children with Epilepsy," *Epilepsia* 48, no. suppl. S9 (December 2007), 6–9.

26. Rixey, *Guarding the Health of Our Presidents*.

27. Leech, 27–8: seeing Dr. Bishop in New York; Joseph N. Bishop, *1898 Medical and Surgical Register of the United States and Canada* (Detroit: R.L. Polk,

1898), 1150; Jay Henry Mowbray, ed., *Representative Men of New York*, vol. 1, "Joseph Norton Bishop" (New York: New York Press, 1898), 50–53.

28. Leech, 27.

29. Braisted and Bell, 35–7.

30. Leech, 99, 577–9.

31. Rixey.

32. Ibid.; Leech, 577–8.

33. Associated Press (to *Los Angeles Times*): "Official Announcements: Bulletins from the Bedside," May 17, 1901. Braisted and Bell, 43–47, 241–3, provides background from Rixey's point of view. Rixey's "Guarding the Health of Our Presidents" attributed Ida McKinley's recovery to the prevailing of "heroic efforts."

34. Rixey.

35. *New York Times*: "Mrs. McKinley's Condition Is Reportedly Grave," June 5, 1901.

36. Leech, 577–9, 583; Braisted and Bell, 47; "Off for Canton Home," *Washington Post*, July 6, 1901.

37. Henry Jr. Gibbons, Obituary, *Journal of the American Medical Association* 57, no. 16 (October 14, 1911), 1300; Clinton Cushing, Obituary: *Journal of the American Medical Association* 42(21), 1369, May 21, 1904; William Fitch Cheney, "Reminiscences of Three Eminent San Francisco Physicians," *California State Journal of Medicine*, no. 8 (August 21, 1923): 325–7.

38. Joseph Oakland Hirschfelder, *Directory of Deceased Physicians*, vol. 1 (Chicago: AMA, 1993), 719.

39. Molly Caldwell Crosby, *The American Plague: The Untold Story of Yellow Fever, the Epidemic That Shaped Our History* (New York: Berkley, 2006), 98, 126–7, 129–30, 136–7, 154, 229; Howard A. Kelly and Walter L. Burrage, *American Medical Biographies* (Baltimore: Norman, Remington, 1920), for William Johnson.

40. Braisted and Bell, 244–5.

41. Ibid., 245.

42. "No Hope for Mrs. McKinley," *New York Times*, May 25, 1907; "Mrs. McKinley Dies in Canton Cottage," *New York Times*, May 27, 1907.

43. Rixey.

44. Ida McKinley, Biography, National First Ladies' Library, http:www.firstladies.org/biographies/firstladies.aspx?biography=25 (accessed June 25, 2010).

45. DeToledo.

46. Leech, 22.

47. DeToledo.

48. Quote is from Herron, 36; Ida McKinley, National First Ladies' Library.

49. Chapter Five.

50. John R. Gates, "Non-Epileptic Seizures: Classification Co-existence with Epilepsy: Diagnosis, Therapeutic Approaches and Consensus," *Epilepsy and Behavior* 3 (2002), 28–33; Vernon M. Neppe, "Pseudoseizures or Somatoform Spells; Hysteroepilepsy or Somatoform Spell Disorder," Pacific Neuropsychiatric Institutes, http://www.pni.org/neuropsychiatry/seizures/epilepsy/pseudo_seizure.html (accessed May 2, 2012).

51. Alan Levenson, personal communication to author, April 18, 2012.

52. Jonathan Davidson, personal communication to author, April 18, 2012.

53. Herron, 36; Ida McKinley, National First Ladies' Library; Leech, 436.

54. Leech, 27–8, 32.

55. Ibid., 120, 129; Herron, 37.

56. Ida McKinley, National First Ladies' Library; Leech, 28.

57. Ida McKinley, National First Ladies' Library; DeToledo.

58. Watson, *The Presidents' Wives*, 195: rated her as 32 of 36 first ladies; Roberts, *Rating the First Ladies* listed her as 32 of 38, xxiv.

59. Watson, 140–3.

60. DeToledo; Herron, 35.

61. Leech, 19.

62. Ida McKinley, National First Ladies' Library.

Chapter Nine

1. Lewis L. Gould, *Helen Taft: Our Musical First Lady* (Lawrence: University Press of Kansas, 2010), 154.

2. Carl Sferrazza Anthony, *Nellie Taft: The Unconventional*

First Lady of the Ragtime Era (New York: Harper, 2005), 25.

3. Ibid., 32.

4. Ibid., 39.

5. Ibid., 47–8, 54–5; Taft, Helen, National First Ladies' Museum, http://www.firstladies.org/biographies/firstladies.aspx?biography=27 (accessed 20 November 2013).

6. Gould, *Helen Taft*, 8.

7. Anthony, 92, 103, 123; William Degregorio, *The Complete Book of U.S. Presidents* (New York: Wings, 1993), 394–5.

8. Anthony; Judith Icke Anderson, *William Howard Taft: An Intimate History* (New York: W.W. Norton, 1981); Gould, *Helen Taft*; Lewis L. Gould, ed., *My Dearest Nellie: The Letters of William Howard Taft to Helen Herron Taft, 1909–1912* (Lawrence: University Press of Kansas, 2011); Helen Herron Taft, *Recollections of Full Years* (New York: Dodd, Mead, 1914).

9. Anthony, 33, 36, 38, 40, 42.

10. Ibid., 10: "It was simply that if I was not busy"; 175: hints of poor health and ennui; 360: her memoir.

11. Anthony, 164, quotes a letter excerpt from Nellie Taft to her husband, written February 1, 1902: "despite her own physical ailments resulting from malaria"; Gould, 19: "fragile looking woman."

12. Chapter Two.

13. Degregorio, 397.

14. Gould, 19.

15. Anthony, 213.

16. Anderson, 154.

17. Anderson, 153, for compliments; Anthony, 228.

18. Anthony, 86–7, 160, regarding Helen's mother; 164, 304, regarding Helen's father.

19. Paula Jerrard-Dunne, Geoffrey Cloud, Ahmad Hassan and Hugh S. Markus: "Evaluating the Genetic Component of Ischemic Stroke Subtypes: A Family History Study," *Stroke* 34 (2003): 1364–1369.

20. Jose Antonio Egido, Olga Castillo, et al., "Is Psycho-Physical Stress a Risk Factor for Stroke? A Case-Control Study," *Journal of Neurology, Neurosurgery, Psychiatry* (10 September 2012): 1136.

21. Anthony, 39, 219, 407; Gould, 18.

22. Edelson, ed.: "Stroke Risk in Women Smokers Goes Up by Each Cigarette," http://health.usnews.com/health-news/family-health/heart/article/2008/08/14/stroke-risk-in-women-smokers (8 September 2012); Philip A. Wolf, Ralph B. D'Agostino, et al., "Cigarette Smoking as a Risk Factor for Stroke," *Journal of the American Medical Association* 259, no. 7 (1988): 1025–1029; Graham A. Colditz, Ruth Bonita, et al., "Cigarette Smoking and Risk of Stroke in Middle-Aged Women," *New England Journal of Medicine* 318 (April 14, 1988): 937–941.

23. Anthony, 258–260, 262.

24. William Taft to Robert Taft, May 18, 1909, "Physicians in William Howard Taft's Life," http:///www.apneos.com/physicians.html (accessed September 8, 2012).

25. "Mrs. Taft's Illness Due to Social Causes," *New York Times*, May 19, 1909; Gould, 50–51; Anthony, 261.

26. "Mrs. Taft Can't Meet Guests," *New York Times*, May 22, 1909; "Mrs. Taft Still Ill; Not At Garden Party," *New York Times*, May 29, 1909.

27. Anthony, 267; Gould, 53.

28. Anthony, 263; Gould, 53.

29. A. McGehee Harvey, Gert H. Brieger, Susan L. Abrams and Victor A. McKusick: *A Model of Its Kind: A Centennial History of Medicine at Johns Hopkins,* vol. 1 (Baltimore: Johns Hopkins University Press, 1989), 44; William H. Taft to Helen Herron Taft, October 31, 1909, "Physicians in William Howard Taft's Life," http:///www.apneos.com/physicians.html (accessed September 8, 2012).

30. Anthony, 275–6.

31. Gould, 63: "she made remarkable progress in the preceding two months"; Anthony, 294, 297.

32. "Apraxia of speech," National Institute on Deafness and Other Communicative Disorders, http://www.nidcd.nih.gov/health/voice/pages/apraxia.aspx (accessed November 23, 2013).

33. Anthony, 304: Daughter Helen's quote; Gould, 123–4; "Mrs. Taft Ill Here, President with Her," *New York Times*, May 15, 1911.

34. Gould, 123–4; "Mrs. Taft Will Rest," *New York Times*, May 20, 1911.

35. Gould, 133, 136: Tafts' twenty-fifth wedding anniversary celebration; Anthony, 346: 1912 Democrat National Convention.

36. Anderson, 167: "During Nellie's Illness Taft Was a Somber and Stricken Man"; Anthony, 264.

37. Anthony, 279.

38. Gould, 51.

39. Anderson, 162.

40. Gould, 154.

41. Anthony, 398–9.

42. Gould, 52; Anthony, 385: quote regarding self-control of stress.

43. Anthony, 385.

44. Anthony, 402, 404. There are suggestions, unconfirmed and medically undocumented, that Nellie Taft had other attacks. In a letter from William Taft to his son Robert at the time of the 1909 stroke, Taft said, "You know she has had these attacks which seem to proceed from nervous exhaustion, and in which her heart functionates [*sic*] very feebly. It is not an organic trouble of the heart, but it seems to be some nervous affection" (Anthony, 262), and "Henry Adams learned from the widow of John Hay that Mrs. Taft's attack in May 1909 was the 'third time she has had something of the kind'" (Gould, 49).

45. Anthony, 408–410; "Mrs. W.H. Taft Dies, President's Widow," *New York Times*, May 22, 1943.

46. *New York Times*, May 22, 1943; "General Delaney Dies, Physician to Taft," *Wilkes-Barre (PA) Record*, November 13, 1936.

47. John C. Lungren and John C. Lungren Jr., *Healing Richard Nixon* (Lexington: University of Kentucky Press, 2003), 162.

48. Paul F. Boller, *Presidential Wives: An Anecdotal History* (New York: Oxford University Press, 1998), 397; Watson, *The Presidents' Wives*, 79.

49. William Safire, "Political Spouse," *New York Times*, June 24, 1993; Donnie Radcliffe, "Appreciation: Pat Nixon; Cloth Coat, Ironclad Devotion," *Washington Post*, June 23, 1993.

50. Julie Nixon Eisenhower, *Pat Nixon: The Untold Story* (New York: Simon & Schuster, 1986), 17–55; Mary C. Brennan, *Pat Nixon. Embattled First Lady* (Lawrence: University Press of Kansas, 2011), 1–14.

51. Eisenhower, 171; Brennan, 71.

52. Brennan, 163: "on several occasions, she even smoked in public"; 173: her answers to reporters were false; Robert B. Semple Jr., "A Stoic Pat Nixon Is Recalled by Aide," *New York Times*, August 14, 1976.

53. Bob Woodward and Carl Bernstein, *The Final Days* (New York: Simon & Schuster, 1976), 32, 164–6, 243–4, 346.

54. Eisenhower, 447–453.

55. Lungren, 159; Jack Jones, "Pat Nixon's Doctors Optimistic," *Los Angeles Times*, July 9, 1976.

56. Lungren, 162; "Therapy Expert Aids Mrs. Nixon," *Los Angeles Times*, July 15, 1976; "Pat Leaves Hospital, Says She 'Feels Fine,'" *Los Angeles Times*, July 23, 1976; Eisenhower, 447–453.

57. Jon Nordheimer, "Doctors Say Mrs. Nixon Is Showing Improvement," *New York Times*, July 10, 1976.

58. "Pat Reading 'That' on the Day of Stroke," *Chicago Tribune*, August 9, 1976.

59. "Standing by for Mrs. Nixon," editorial, *Chicago Tribune*, July 10, 1976.

60. Lungren, 162.

61. Brennan, 175; "Pat Nixon Suffers Stroke, Spends 5 Days in Hospital," *Los Angeles Times*, August 22, 1983; "Pat Nixon Returns Home After Stroke," *Los Angeles Times*, August 23, 1983.

62. Brennan, 176; "Pat Nixon, Former First Lady, Dies at 81," *New York Times*, June 23, 1993.

Chapter Ten

1. "Mrs. Wilson Dies in the White House," *Los Angeles Times*, August 7, 1914; "Mrs. Wilson Dies in White House," *New York Times*, August 7, 1914.

2. August Heckscher, *Woodrow Wilson: A Biography* (New York: Macmillan, 1991), 280–1.

3. Kendrick A. Clements, *Woodrow Wilson: World Statesman* (Boston: Twayne, 1987), 97.

4. Heckscher, 289–1.

5. Eleanor Wilson McAdoo, *The Woodrow Wilsons* (New York: Macmillan, 1937), 229–230.

6. Sina Dubovoy, *Ellen A. Wilson: The Woman Who Made a President* (New York: Nova History, 2003), 248; Roberts, *Rating the First Ladies*, 197: "There were five hundred guests at the ceremony.

7. Dubovoy, 228, and Edwin A. Weinstein, *Woodrow Wilson: A Medical and Psychological Biography* (Princeton, NJ: Princeton University Press, 1981), 254: cancellation of the inaugural ball; Heckscher, 333: Jesse's wedding.

8. Dubovoy, 234–5, and Clements, 97: Ellen Wilson's cause was the Alley slums in Washington; McAdoo, 235–6: "often taking groups of Congressmen with her"; Francis Wright Saunders, *Ellen Axson Wilson: First Lady Between Two Worlds* (Chapel Hill: University of North Carolina Press, 1985), 248: illness forced her to abandon her crusade; McAdoo, 236: passage of the Alley Clearing bill.

9. Watson, *The Presidents' Wives*, 140, 143, 189.

10. Roberts, xxiii–xxiv.

11. Craig Hart, *A Genealogy of the Wives of American Presidents and Their First Two Generations of Descent* (Jefferson, NC: McFarland, 2004), 244.

12. Saunders, 67; letters from cousin Mary E. Hoyt (Rome, Georgia) to Ellen A. Wilson (Bryn Mawr, Pennsylvania): "very unwell" October 9, 1885; "are so sick," November 7, 1885. Her aunt Louise sympathized: "been so sick"; Louisa Hoyt Brown (Gainesville, Georgia), letter to Ellen Axson Wilson (Bryn Mawr, Pennsylvania), November 20, 1885.

13. Dubovoy, 69.

14. Eleanor Wilson McAdoo, *The Priceless Gift: The Love Letters of Woodrow Wilson and Ellen Axson Wilson* (Westport, CT: Greenwood, 1962), 148.

15. Dubovoy, 72–4; Heckscher, 85–6.

16. James W. Bailey, Obituary, *Journal of the American Medical Association* 54, no. 15 (April 9, 1910): 1229.

17. Louisa Hoyt Brown (Gainesville, Georgia), letters to Woodrow Wilson (Bryn Mawr, Pennsylvania), April 16, 17, 1886.

18. McAdoo, *The Priceless Gift*, 155.

19. Leon C. Chesley, "The Origin of the Word 'Eclampsia,'" *Obstetrics and Gynecology* 39, no. 5 (May 1972): 802–4: "Toxemia: Pre-eclampsia and Hypertension in Pregnancy," http://www.pregnancycrawler.com/toxemia.html (June 8, 2012; Howard Lein, personal correspondence, November 18, 2009; Bjorn Egil Vikse, Lorentz M. Irgens, et al.: "Pre-eclampsia and the Risk of End-Stage Renal Disease"; *New England Journal of Medicine* 359 (2008): 800–9: all references for eyelid edema; George Howe, letter to Ellen Axson Wilson (Gainesville, Georgia), May 2, 1886.

20. Edwin A. Weinstein, *Woodrow Wilson*, 86: Travel to Georgia for her second delivery; Dubovoy, 78, and the following letters for Ellen's distress: Mary E. Hoyt (Rome, Georgia), letters to Ellen A. Wilson (Bryn Mawr, Pennsylvania), February 23, 1887, March 13, 1887: "you are suffering so"; Ellen Axson (Savannah, Georgia), letter to Ellen Axson Wilson (Bryn Mawr, Pennsylvania), April 1, 1887: "were sick again"; Mary E. Hoyt (Rome, Georgia), letter to Woodrow Wilson (Bryn Mawr, Pennsylvania), August 30, 1887: "I knew Ellen had been very unwell during the summer"; McAdoo: *The Priceless Gift*, 160: for Aunt Louise's postpartum care.

21. Saunders, 78; Heckscher, 93.

22. Saunders, 78.

23. Ibid.

24. Ibid., 80; Weinstein, 98–9; Dubovoy, 82–4.

25. Saunders, 80.

26. Dubovoy, 82–4; Anne Taylor Kirschmann, *A Vital Force: Women in American Homeopathy* (New Brunswick, NJ: Rutgers University Press, 2004), 33, 123; *Taft, Florence: Puerperal Eclampsia: Proceedings of the Annual Session of the International Hahnemannian Association* (1895): 279–288.

27. "Toxemia: Pre-eclampsia and Hypertension in Pregnancy," http://www.pregnancycrawler.com/toxemia.html (June 8, 2012); Chesley, "The Origin of the Word 'Eclampsia,'" 802–4.

28. Saunders, 107, 115–6, 119; Dubovoy, 101; Weinstein, 150; Stockton Axson to Ellen Axson Wilson, letter November 7, 1897: "When I learned from Dr. Van Valzah that you had been at his office yesterday … I am glad to hear from the doctor that you and Brother Woodrow are both doing nicely in health." "Mrs. Wilson Dies in White House," *New York Times*, August 7, 1914: "Edward Parke Davis of Philadelphia, who had attended the Pres. and Mrs. Davis while they were residents of Philadelphia."

29. Weinstein, 149.

30. Van Valzah, *Directory of Deceased Physicians, 1804–1929*, vol. 2 (Chicago: American Medical Association, 1993), 1582; "Van Valzah Renounces Allopathy," *New York Times*, November 29, 1882; Van Valzah.

31. Eleanor Wilson McAdoo, *The Woodrow Wilsons* (New York: Macmillan, 1937), 56.

32. Saunders, 157: "Health-Wise She Never Felt Better"; Saunders, 174; Weinstein, 164.

33. Saunders, 254: "mother was less animated"; Dubovoy, 211, 216: "that something was very wrong with Ellen"; Saunders, 225: "walking slowly and wearily."

34. Lein, personal communication; Bjorn Egil Vikse, Lorentz M. Irgens, et al.: "Preeclampsia and the Risk of End-Stage Renal Disease," *New England Journal of Medicine* 359 (2008): 800–9; Weinstein, 254: Colonel House's comment; Dubovoy, 228: cancellation of the inaugural ball.

35. Deppisch, *The White House Physician*, 90–1.

36. Cary Grayson, *Woodrow Wilson: An Intimate Memoir*, 2d ed. (Washington: Potomac, 1960), ix, lists this date; McAdoo: *The Woodrow Wilsons*, 210–211. Daughter Eleanor also claims that the Wilsons met Grayson for the first time at tea with the Tafts the day before Wilson's inauguration. Grayson had taken care of Aunt Annie; Weinstein, 250; Grayson, 1–2; Gene Smith, *When the Cheering Stopped: The Last Years of Woodrow Wilson* (New York: William Morrow, 1964), 5; McAdoo, 210–11: all record the medical attention provided to Aunt Annie Howe, although the date of the event, either the day before or the day of the inauguration, is not uniformly stated; Grayson, 1, called the circumstances of his attendance upon Wilson's aunt "providential"; Grayson, 1–2, describes his official appointment; Grayson, 1–2, and Smith, 7, describe Ellen's involvement in Grayson's appointment; Weinstein, 250, states that Grayson was recommended by outgoing President Taft.

37. Dubovoy, 236: "It escaped no one's notice … that Ellen was taxing her strength to the limit"; "Mrs. Wilson Needs Rest," *New York Times*, June 21, 1913.

38. Saunders, 262; Weinstein, 254–5.

39. Saunders, 262: being tired with the necessity of rest breaks; Dubovoy, 249: lost weight; McAdoo, *The Priceless Gift*, 314: "lovely color in her cheeks disappeared."

40. Weinstein, 255: "a triad of symptoms typical of chronic nephritis"; Saunders, 270–1; Dubovoy, 253–4.

41. Edward Parker Davis, *The Man and the Hour* (privately published, 1919), was a slim volume of poems dedicated to Woodrow Wilson; "Mrs. Wilson Dies in White House," *New York Times*, August 7, 1914: "who had attended the President and Mrs. Wilson while they were residents of Princeton"; Davis to Grayson, July 22, 1913: "I think your present program is an excellent one." Edward P. Davis to Dr. Cary T. Grayson, February 12, February 24, April 7, 1914; *Medical and Surgical Register of the United States and Canada* (Detroit: R.L. Polk, 1917), 1388–9, and Pascal Brooke Bland, "Edward Parker Davis," in Jefferson Medical College Yearbook, 1937. After his Princeton graduation, Davis's academic journey took a peculiar route: graduation from two medical schools, Rush Medical College in 1882 and Jefferson Medical College in 1888. He became chief of obstetrics and gynecology at Jefferson in 1898 and remained in that position until his retirement in 1925. Davis authored several standard textbooks, including *A Treatise on Obstetrics for Students and Practitioners*, and was a special representative of the United States to the 1910 meeting of the International Obstetrical and Gynecological Society in Saint Petersburg, Russia.

42. Saunders, 270–1; Dubovoy, 254, speculated that the surgery was for a gynecological problem; Edward P. Davis (Philadelphia) to Dr. Cary T. Grayson (The White House), May 16, 1914: Davis informed Grayson that Dr. Widdowson, the anesthesiologist, had sent his bill to Mrs. Wilson, who took care of the Wilson family accounts. Davis wished Grayson to explain the reason for this bill to Mrs. Wilson. Widdowson was "an expert in anesthesia, and … he took considerable time to come to Washington to do what he did."

43. Saunders, 270–1: "distressingly ill"; Dubovoy, 254; Davis to Grayson letter, April 7, 1914.

44. Saunders, 270–1; Dubovoy, 255; Weinstein, 256.

45. Dubovoy, 255; McAdoo: *The Priceless Gift*, 315.

46. Weinstein, 253–4.

47. Harvey, A. McGehee, "Medical Students on the March: Brown, MacCallum and Opie," *Johns Hopkins Medical Journal* 134 (June 1974), 330–4.

48. Saunders, 273–6.

49. "Mrs. Wilson Dies in the White House," *Los Angeles Times*, August 7, 1914; "Mrs. Wilson Dies in White House," *New York Times*, August 7, 1914; Kristie Miller, *Ellen and Edith: Woodrow Wilson's First Ladies* (Lawrence:

University Press of Kansas, 2010), 89–90; Dubovoy, 258; Certificate of Death, District of Columbia, for Ellen Axson Wilson, August 6, 1914, reproduction issued August 8, 1969, and certified by John H. Crandall, chief of Vital Records Division.

50. McAdoo, *The Priceless Gift*, 315; Ray Stannard Baker, interviews with Cary T. Grayson, February 18–19, 1926, RSB Collection; Weinstein, 99, 254–5; Albert S. Lyons and R. Joseph Petrucelli II, *Medicine: An Illustrated History* (New York: Harry C. Abrams, 1987), 516: Bright's disease is named after the Edinburgh and Guy's Hospital 19th-century physician Richard Bright, who studied diseases of the kidney and may have been the first recognized nephrologist.

51. Dubovoy, 257; Woodrow Wilson to J.R. Wilson, August 6, 1914.

52. Dubovoy, 258.

53. Grayson, 232–5.

54. Weinstein, 256; Saunders, 273–6: "now in its late stages, yet could not bring himself to tell the president that her condition was helpless."

55. Cary Grayson letter to Col. House, August 20, 1914 (House papers).

56. Woodrow Wilson to Mary Allen Hulbert, June 21, 1914: "but that fear, thank God, is past and she is coming along slowly, but surely"; Woodrow Wilson to Alfred P. Wilson, July 23, 1914: "Ellen is making good progress, though painfully slow"; Woodrow Wilson to E.P. Davis, July 26, 1914: "at present to be making little progress, and yet it still seems certain that there is nothing wrong with her."

57. *New York Times*, August 7, 1914,

58. Weinstein, 258–9; Sigmund Freud and William C. Bullitt, *Thomas Woodrow Wilson: A Psychological Study* (Boston: Houghton Mifflin, 1966), 156.

59. Freud, 155; Weinstein, 258–9: Wilson's depression.

60. Grayson, 35–6; Miller, *Ellen and Edith* (Lawrence: University Press of Kansas, 2010), 97: confession to Colonel House.

61. Edmund: Morris, *Colonel Roosevelt* (New York: Random House, 2010), 384, 398.

62. Grayson, 48; Freud and Bullitt, 214: "a nervous collapse."

63. Miller, 99, 108; Grayson, 50–1.

64. Edith Bolling Wilson, *My Memoir* (Indianapolis: Bobbs-Merrill, 1938, 1939), 127.

65. Miller, *Ellen and Edith*, 129–130: Wilson's marriage to Edith; 108–110: whirlwind courtship; 11,34, 97: dependency and need for women; Freud and Bullitt, 157–8.

66. Miller, 118: Even when engaged, Wilson passed along to Edith all sorts of confidential information and papers; Miller, 128: reviewed speeches and saw diplomatic communiqués before wedding; Miller, 114: Edith encouraged Wilson to accept Bryan's resignation as secretary of state.

67. Miller, 99: "She personally made high-level governmental decisions, guessing at what Wilson would have wanted. Sometimes she refused to make necessary decisions and prevented others from making them. She did not hesitate to push out longtime Wilson advisers and appointees. Unquestionably she lied"; Miller, 171: Edith with Woodrow Wilson in Europe for Treaty negotiations; Wilson, 151: coded and decoded messages from House in Europe; Anthony, *First Ladies*, 352–3, 356, 359, 371, 376, 379.

68. Miller, 178–215, Anthony, 371–380, and Weinstein, 348–366: narratives of Edith's role during Wilson's disability; Miller, 186: "Edith made a crucially important decision."

69. James S. McCallops, *Edith Bolling Galt Wilson: The Unintended President* (New York: Nova History, 2003).

70. Roberts, *Rating the First Ladies*, 205–6.

71. Miller, 152: September 22, 1917–She was seriously ill with a respiratory infection and took to her room for two weeks. Wilson postponed an important meeting with Colonel House; Wilson, 144: In summer, 1917, Edith awoke

with high fever, aching all over. Grayson was away and Ruffin was sent for and he pronounced the ailment grippe. Since Grayson was gone for a month, Altrude, Edith's close companion and Grayson's wife, stayed at the White House: "I was in my room more than two weeks."

72. *Dorland's Illustrated Medical Dictionary*, 23rd ed. (Philadelphia: W.B. Saunders, 1957); McCallops, 42: alleged that Edith Wilson contracted an early case of the pandemic influenza; John M. Barry, *The Great Influenza* (New York: Penguin, 2004), 93, 96: references to Kansas locations, 383–8: Woodrow Wilson's bout with the flu in Paris.

73. Miller, 174; Wilson, 260.

74. *New York Times*, January 31, 1924: "well known as a diagnostician"; Anthony, 119–120: "one of the city's better physicians"; Obituary of Sterling Ruffin, *Transactions of the American Clinical and Climatological Association*: "a man of distinguished appearance, of great dignity of manner, and of outstanding ability."

75. Miller, 239; Wilson, 288, 291, 359; Anthony, 119–120, for Dr. Ruffin's treatment of Florence Harding.

76. Miller, 239: Ruffin an "old friend"; Wilson, 85: documented his attendance at the Galt-Wilson wedding; *New York Times*, October 2, 1925: related the romantic rumors between the widow Edith and Dr. Ruffin.

77. Edith Bolling Wilson Birthplace and Museum: "The Genealogy of Edith Bolling Wilson," http://edithbollingwilson. org/the-genealogy-of-edith-bolling-wilson/ (March 4, 2013); Anthony, 356, for campaign discussion of Indian heritage.

78. Miller, 103–5.

79. Miller, 104–6; Wilson, 29, 51–3, 100.

80. Wilson, 51: Grayson "a long and valued acquaintance of mine"; Miller, 117: "my dear boy" and successful lobbying for Grayson's promotion.

81. Miller, 135; Watson, 140.

82. Miller, 238; Wilson, 351, 358.

83. Miller, 261.
84. Ibid., 242.
85. Ibid., 257, 260–1.

Chapter Eleven

1. Carl Sferrazza Anthony, *Florence Harding: The First Lady, the Jazz Age, and the Death of America's Most Scandalous President* (New York: William Morrow, 1998), xiv.

2. Cynthia Bittinger, *Grace Coolidge: Sudden Star* (New York: Nova History, 2005), 87–8.

3. Ludwig M. Deppisch, "Homeopathic Medicine and Presidential Health," *PHAROS* 60, no. 4 (Fall 1997), 5–10.

4. Ibid.; Chapter Ten, for Van Valzah.

5. Deppisch, *The White House Physician*, 78.

6. Deppisch, "Homeopathic Medicine."

7. Ibid.

8. Anthony, 64, 516–18, 522.

9. Ibid., 55.

10. John J. Bell, "Nephroptosis: Its Causation, Symptoms and Radical Cure," *British Medical Journal* (May 26, 1923): 889–892; Douglas L. McWhinnie and David N.H. Hamilton: "The Rise and Fall of Surgery for the 'Floating' Kidney," *British Medical Journal* 288 (March 17, 1984): 845–7.

11. Anthony, 79–80.

12. "Mrs. Harding Worse; Recovery Not Sure; Specialists Called," *New York Times*, September 8, 1922; George Paulson, *James Fairchild Baldwin, MD (1850–1930): An Extraordinary Surgeon, House Call, Medical Heritage Center, at Ohio State University* 9 no. 1 (Fall 1905), 1–2.

13. Anthony, 86.

14. Ibid., 103.

15. Stuart J. Koblentz, "The Sawyers in Marion," 59–72, in *Marion* (Charleston, SC: Arcadia, 2004), for White Oaks description; Anthony, 102: "rigorous outdoor exercise, light therapy, hydrotherapy, massage and electrotherapy."

16. Anthony, 103; Carl Sawyer, *Polk's Medical Registry and Directory*, 1917; Sawyer, Carl, Obituary, *Journal of the American Medical Association* 196, no. 3 (June 27, 1966): 154.

17. Anthony, 107; Francis Russell, *The Shadow of Blooming Grove: Warren G. Harding in His Times* (New York: McGraw-Hill, 1968), 237.

18. Anthony, 115; "Mrs. Harding Worse; Recovery Not Sure; Specialists Called," *New York Times*, September 8, 1922.

19. Anthony, 119–121.

20. Ibid., 154; Russell, 310; Bernard Lauriston Hardin, Obituary, *Journal of the American Medical Association* 107, no. 2 (July 11, 1936), 145; B.L. Hardin to Florence Harding, December 11, 1922; B.L. Hardin to Florence Harding, undated.

21. Deppisch: *The White House Physician*, 83.

22. Anthony, 375–383; Russell, 549–550.

23. *New York Times*, September 7, 1922: "an ailment neither alarming nor serious"; Milton F. Heller, Jr.: *The Presidents' Doctor: An Insider's View of Three First Families* (New York: Vantage, 2000), 39–43: Boone summoned; Russell, 549: "I am afraid that Florence is going."

24. John Milton Cooper, Jr.: *Woodrow Wilson. A Biography* (New York: Random House, 2009), 535–540.

25. Anthony, 376–7.

26. J.M.T. Finney: *A Surgeon's Life: The Autobiography of J.M.T. Finney* (New York: G.P. Putnam's Sons, 1940), 264–7.

27. Ibid.

28. Florence Harding to Evalyn McLean, February 5, 1923; Harry Daugherty to Florence Harding, February 16, 1923.

29. Charles H. Mayo, Obituary, *British Medical Journal* 159–160 (June 3, 1939).

30. John Miller Turpin Finney, Obituary, *Annals of Surgery* 119, no. 4 (April 1944): 616–621.

31. Finney, 264–7.

32. Robert H. Ferrell, *The Strange Deaths of President Harding* (Columbia: University of Missouri Press, 1996).

33. "Mrs. Harding Back in Washington," *New York Times*, January 3, 1924.

34. Anthony, 516–518.

35. Ibid., 522.

36. Ibid., 524–5; "Harding's Widow Is Seriously Ill," *New York Times*, November 3, 1924.

37. Burke A. Hinsdale and Isaac Newton Demmon, *History of the University of Michigan* (Ann Arbor: University of Michigan Press, 1906), 272: biography of Dr. James Craven Wood; "Perform Operation on Mrs. Harding," *New York Times*, November 8, 1924; "Mrs. Harding Dies After Long Fight," *New York Times*, November 22, 1924; Anthony, 524–5.

38. Milton F. Heller, Jr.: *The Presidents' Doctor: An Insider's View of Three First Families* (New York: Vantage, 2000), 5–7; Charles A. Roos, "Physicians to the Presidents, and Their Patients: A Bibliography," *Bulletin of the Medical Library Association* 49 (1961).

39. Cynthia Bittinger, *Grace Coolidge: Sudden Star* (New York: Nova History, 2005), 8; Grace Coolidge, *Grace Coolidge: An Autobiography*, ed. Lawrence Wilander and Robert Ferrell (Worland, WY: High Plains, 1992), ix, 79, 111.

40. Coolidge, *Grace Coolidge*, ix; Bittinger, 5, 8; Ishbel Ross, *Grace Coolidge and Her Era* (Plymouth, VT: Calvin Coolidge Memorial Foundation, 1988), 4.

41. Bittinger, 8: "She needed to improve her health"; Ross, 4: "Grace definitely liked long walks."

42. Coolidge *Grace Coolidge*, x.

43. Ibid., 32.

44. Ross, 11–12: "They made an uncommon pair"; Robert E. Gilbert, *The Tormented President: Calvin Coolidge, Death and Clinical Depression* (Westport, CT: Praeger, 2003), 13: "shy disposition, somber demeanor, and conscientious devotion to duty."

45. Bittinger, 51.

46. Robert H. Ferrell, *Grace Coolidge: The People's Lady in Silent Cal's White House* (Lawrence: Vantage, 2008), 6: eye for style, 72: great charm, poise and grace; Bittinger, 73: her personality was her strongest point.

47. Bittinger, 93.
48. Ross, 102.
49. Joel Boone, Boone Diary, Library of Congress, Boone Collection, Box 40.
50. Ibid.
51. Ibid.
52. Ibid.; Heller, 112–3.
53. Ross, 238.
54. Boone, Boone Diary; Heller, 112–3.
55. Boone, Boone Diary: Coolidge's evaluation of Coupal's professional ability; Heller, 124: Boone's assessment of Coupal's medical ability.
56. J. Morton Boice, "Benzyl Benzoate," *New York Medical Journal* (December 13, 1919): 977–982; Boone, Boone Diary: his opinion of Coupal's therapy, Dr. Young's approval.
57. Ross, 242–3; Bittinger, 87.
58. Bittinger, 87.
59. "Capital Society Events," *Washington Post*, February 15, 1928: "prevented from attending by illness"; February 22, 1928: "recovery from recent illness"; March 4, March 14, 1928: "Mrs. Coolidge was unable to attend."
60. Hugh Young, *Hugh Young: A Surgeon's Autobiography* (New York: Harcourt, Brace, 1940), 398–403.
61. Chapter Five, for the Pierce and Lincoln deaths; see below for the Kennedy death.
62. Bittinger, 63.
63. Heller, 84.
64. "President's Son Is Seriously Ill; Foot Is Poisoned," *Atlanta Constitution*, July 5, 1924; "Calvin Coolidge Jr. Is Seriously Ill," *New York Times*, July 5, 1924; "Condition of Coolidge Boy Is Unchanged, But Serious," *Washington Post*, July 5, 1924.
65. "President's Son Is Seriously Ill," *Atlanta Constitution*; "Calvin Coolidge Jr. Is Seriously Ill," *New York Times*.
66. "Operation on President's Son Called Success: Father and Mother Spent Night at Hospital," *Atlanta Constitution*, July 6, 1924.
67. Ross, 117–120; Bittinger, 65–9; Heller 83–87.
68. "Operate on Calvin, Jr. Doctors Battle for Boy's Life," *Los Angeles Times*, July 6, 1924; "Calvin Coolidge Jr. Dies of Blood Poisoning," *Atlanta Constitution*, July 8, 1924; "Services Today For President's Son," *New York Times*, July 9, 1924; "Funeral for Coolidge's Son at 4 p.m. Today," *Chicago Daily Tribune*, July 9, 1924; "Coolidges Depart for a Sunday Cruise," *New York Times*, July 20, 1924.
69. Gilbert, 165: "not believing that death has occurred"; 170: President Coolidge's change in personality.
70. Ibid., 213–4.
71. Ibid., 123, 165; Bittinger, 72–3, and Ross, 123: wearing of white clothes.
72. Ross, 138, 335.
73. Bittinger, 49.
74. Gilbert, 169.
75. Bittinger, 62.
76. Coolidge: *Grace Coolidge*, 33–5.
77. Ibid., 109: death of Calvin Coolidge; Bittinger, xi: Grace Coolidge's retirement.
78. Bittinger, 116: walking habit; Ross, 334: cessation of walking habit in 1952.
79. Bittinger, 117; Coolidge: *Grace Coolidge*, 115; Ross, 341.
80. Ross, 341.

Chapter Twelve

1. "Mrs. Eisenhower and a Rumor," *New York Times*, November 3, 1973; Susan Eisenhower, *Mrs. Ike* (New York: Farrar, Straus and Giroux, 1996), 270, has an additional Mamie Eisenhower quote from the same interview regarding her rumored alcoholism: "It never bothered me if people thought that. I lived with myself. I knew it wasn't so. And my friends knew it was not"; Wikipedia: "Dipsomania" is a historical term describing a medical condition involving an uncontrollable craving for alcohol.
2. Catherine Clinton, *Mrs. Lincoln: A Life* (New York: HarperCollins, 2009), 154: "Charges of treason and adultery were part and parcel of the smear tactics employed to bring down the controversial Mrs. Lincoln."
3. Eisenhower, *Mrs. Ike*, 196–7.
4. Stephen E. Ambrose, *Eisenhower: Soldier, General of the Army, President-Elect 1890–1952* (New York: Simon & Schuster, 1983), 52: Taft campaign; Eisenhower, *Mrs. Ike*, 269–270: embassy party; Lester David and Irene David, *Ike and Mamie* (New York: G.P. Putnam's Sons, 1981), 183.
5. Ambrose, 532.
6. National First Ladies' Library, http://www.firstladies.org/personalinterests.aspx.
7. Marilyn Irvin Holt, *Mamie Doud Eisenhower: The General's First Lady* (Lawrence: University Press of Kansas, 2007), 114–5.
8. Mamie Eisenhower, National First Ladies' Library, http://www.firstladies.org/biographies/firstladies.aspx?biography=35.
9. David and David, 263–4.
10. National First Ladies' Library, http://www.firstladies.org/personalinterests.aspx.
11. Mamie Eisenhower Medical Record, Walter Reed Army Medical Center, January 4, 1946, George P. Robb, M.D.; Susan Eisenhower, 195, David and David, 160–1: only one Old Fashioned; David and David: "had virtually ceased many years earlier"; Susan Eisenhower, 195, and David and David, 160–1, 265–6: Milton Eisenhower, Maxwell Rabb, and others affirmed that she was not an alcoholic.
12. Mamie Eisenhower Medical Record, Walter Reed Army Medical Center, January 4, 1946, George P. Robb M.D.
13. David and David, 264: Sterrett diagnosis; Mamie Eisenhower, interview by John Wickman, August 15, 1972, for the Eisenhower Library, Abilene, KS: OH #12, 92–3: "For twenty-five years or more than that I carried this equilibrium problem, which is carotid sinus."
14. Shona J. McIntosh and Rose Anne Kenny, "Carotid Sinus Syndrome in the Elderly," *Journal of the Royal Society of Medicine* 187 (December 1994), 798–800; Mevan N. Wijetunga and Irwin J. Schatz, "Carotid Sinus Hypersensitivity," http://emedicine.medscape.com/article/153312-overview (accessed May 11, 2010).

15. Julie Nixon Eisenhower, *Special People* (New York: Simon & Schuster, 1977), 208; the record of this diagnosis could not be located in a review of Mrs. Eisenhower's Walter Reed medical file.

16. Susan Eisenhower, 196–7: The doctors made the diagnosis of Menière's sometime after the war; David and David, 264: testing confirmed, probably at Walter Reed.

17. Susan Eisenhower, 169–70; David and David: Dr. Sterrett's diagnosis.

18. Peter C. Weber and Warren Y. Adkins Jr.: "The Differential Diagnosis of Menière's Disease," *Otolaryngologic Clinics of North America* 30, no. 6 (December 1997): 977–986.

19. Venita Jay, "A Portrait in History: Prosper Menière," *Archives of Pathology* (February 2000), 124, 192.

20. N.J. Beasley and N.S. Jones: "Menière's Disease: Evolution of a Definition," *Journal of Laryngology and Otology* 110, no. 12 (December 1996): 1107–13.

21. L.R. Lustig and A. Lalwani: "The History of Menière's Disease," *Otolaryngologic Clinics of North America* 30, no. 6 (December 1997): 917–45.

22. David and David, 264; Holt, 21: symptoms while descending the Alps; Susan Eisenhower, 196–7: "pitching sensation" in the Philippines.

23. Holt, 40: "more acute than anything experienced in the Philippines"; Susan Eisenhower, 197: "couldn't even hail a taxi"; Mamie Eisenhower, interview by Dr. John Wickman for the Eisenhower Library, August 15, 1972: OH #12, 92–3: could not drive a car; smelling salts; Dwight D. Eisenhower (Versailles) to Mamie Eisenhower (Washington), September 23, 1944.

24. David and David, 265.

25. A.C. Sodeman, J. Moller, et al.: "Stress as a Trigger of Attacks in Menière's Disease," *Laryngoscope* 10 (October 2004): 1843–8; "Stress Management Therapy for Menière's Disease," http:///www.clinical trails.gov/ct2/show/NCT01099046 (accessed March 19, 2013); Menière's

Society: "Managing Menière's Disease," http://www.menieres.org.uk/managing_md_the_task.html (accessed March 19, 2013); Menière's Disease: http://www.entnet.org/HealthInformation/menieresDisease.cfm (accessed March 19, 2013); "What is Menière's Disease? What Causes Menière's Disease?" *Medical News Today*, http://www.medicalnewstoday.com/articles/163888.php (accessed March 19, 2013).

26. Susan Eisenhower, 83, 90.

27. Mamie Eisenhower: Pueblo Hospital Medical Records, 1931.

28. Susan Eisenhower, 145; Holt, 26; David and David, 111–3.

29. Julie Eisenhower, 202; Ambrose, 244–5, 414; Susan Eisenhower, 187; David and David, 111–.

30. Holt, 94.

31. Howard Snyder Papers, Eisenhower Library; Mamie Eisenhower Medical Records, Walter Reed Army Medical Center, Thomas Mattingly, 1951–57.

32. Eisenhower Medical Record, Walter Reed Army Hospital, Susan Eisenhower, 20: for discussion of childhood rheumatic attack; Clarence G. Lasby, *Eisenhower's Heart Attack* (Lawrence: University Press of Kansas, 1997), 29: for heart complications of rheumatic disease.

33. Lasby, 29.

34. Lasby, 29, Ambrose 244–5, 271: medical condition during World War II; Holt, 65: 1946 examination; Taylor letter to Snyder: progression of heart disease; Ambrose, 496: Eisenhower regarding NATO.

35. Holt, 65, Walter Reed Medical Records: Mattingly; Walter Reed Medical Records, for Mattingly Consultations.

36. Walter Reed Medical Records (Mattingly file); Holt, 143.

37. Susan Eisenhower, 277; Holt, 65–7.

38. Susan Eisenhower, 279.

39. Holt, 65–7; Julie Eisenhower, 205; Watson, *The Presidents' Wives*, 141.

40. Watson, 141; Julie Eisenhower, 189: role as emotional support of her husband, 201: thirty-four moves, 203: "I never

pretended to be anything but Ike's wife."

41. Watson, 141; Julie Eisenhower, 204: advice sought for re-election campaign.

42. Susan Eisenhower, 298, and Holt, 92: hysterectomy.

43. Snyder book notes, 1–10; Deppisch, *The White House Physician*, 98–9.

Chapter Thirteen

1. Annette Dunlap, *Frank: The Story of Frances Folsom Cleveland, America's Youngest First Lady* (Albany: State University of New York Press, 2009), 17.

2. Ibid., 34.

3. C. David Heymann, *A Woman Named Jackie* (New York: Carol, 1994), 190.

4. Jacqueline Kennedy Biography, National First Ladies' Library, http://www.firstladies.org/biographies/firstladies.aspx?biography=36 (accessed April 15, 2013).

5. Hugh Smith, interview, April 19, 2013.

6. Heymann, 145.

7. Jack Anderson, "Kennedy's Most Pressing Date," *Los Angeles Times*, August 6, 1963, p. 6.

8. Thomas Reeves, *A Question of Character: A Life of John F. Kennedy* (New York: Free Press/ Macmillan, 1991), 137–8: "Jack might have spent some time with his wife, offering sympathy and companionship, but instead, he went on his own way"; "Jack only agreed to return home three days later, after Smathers convinced him that a shattered marriage would harm his political career"; C. David Heymann, *Bobby and Jackie: A Love Story* (New York: Atria, 2009), 22–4: "On August 23, two days after learning of her husband's infidelity, Jackie experienced severe stomach cramps and soon began to hemorrhage"; "She thought that Jack should have been there for her and not off on a pleasure cruise with a trio of young, sexy bimbos."

9. Reeves, 137–8; Heymann: *A Woman Named Jackie*, 190–2.

10. "Wife of Sen. Kennedy

Loses Unborn Baby," *Chicago Daily Tribune*, August 24, 1956.

11. "Kennedy Reaches Ill Wife's Side," *Washington Post and Times Herald*, August 29, 1956: He arrived by plane from Paris five days after the miscarriage. Mrs. Kennedy's condition was "fine."

12. Heymann: *A Woman Named Jackie*, 191–2.

13. Jackie Kennedy, Female Celebrity Smoking List, http://smokingsides.com/asfs?K/Kennedy.html (accessed April 26, 2013): her smoking habit; Smoking tied to miscarriage risk, http://www.abs-cbnnews.com/lifestyle/01/01/11/smoking-tied-miscarriage (accessed April 22, 2013).

14. Heymann, 200; "Kennedys Have Daughter," *Washington Post*, November 28, 1957.

15. Sally Bedell Smith, *Grace and Power: The Private World of the Kennedy White House* (New York: Random House, 2004), 54.

16. "Jacqueline and Baby 'Doing Fine,'" *Washington Post*, November 26, 1960.

17. Reeves, 219–220.

18. "Mrs. Kennedy Bears Son," *Chicago Daily Tribune*, November 25, 1960; "Jacqueline and Baby 'Doing Fine,'" *Washington Post*, November 26, 1960; "Kennedy Alters Schedule to Stay Close to New Son," *New York Times*, November 26, 1960.

19. Laurence Leamer, *The Kennedy Women* (New York: Villard, 1994), 512–15.

20. Clint Hill, *Mrs. Kennedy and Me* (New York: Gallery, 2012), 31.

21. Leamer, 518, 521–2; Barbara Leaming, *Mrs. Kennedy: The Missing History of the Kennedy Years* (New York: Free, 2001), 23–4: "alone and terrified," 31.

22. Jacqueline Kennedy, *Historic Conversations with Arthur Schlesinger, Jr., 1964* (New York: Hyperion, 2011), 153. Dexedrine is a brand name for dextroamphetamine.

23. Leamer, 21: in bed for a week; Leaming, 51: engagements cancelled; 100: secluded in a bedroom with depression.

24. Leaming, 103: Kennedy friend Chuck Spalding intro-duced JFK to "Dr. Feelgood." Jacobson injected Kennedy just prior to the first Nixon-Kennedy television debate, 104: description of Feelgood's procedure and results.

25. Heymann: *A Woman Named Jackie*, 312.

26. "Postpartum depression," MayoClinic.com, http://www.mayoclinic.com/health/postpartum-depression/DS00546 (accessed April 25, 2013).

27. Richard A. Lertzman and William J. Birnes, *Dr. Feelgood* (New York: Skyhorse, 2013), xiv, 9.

28. Smith, 202–3; Leaming, 105: dry mouth a side effect of amphetamines.

29. Leaming, 105, 106, 108, 109, 110, 116, 117; Leamer, 534, 535, 537; Smith, 202–204.

30. Heymann, *Jackie and Bobby*, 12–3.

31. "Newborn Kennedy Son Ill," *Chicago Tribune*, August 8, 1963.

32. Hill, 237–8; *Chicago Tribune*, August 8, 1963, regarding the upgrade of the Otis maternity unit.

33. Anderson.

34. Smith, 390.

35. Ibid., 393; *Chicago Tribune*, August 8, 1963; "2d Son Born to Kennedys; Has Lung Illness," *New York Times*, August 8, 1963; "Kennedy Baby Dies at Boston Hospital; President at Hand," *New York Times*, August 9, 1963.

36. Jerome Groopman, "A Child in Time," *New Yorker*, October 24, 2011.

37. "First Lady Quits Hospital Today," *New York Times*, August 13, 1963; Hugh Smith interview.

38. "Mrs. Kennedy Told to Curb Her Activities," *Chicago Tribune*, August 14, 1963; "Mrs. Kennedy Rests at Home," *Washington Post*, August 16, 1963.

39. Smith, 396–7; Hill, 251.

40. Ibid., 264.

41. Smith, 449; Heymann: *Jackie and Bobby*, 8.

42. "John W. Walsh, 87, Kennedy Obstetrician," Obituary, *New York Times*, November 25, 2000.

43. Allan Nevins, *Grover Cleveland: A Study in Courage* (New York: Dodd, Mead, 1948), 522.

44. William Degregorio, *The Complete Book of U.S. Presidents* (New York: Wings, 1993), 320–3; Craig Hart, *A Genealogy of the Wives of American Presidents and Their First Two Generations of Descent* (Jefferson, NC: McFarland, 2004), 56; Francis Cleveland Biography, National First Ladies' Library, http://www.firstladies.org/biographies/firstladies.aspx?biography=23 (accessed December 16, 2013).

45. Annette Dunlap, *Frank: The Story of Frances Folsom Cleveland, America's Youngest First Lady* (Albany: State University of New York Press, 2009), 29: quote, 32, 85: for social grace and poise.

46. Ibid., 99.

47. Ibid., 32, 87–90; Ludwig M. Deppisch, "President Cleveland's Secret Operation," *PHAROS* 58, no. 3 (Summer 1995), 11–16: circumstances surrounding Cleveland's operation.

48. Dunlap, 93.

49. Nevins, 522.

50. Ibid.; Dunlap, 94.

51. Joseph Decatur Bryant, "Deaths," *Journal of the American Medical Association* 62 (1914): 1185, for Dr. Bryant's professional accomplishments and friendship with the Clevelands; "Grover's Baby," *Atlanta Constitution*, December 4, 1891; "If It Only Were a Boy!," *Chicago Daily Tribune*, October 4, 1891; "Mrs. Cleveland a Mother," *Washington Post*, October 4, 1891: Bryant's delivery of Ruth Cleveland; Dunlap, 113–14: Bryant at the death of Baby Ruth Cleveland; Dunlap, 121: years later Frances Cleveland was the plaintiff in a fraud suit over a newspaper article. Her case was prosecuted "with help [from] her longtime friend and family physician, Dr. Joseph Bryant."

52. Dunlap, 73–4: "rather a long labor—but not at all severe"; Dunlap, 101: "and I feel that it is only fair to their father to have them as young as he can"; Hart, 55–6: for the births and deaths of the five Cleveland children.

53. Dunlap, 131–2.

54. Ibid., 165.

55. Sylvia Jukes Morris, *Edith Kermit Roosevelt: Portrait of a First Lady* (New York: Coward, McCann and Geoghegan, 1980), 249–50.

56. Ibid., 62, 64, 74; "Alice Hathaway Lee Roosevelt," Theodore Roosevelt Center at Dickinson State University, http://www.theodorerooseveltcenter.org/Learn-About-TR/Themes (accessed December 18, 2013).

57. Morris, 88, 91, 94, 100.

58. "Teddy Roosevelt's Widow Dies at 87," *Chicago Daily Tribune*, October 1, 1948: "a brilliant social regime"; "Mrs. T. Roosevelt Dies at Oyster Bay," *New York Times*, October 1, 1948: "she presided as mistress of the White House (1901–1909), with grace and distinction.... She was an excellent conversationalist and a musician of more than ordinary attainments."

59. Morris, 372–3.

60. *New York Times*, October 1, 1948, for hip fracture; Morris, 516.

61. Morris, 111–3, 120, 136, 150, 168.

62. Ibid., 111–3.

63. Ibid., 170, 172.

64. Edith Carow Roosevelt, Biography. National First Ladies' Library, http://www.firstladies.org/biographies/firstladies.aspx?biography=26 (accessed December 18, 2013); H.W. Brands, *TR: The Last Romantic* (New York: Basic, 1997), 217.

65. Morris, 249–50.

66. Carl Sferrazza Anthony, *First Ladies: The Saga of the Presidents' Wives and Their Power, 1789–1961*, vols. 1, 2 (New York: William Morrow, 1990), 307: As first lady, Edith twice became pregnant, although miscarriage intervened; Edith Roosevelt Biography, National First Ladies' Library; Morris, 238: letter to sister.

67. Morris, 265.

68. Anthony, 128.

69. Julia Tyler, Biography. National First Ladies' Library, http://www.firstladies.org/biographies/firstladies.aspx?biography=11 (accessed December 19, 2013).

70. Chapter Three.

71. Anthony, 124.

72. Julia Tyler Biography, National First Ladies' Library: explosion aboard the *Princeton*; Julia Gardner Tyler, *American President: A Reference Resource*, http://millercenter.org/president/tyler/essay/firstlady/julia tyler (accessed April 2, 2013): Dolley Madison a mentor.

73. Anthony, 126–9.

74. Hart, 124–7.

Chapter Fourteen

1. Anthony, *First Ladies: The Saga of the Presidents' Wives and Their Power, 1789–1961*, vols. 1, 2 (New York: William Morrow, 1990), 431.

2. Ibid, 435, 445; John B. Roberts, II: *Rating the First Ladies* (New York: Citadel, 2003), 231; Lou Hoover, National First Ladies' Library, http://www.firstladies.org/biographies/firstladies.aspx?biography=32 (accessed May 8, 2013).

3. Anthony, 436.

4. Lou Hoover, First Ladies' Library; Roberts, *Rating the First Ladies*, 236.

5. "Mrs. Hoover Dies of Heart Attack," *New York Times*, January 8, 1944.

6. Craig Hart, *A Genealogy of the Wives of American Presidents and Their First Two Generations of Descent* (Jefferson, NC: McFarland, 2004), 129–30.

7. Milton F. Heller, Jr.: *The Presidents' Doctor: An Insider's View of Three First Families* (New York: Vantage, 2000), 56: taught Lou Hoover how to dance; 118: advice regarding prep school.

8. Ibid., 140–1.

9. "Herbert Hoover Jr. to Convalesce at Asheville," *Lewiston Star*, October 16, 1930.

10. Heller, 139.

11. Margaret Truman, *First Ladies* (New York: Random House, 1995), 57.

12. Ibid., 56–71. The chapter "The Lost Companion" incisively details the personal dynamics of President and Mrs. Roosevelt by someone who was a very astute observer of presidential couples.

13. Roberts, *Rating the First Ladies*, xxiii; Watson, *The Presidents' Wives*, 189.

14. Joseph P. Lash, *Eleanor and Franklin* (New York: W.W. Norton, 1971), 83.

15. Ibid., 154, 159, 163, 166, 193–4.

16. Ibid., 178.

17. Joseph P. Lash, *Eleanor: The Years Alone* (New York: W.W. Norton, 1972), 305.

18. David Gurewitsch, "The Eleanor Roosevelt Papers Project," http://www.gwu.edu/~erpapers/teachinger/glossary/gurewitsch-david.cfm (accessed June 20, 2013).

19. Lash, *Eleanor*, 321–2.

20. Ibid., 331, quotes letter from son-in-law Dr. James Halsted to son James Roosevelt; last illness, 330–2.

21. Barron H. Lerner, "What Can We Learn from Eleanor Roosevelt's Death?" http://www.huffingtonpost.com/barron-h-lerner/eleanor-roosevelt-end.html (June 18, 2013).

22. Sara L. Sale: *Bess Wallace Truman: Harry's White House "Boss"* (Lawrence: University Press of Kansas, 2010), 33.

23. Ibid., 19: for Truman wedding; Bess Truman, Biography, National First Ladies' Library and Museum, http://www.firstladies.org/biographies/firstladies.aspx?biography=34 (accessed May 28, 2013): for the longevity of the Truman marriage.

24. Sale, 22: "and made a bed for her in a bureau drawer"; Margaret Truman, *Bess W. Truman* (New York: Macmillan, 1986), 84: Bess Truman's concern over age at pregnancy.

25. Sale, 103.

26. Ibid., 33.

27. "Mrs. Truman Retires With Nation's Esteem," *Los Angeles Times*, January 18, 1953.

28. Bess Truman, Biography, First Ladies.'

29. "Mrs. Truman/ Cheerfulness Reason Plain," *Los Angeles Times*, March 30, 1952; "First Lady Ready for Folksy Ways," *New York Times*, March 30, 1952.

30. Sale, 65–6; M. Truman, 338–9, 347.

31. Deppisch, *The White*

House Physician, 106–108, for a discussion of Dr. Wallace Graham's career; "Ex-1st Lady OK After Hip Surgery," *Chicago Tribune*, May 8, 1981.

32. Sale, 133.

33. "Bess Truman in Hospital," *Los Angeles Times*, November 22, 1978.

34. Sale, 130.

35. "Ex-1st Lady OK After Hip Surgery," *Chicago Tribune*, May 8, 1981; "Bess Truman Home, Happy," *Los Angeles Times*, June 22, 1981.

36. "Stroke Hospitalizes Mrs. Truman," *Los Angeles Times*, September 28, 1981.

37. Sale, 130: for Mrs. Truman's symptoms, reasons for delayed treatment and difficult recovery; "Mrs. Truman Has Operation. Tumor Removed from Left Breast," *Chicago Daily Tribune*, May 19, 1959; "Good News— Twice for Harry Truman," United Press International, May 19, 1959: benign, an "unusual type of tumor known medically as a benign myxoma"; "Mrs. Truman Home in 'Excellent' Condition," *Chicago Daily Tribune*, June 4, 1959; G. Magro, et al.: "Clinico-Pathological Features of Breast Myxoma: Report of a Case with Histogenetic Considerations," *Virchow's Arch.* 456, no. 5 (May 2010): 581–6: If the diagnosis of benign myxoma was correct, it indeed was a very rare tumor. Mrs. Truman's tumor-free survival of twenty-three years proved that the tumor was certainly benign and definitely not malignant.

38. "Truman's Widow Bess Dead at 97," *Chicago Tribune*, October 19, 1982.

39. "Lady Bird Johnson, 94, Dies; Eased a Path to Power," *New York Times*, July 12, 2007.

40. Margaret Truman, *First Ladies* (New York: Random House, 1995), 6: advice given by former First Lady Lou Hoover to incoming First Lady Bess Truman.

41. Lewis L. Gould, *Lady Bird Johnson: Our Environmentalist First Lady* (Lawrence: University Press of Kansas, 1999), 10, 14.

42. David Murphy, *A Texas Bluebonnet: Lady Bird Johnson* (New York: Nova Science, 2011), 99.

43. Gould, 126; Murphy, 99.

44. Gould, ix.

45. Watson, *The Presidents' Wives*, 188–9; Roberts, *Rating the First Ladies*, xxiii.

Chapter Fifteen

1. BreastCancer.org, http://www.breastcancer.org/symptoms/understand_bc/statistics (accessed December 22, 2013): About 1 in 8 U.S. women (just under 12 percent) will develop invasive breast cancer over the course of her lifetime. In 2013, an estimated 232,340 new cases of invasive breast cancer were expected to be diagnosed in women in the United States, along with 64,640 new cases of noninvasive (in situ) breast cancer.

2. Center for Disease Control and Prevention, "Leading Causes of Death in Females United States, 2010," http://www.cdc.gov/women/lcod/2010/index.htm (accessed December 22, 2013).

3. Woody Holton, *Abigail Adams* (New York: Free, 2009): for Nabby Adams Smith's three-year battle with cancer of the breast, 365–371, 373, 376, 385–8; Chapter Eleven, for Mrs. Truman's benign breast tumor.

4. John Robert Greene, *Betty Ford: Candor and Courage in the White House* (Lawrence: University Press of Kansas, 2004), 106.

5. Betty Ford with Chris Chase, *The Times of My Life* (New York: Ballantine, 1978), birth, 5–6, first marriage and divorce, 40, 45.

6. Ibid., 57: for second marriage, 77: for her pregnancies; Hart, 90.

7. Greene, 51–2.

8. Ibid., 45–7.

9. "Mrs. Ford Faces a Breast Biopsy," *New York Times*, September 28, 1974: report of a previous gynecological examination; K.J. Robson, "Advances in Mammographic Imaging," *British Journal of Radiology* (2010), 83, 273–275; for first mammogram machine; "Chronological History of ACS Recommendations for the Early Detection of Cancer," http://www.cancer.org/healthy/findcancerearly/cancerscreening-guidelines.html (accessed July 19, 2013): for the American Cancer Society's guidelines.

10. Greene, 45–7: for the sequence of events; "Mrs. Ford Faces a Breast Biopsy," *New York Times*, September 28, 1974.

11. Greene, 45–7; "The Most Feared of Tumors," *Time*, October 7, 1974, specified the location of the cancer and added details of Dr. Fouty's experience.

12. "The Most Feared of Tumors," *Time*.

13. "Mrs. Ford Ready to Leave Hospital," *New York Times*, October 11, 1974; "Mrs. Ford Resumes Her Role as Hostess," *New York Times*, October 24, 1974.

14. Ford with Chase, 204, 210.

15. Greene, 49, enumerated 45,000 letters and cards; Jeffrey S. Ashley, "The Social and Political Influence of Betty Ford: Betty Bloomer Blossoms," *White House Studies* 101, no. 8 (Winter 2001), estimated 55,000 cards and letters; Greene, 49: Happy Rockefeller.

16. Ashley.

17. Tasha N. Dubriwny, "Constructing Breast Cancer in the News: Betty Ford and the Evolution of the Breast Cancer Patient," *Journal of Communication Inquiry* 33, no. 2 (April 2009), 104–125; "New Attitudes Ushered in by Betty Ford," *New York Times*, October 17, 1987.

18. Greene, 52.

19. Ford with Chase, *The Times of My Life*; Betty Ford with Chris Chase, *Betty: A Glad Awakening* (New York: Jove, 1988).

20. Ford with Chase: *Betty: A Glad Awakening*, 37; Greene, 3–4: father and brother were alcoholics; Ford with Chase, *The Times of My Life*, 41–5; Greene, 12–13; first husband was a heavy drinker.

21. Ford with Chase, *Betty: A Glad Awakening*, 38: "In Washington there is more alcohol consumed per capita than in any other city in the United States."

22. Ford with Chase, *The Times of My Life*, 10.

23. Ibid., 134: "quit drinking for a couple of years"; Greene, 25: "I don't remember when I went from being a social drinker to being preoccupied with drinking, but I am sure it was pretty gradual."

24. Ford, Betty, http:///www.fofweb.com/Hiytory/HistRefMain.asp?Pin=firstladies34 (accessed July 26, 2013; Ford with Chase, *Betty: A Glad Awakening*, 43–4: "I was hospitalized for stomach trouble. The doctors checked stomach, gallbladder, kidneys, and they couldn't find anything wrong. Then they brought in a specialist who diagnosed my illness as pancreatitis. He said: 'Young lady, if I were you, I would just stay on the other side of the room from the bar for a while.' I don't even remember how or why I started drinking again."

25. Ford with Chase, *Betty: A Glad Awakening*, 128–9, 131, 133; Greene, 24.

26. Greene, 3.

27. Ford with Chase, *The Times of My Life*, 135–6.

28. Greene, 68.

29. Ford with Chase, *Betty: A Glad Awakening*, 45: "It was better in the White House"; Greene, 69–70: drinking in the White House.

30. Greene, 102–4.

31. Ibid., 104–8.

32. Ibid., 108.

33. "Betty Ford, Former First Lady, Dies at 93," *New York Times*, July 8, 2011.

34. Nancy Reagan, Biography, National First Ladies' Library and Museum, http://www.firstladies.org/biographies/firstladies.aspx?biography=41 (accessed July 17, 2013).

35. Craig Hart, *A Genealogy of the Wives of American Presidents and Their First Two Generations of Descent* (Jefferson, NC: McFarland, 2004), 181: Nancy Reagan's parents and birth; Nancy Reagan, National First Ladies' Museum: for her mother's career, second marriage and death.

36. Nancy Reagan Biography, National First Ladies' Library;

Nancy Reagan with William Novak, *My Turn: The Memoirs of Nancy Reagan* (New York: Random House, 1989), 63.

37. "Chronological History of ACS Recommendations for the Early Detection of Cancer," http://www.cancer.org/healthy/findcancerearly/cancerscreeningguidelines.html (accessed July 19, 2013): American Cancer Society guidelines.

38. James G. Benze, Jr., *Nancy Reagan* (Lawrence: University Press of Kansas, 2005), 111–2; Reagan, *My Turn*, 285.

39. Reagan, *My Turn*, 286–7.

40. Thomas R. Russell, "Remembering Oliver H. Beahrs," *Oncology Times* 28, no. 7 (April 10, 2006): 33–34, for Beahrs' biography; Reagan, *My Turn*, 286, for Nancy Reagan's comfort with him as a physician.

41. Oliver H. Baehrs, "The Medical History of President Ronald Reagan," *Journal of the American College* 178 (January 1994), 86–96; "President Is Well After Operation to Ease Prostate," *New York Times*, January 6, 1987.

42. Reagan, *My Turn*, 292, for discussion with Marlin Fitzwater, the presidential press secretary.

43. "Mastectomy Seen as Extreme for Small Tumor," *New York Times*, October 18, 1987, for specifics regarding Mrs. Reagan' cancer; Reagan, *My Turn*, 296: Involvement of John Hutton; "In Breast Cancer, Treatment Dilemma Persists," *Washington Post*, October 20, 1987: Prognosis close to 100 percent.

44. "More Women Seek X-Rays of Breasts," *New York Times*, November 1, 1987, reported the 30 percent to 50 percent estimate; Dorothy S. Lane, Anthony P. Polednak and Mary Ann Burg, "The Impact of Media Coverage of Nancy Reagan's Experience on Breast Cancer Screening," *American Journal of Public Health* 70, no. 11 (November 1989): 1551–2. This article with a two-year retrospective determined a more modest 12 percent increment; "Nancy Reagan Urges Breast Checkups," *Chicago Tribune*, October 21, 1987. Spokeswoman Elaine Crispen released the statement.

45. "First Lady Welcomed Home by Crowd, Jazz Combo," *Los Angeles Times*, October 23, 1987; "First Lady Marks First Year Since Cancer Surgery," *Los Angeles Times*, October 18, 1988.

46. "Mastectomy Seen as Extreme for Small Tumor," *New York Times*, October 18, 1987. Rose Kushner, executive director of the Breast Cancer Advisory Center in Kensington, Maryland, added, "I am not recommending that anyone do it her way"; "In Breast Cancer, Treatment Dilemma Persists," *Washington Post*, October 20, 1987, pointed out that the recommended surgery was a lumpectomy; Letter to the editor, "Mastectomy Is Not the Only Choice," *Chicago Tribune*, October 31, 1987.

47. "Nancy Reagan Defends Her Decision to Have Mastectomy," *New York Times*, March 5, 1988.

48. Ann Butler Nattinger, et al.: "Effect of Nancy Reagan's Mastectomy on Choice of Surgery for Breast Cancer by U.S. Women," *Journal of the American Medical Association* 279, no. 10 (1998): 762–766.

49. "Nancy Reagan Has Tumor Removed from Her Face," *New York Times*, August 30, 1990; "Nancy Reagan Hospitalized with Broken Pelvis," *People*, October 15, 2008; Paula Spencer Scott, "Nancy Reagan's Fall Wasn't Her First," http://www.caring.com/blogs/fyi-daily/nancy-reagans-fall-wasnt-her-first (accessed July 14, 2013); "Frail Nancy Reagan Soldiers On," *National Enquirer*, March 4, 2013.

50. "Doctors Remove Benign Lump from Breast of Rosalynn Carter," *Toledo Blade*, April 29, 1977.

51. "Mrs. Carter 'Just Fine' Following Minor Surgery," *Ellensburg Daily Record*, August 15, 1977.

Chapter Sixteen

1. Barbara Bush, *Barbara Bush: A Memoir* (New York: Scribner, 1994), 283.

2. George W. Bush, *Decision Points* (New York: Crown, 2010).

3. B. Bush, *A Memoir*, 27, 36, 38, 47, 53–4.

4. Ibid., 39–49.

5. Thyroid Newsmakers: Barbara Bush, http.//www.coulditbemythyroid.com/Book-Experts/nsmaker-BBush.html (April 18, 2011).

6. B. Bush, *A Memoir*, 283.

7. "Barbara Bush Says Thyroid Condition Caused Weight Loss," *New York Times*, March 30, 1989: "big, puffy, horrible eyes"; B. Bush, *A Memoir*, 283, for Dr. Lee's reaction. "I did not want pop eyes."

8. *New York Times*, March 30, 1989, "wacko"; B. Bush, *A Memoir*, 283: "berserk."

9. B. Bush *A Memoir*, 284; *New York Times*, March 30, 1989; "Barbara Bush Being Treated for Graves' Disease, a Thyroid Disorder," *Los Angeles Times*, March 30, 1989.

10. "Form of Cortisone Prescribed for First Lady's Eye Ailment," *New York Times*, August 23, 1989.

11. Graves' disease, Diffuse thyrotoxic goiter, PubMed Health, http://www.nlm.nih.gov/pubmedhealth/PMH0001398/ (accessed June 5, 2011); Rebecca Bahn, "Unlocking the Mysteries of Graves' Ophthalmopathy," *Newsletter of the Graves' Disease Foundation* (Fall 2009); Seema Kumar, Sarah Nadeem, et al: "A Stimulatory TSH Receptor Antibody Enhances Adipogenesis Via Phosphoinositide 3-Kinase Activation in Orbital Preadipocytes from Patients with Graves' Ophthalmopathy," *Journal of Molecular Endocrinology* 46, no. 3 (June 2011), 156–163.

12. Peter Smyth, PA: "Graves, Robert James (1796–1853)," *Milestones in European Thyroidology*. European Thyroid Association, http://www.eurothyroid.com/about/met/graves.php (accessed June 9, 2011).

13. *New York Times*, August 23, 1989.

14. "Stable, Barbara Bush Learned, After Two Hours of Tests," *Orlando Sentinel*, November 29, 1989; "Radiation Therapy Is Weighed for Mrs. Bush," *New York Times*, December 1, 1989.

15. B. Bush, *A Memoir*, 353.

16. "First Lady Begins Radiation Treatment," *Washington Post*, January 4, 1990; "First Lady Starts Radiation Therapy for Eyes," *New York Times*, January 4, 1990.

17. B. Bush, *A Memoir*, 264–89.

18. Devin Dwyer, "Barbara Bush May Be Released from Hospital," *ABC News*, March 30, 2010; Devin Dwyer, Ann Compton and Gina Sunseri: "Former First Lady Barbara Bush Had 'Mild Relapse' of Graves' Disease," *ABC News*, March 31, 2010.

19. Lawrence Altman, "Every Time, Bush Says 'Ah,' Second Guessers of His Doctor Cry 'Aha,'" *New York Times*, February 18, 1992; "Bush's Physicians Say Thyroid Gland Disrupted Heart," *New York Times*, May 8, 1991.

20. Dennis Breo, "Tough Talk from the President's Physician," *Journal of the American Medical Association* 262, no. 9 (November 17, 1989): 2742–5.

21. B. Bush, *A Memoir*, 411–2.

22. "Barbara Bush to Aid Group in Boston Speech Planned for Thyroid Fund," *Boston Globe*, July 21, 1992.

23. Graves' Disease Foundation: Onsite Support Bulletin Board, post by Dianne Smith November 15, 1996, http://www.ngdf.org/phpBB/ngdf/viewtopic.php?f+4&t+372 (accessed June 7, 2011): "They both do public service announcements for the Thyroid Society here in Houston"; Nancy Hord Patterson, telephone interview, June 13, 2011: information regarding the Graves' Disease Foundation. Both Bushes were made honorary members while they still inhabited the White House.

24. Graves' Disease Foundation: Onsite Support Bulletin Boards, posts by Gwen Shannon, June 8, 1997, http:/ngdf.org/phpBB/ngdf/viewtopic.php?f=4&t=3185 (accessed June 7, 2011); Nancy Hord Patterson, telephone interview, June 13, 2011.

25. Barbara Bush, *Reflections: Life After the White House* (New York: Scribner, 2003).

26. Ibid., 11–12.

27. Ibid., 12.

28. Ibid., 35: for Dr. Orton; "Barbara Bush Hospitalized for Pneumonia in Texas," *New York Times*, December 31, 2013: for miscellaneous hospitalizations at Houston's Methodist Hospital.

29. Connie Mariano, *The White House Doctor: My Patients Were Presidents: A Memoir* (New York: St. Martin's, 2010), 190.

30. Hillary Clinton, *Living History* (New York: Scribner, 2003), 258–259.

31. Ibid., 148.

32. "Court Rules That First Lady Is 'De Facto' Federal Official," *New York Times*, June 23, 1993.

33. Clinton, 84.

34. Mariano, 188–190.

35. Clinton, 482.

36. Mariano, 188–190.

37. Ibid.; Clinton, 482.

38. Deep vein thrombosis (DVT), Mayo Clinic, http://www.mayoclinic.com/health/deep-vein-thrombois/DS01005 (accessed August 26, 2013); "Deep Vein Thrombosis Overview," Society of Interventional Radiology, http://www.sirweb.org/patients/deep-vein-thrombosis/ (accessed August 26, 2013).

39. Clinton, 482; Deep Vein thrombosis (DVT): Mayo Clinic listed causes of DVT.

40. Clinton, 482; Mariano, 188–190.

41. Mariano, 190.

42. Mariano, personal communication, July 1, 2013.

43. Deppisch, *The White House Physician*. For a review of the White House Medical Unit, read Chapter 11, 150–158.

44. Richard Tubb, personal interview, August 11, 2011.

45. Mariano, personal communication.

46. "Fear for Hillary Clinton as She Is Rushed to Hospital with Blood Clot Just Three Weeks After Suffering Concussion," *London Daily Mail* December 31, 2012; "Hillary Clinton Recovering at Home Following Concussion Caused by Fall," *London Guardian*, December 15, 2012; "Hillary Clinton Making 'Excellent Progress' Doctors Say," *USA Today*, January 1, 2013.

47. "Laura Bush: Skin Cancer 'No Big Deal,'" *Washington Post*, December 19, 2006.

48. Laura Bush, *Spoken from the Heart* (New York: Scribner, 2010), 4–6, for her mother's pregnancy history, 90, for Laura Bush's professional career.

49. Ibid., 105.

50. Ibid., 106–7.

51. Jim Rutenberg, "The First Lady's Skin Cancer," *Caucus*, http://thecaucus.blogs.nytimes.com/2006/12/19/the-first-ladys-skin-cancer (accessed August 31, 2013); James Joyner, "Laura Bush Skin Cancer Flap," Outside the Beltway, December 19, 2006, http://www.outsidethebeltway.com/laura_bush_skin_cancer_flap/ (accessed June 19, 2011); "White House Stayed Quiet on Laura Bush Cancer Surgery," *(UK) Independent*, December 20, 2006; "Laura Bush: Skin Cancer 'No Big Deal,'" *Washington Post*, December 19, 2006; Bush, *Spoken from the Heart*, 182.

52. *UK Independent*, December 20, 2006.

53. *Washington Post*, December 19, 2006.

54. Rutenberg.

55. *Face the Nation*, CBS, December 24, 2006.

56. Bush, *Spoken from the Heart*, 382.

57. "First Lady Cancels Trip to Australia," *Los Angeles Times*, August 27, 2007.

58. "Laura Bush Has Surgery for Pinched Nerve," *New York Times*, September 8, 2007; "Successful Neck Surgery for First Lady Laura Bush," *Fox News*, September 8, 2007; Richard Tubb, personal interview.

59. Bush, *Spoken from the Heart*, 382; *Fox News*, September 8, 2007; *New York Times*, September 8, 2007; quote in personal communication with Emanuel Husu, M.D.

60. Chapter Fifteen.

61. *Fox News*, September 7, 2007.

Chapter Seventeen

1. Learning Center, American Diagnostic Corporation, "History of the Sphygmomanometer," http://adctoday.com/learning-center/about-sphygmomanometers/history-sphygmomanometer (accessed January 7, 2014).

2. Elizabeth G. Nabel and Eugene Braunwald, "A Tale of Coronary Artery Disease and Myocardial Infarction," *New England Journal of Medicine* 366 (January 5, 2012): 54–63.

3. "Cancer Facts and Figures for 2013," American Cancer Society, http://www.cancer.org/acs/groups/content/@epidemiologysurveilance/documents/document/acspc-036845.pdf (accessed January 7, 2014).

4. Steven W. Pray, "Meniere's Disease," Medscape Multispecialty, http://www.medscape.com/viewarticle/509085_2?pa=SYenn1R3OKikkgP%2FeFKQuu%2BC525D2cB2h2t4%2BvRiMnghdgfPvHvy8Pq7ORlu7IzpyDBGK1Oqidp4D2%2FHGprWCA%3D%3D (accessed January 7, 2014).

5. Jim Yeung Sai-Ching, "Graves' Disease," Medscape, http://emedicine.medscape.com/article/120619-overview#a0199 (accessed January 7, 2014).

6. Myra G. Gutin, *Barbara Bush: Presidential Matriarch* (Lawrence: University Press of Kansas, 2008), 20.

7. "Medical Ethics: Confidentiality and Duty to Report," University of Illinois at Chicago College of Medicine, Ethics in Clerkships, http://www.uic.edu/depts/mcam/ethics/confidentiality.htm (accessed January 3, 2014).

8. Connie Mariano, personal communication, August 12, 2011.

9. "Laura Bush: Skin Cancer 'No Big Deal,'" *Washington Post*, December 19, 2006.

10. James Joyner, "Laura Bush Skin Cancer Flap," Outside the Beltway, December 19, 2006, http://www.outsidethebeltway.com/laura_bush_skin_cancer_flap/ (accessed June 19, 2011).

11. "Medical Ethics, Confidentiality and Duty to Report."

12. Joyner.

13. Robert Pear, "Court Rules That First Lady Is 'De Facto' Federal Official," *New York Times*, June 23, 1993.

14. Carl Anthony, personal communication, July 28, 2013.

15. "Obama's NSA Plan to Pre-Empt Privacy Board," *USA Today*, January 9, 2014; Scott Horsley, NPR, "Civil Liberties Groups Call for Obama to Enact NSA Changes," http://www.npr.org/2013/12/19/25559764/civil-liberties-groups-call (accessed January 1, 2014); "N.Y. Judge: NSA Spying 'Imperils Civil Liberties of Every Citizen' but 'Legal,'" *New American*, December 27, 2013.

16. "Patient Privacy Goes Out the Window and into the Obamacare Data Hub," *American Thinker*, November 9, 2013; "Obamacare and Confidentiality," *Patheos*, September 18, 2013.

Bibliography

Books, Journals, Periodical Articles and Websites

"Absence Seizure." "Petit Mal Seizure." Mayo Clinic; http://www.mayoclinic.com/health/petit-mal-seizure/DS00216/DSEC (accessed April 5, 2012).

Adams, Abigail. Biography. http://www.first ladies.org/biographies/firstladies.aspx?bio graphy=2 (accessed October 10, 2013).

Adams, Anne. "Elizabeth Monroe: Elegance in the White House." History's Women, http://www.historyswomen.com/1stWomen/elizabeth monroe.html (accessed November 3, 2012).

Adams, Louisa. *The Adventures of a Nobody: Autobiographical Sketch Begun 1 July 1840.* Boston: Massachusetts Historical Society, 1956.

Adams, Louisa Catherine. *Diary and Biographical Writings of Louisa Catherine Adams.* Edited by Judith Graham, et al. Cambridge MA: Belknap Press, 2012.

Adams, Louisa Catherine Johnson. *Our White House: Looking In, Looking Out.* http://www.ourwhitehouse.org/flpages/ladams.html, (accessed January 3, 2012).

Allgor, Catherine. *Parlor Politics: In Which the Ladies of Washington Help Build a City and a Government.* Charlottesville: University of Virginia Press, 2000.

_____. *A Perfect Union: Dolley Madison and the Creation of the American Nation.* New York: Henry Holt, 2006.

Ambrose, Stephen E. *Eisenhower: Soldier, General of the Army, President-Elect, 1890–1952.* New York: Simon & Schuster, 1983.

American President: A Reference Resource. The Miller Center, University of Virginia. http://millercenter.org/president/events/12_06 (accessed October 19, 2011).

Ammon, Harry. *James Monroe: The Quest for National Identity.* Charlottesville: University of Virginia, 1990.

Anderson, Judith Icke. *William Howard Taft: An Intimate History.* New York: W.W. Norton, 1981.

Anthony, Carl Sferrazza. *America's First Families: An Inside View of 200 Years of Private Life in the White House.* New York: Simon & Schuster, 2000.

_____. *First Ladies: The Saga of the Presidents' Wives and Their Power, 1789–1961.* Vols. 1 and 2. New York: William Morrow, 1990.

_____. *Florence Harding: The First Lady, the Jazz Age, and the Death of America's Most Scandalous President.* New York: William Morrow, 1998.

_____. *Ida Saxton: The Early Life of Mrs. McKinley.* Canton, OH: National First Ladies' Library, 2007.

_____. *Nellie Taft: The Unconventional First Lady of the Ragtime Era.* New York: Harper, 2005.

_____, ed. *This Elevated Position: A Catalogue and Guide to the National First Ladies' Library.* Canton, OH: National First Ladies' Library, 2003.

Anthony, Catharine. *Dolly Madison: Her Life and Times.* Garden City, NY: Doubleday, 1949.

"Apraxia of Speech." National Institute on Deafness and Other Communicative Disorders. http://www.nidcd.nih.gov/health/voice/pages/apraxia.aspx (accessed November 23, 2013).

Ashley, Jeffrey S. "The Social and Political Influence of Betty Ford: Betty Bloomer Blossoms." *White House Studies* 101, no. 8 (Winter 2001).

Auchampaugh, Philip Gerald. *Robert Tyler: Southern Rights Champion, 1846–1866.* Duluth, MN: Himan Stein, 1934.

Baehrs, Oliver H. "The Medical History of President Ronald Reagan." *Journal of the American College* 178 (January 1994): 86–96.

Baharoon, Salim. "Tuberculosis of the Breast." *Annals of Thoracic Medicine* 3 (July–September): 110–114.

Bahn, Rebecca. "Unlocking the Mysteries of Graves' Ophthalmopathy." *Newsletter of the Graves' Disease Foundation* (Fall 2009).

"Bailey, James W." Obituary. *Journal of the Amer-*

ican Medical Association 54, no. 15 (April 9, 1910), 1229.

Baker, Ray Stannard. Interview with Cary Grayson, February 18–19, 1926. Ray Stannard Baker Collection.

Barry, John M. *The Great Influenza*. New York: Penguin, 2004.

Barton, David. *Benjamin Rush*. Aledo, TX: Wallbuilder, 1999.

Bauer, K. Jack. *Zachary Taylor*. Baton Rouge: Louisiana State University Press, 1985.

Beasley, N.J., and N.S. Jones. "Menière's Disease: Evolution of a Definition." *Journal of Laryngology and Otology* 110, no. 12 (1996 December): 1107–13.

Beidler, Anne E. *The Affliction of Mary Todd Lincoln*. Seattle: Coffeetown, 2009.

Bell, John J. "Nephroptosis: Its Causation, Symptoms and Radical Cure." *British Medical Journal* (May 26, 1923): 889–892.

Benze, James G., Jr. *Nancy Reagan*. Lawrence: University Press of Kansas, 2005.

"Bilious Fever." http://www.rootsweb.ancestry. com/~memigrat/diseases.html (accessed October 27, 2013).

Bishop, Joseph N. *1898 Medical and Surgical Register of the United States and Canada*. Detroit: R.L. Polk, 1898.

Bittinger, Cynthia D. *Grace Coolidge: Sudden Star*. New York: Nova History, 2005.

Bland, Pascal Brooke. "Edward Parker Davis." Jefferson Medical College Yearbook, 1937.

Blanton, Wyndham Bolling. *Medicine in Virginia in the Nineteenth Century*. Richmond: Garrett and Massie, 1933.

Boas, Norman F. *Jane M. Pierce, 1806–1863: The Pierce-Aiken Papers; Letters of Jane M. Pierce, Her Sister Mary M. Aiken, Their Family and President Franklin Pierce, with Biographies of Jane Pierce, Other Members of Her Family, and Genealogical Tables*. Stonington, CT: Seaport Autographs, 1983.

Boice, J. Morton. "Benzyl Benzoate." *New York Medical Journal* (December 13, 1919): 977–982.

Boller, Paul F. *Presidential Wives: An Anecdotal History*. New York: Oxford University Press, 1998.

Boller, Paul F., Jr. *Presidential Campaigns*. New York: Oxford University Press, 1985.

Boone, Joel. Boone Diary. Library of Congress, Boone Collection, Box 40.

Borneman, Walter R. *Polk: The Man Who Transformed the Presidency and America*. New York: Random House, 2008.

Brady, Patricia. *Martha Washington: An American Life*. Google Books. http://books.google.com/ books?id=vqCIBnJOwsC&pg=PT170&lpg (accessed October 11, 2011).

"Brain Hemorrhage." "Intracranial Bleeds." Johns Hopkins Symptoms and Remedies. http:// hopkins.portfolio.crushlovely.com/reference/ article/brain-hemorrhage-intracranial-bleeds (accessed October 29, 2012).

Braisted, William C., and William H. Bell. *The Life Story of Presley Marion Rixey*. Strasburg, VA: Shenandoah, 1930.

Brands, H.W. *TR: The Last Romantic*. New York: Basic, 1997.

BreastCancer.Org. http://www.breastcancer.org/ symptoms/understand_bc/statistics (accessed December 22, 2013).

Brennan, Mary C. *Pat Nixon: Embattled First Lady*. Lawrence: University Press of Kansas, 2011.

Breo, Dennis. "Tough Talk from the President's Physician." *Journal of the American Medical Association* 262, no. 9 (November 17, 1989): 2742–5.

Brodsky, Alyn. *Benjamin Rush: Patriot and Physician*. New York: St. Martin's, 2004.

Brown, Harry James, and Frederick D. Williams, eds. *The Diary of James A. Garfield*. Vol. 4, 1878–1881. Lansing: Michigan State University Press, 1981.

"Brown, Thomas Richardson." Obituary. *Transactions of the Association of American Physicians* 64 (1951): 5–6.

Bryan, Helen. *Martha Washington: First Lady of Liberty*. New York: John Wiley, 2002.

Bryant, Joseph Decatur. "Deaths." *Journal of the American Medical Association* 62 (1914): 1185.

Bumgarner, John R. *Sarah Childress Polk: A Biography of a Remarkable First Lady*. Jefferson, NC: McFarland, 1997.

Bumgarner, John R., M.D. *The Health of the Presidents: The 41 United States Presidents Through 1993 from a Physician's Point of View*. Jefferson, NC: McFarland, 1994.

Busey, Samuel. *Personal Reminiscences and Recollections of Forty-Six Years' Membership in the Medical Society of the District of Columbia*. Washington, D.C., 1895.

Bush, Barbara. *Barbara Bush: A Memoir*. New York: Scribner, 1994.

Bush, Barbara. *Reflections: Life After the White House*. New York: Scribner, 2003.

Bush, George W. *Decision Points*. New York: Crown, 2010.

Bush, Laura. *Spoken from the Heart*. New York: Scribner, 2010.

Busowki, Mary T., Burke A. Cunha, et al. *Yellow Fever*. http://emedicine.medscape.com/article/ 232244 (accessed October 20, 2011).

Byrd, Robert. "The Greenbrier." *Congressional Record*, 106th Congress, 1999–2000. http:// thomas.loc.gov/cgi-bin/query/z?r106:S10JY0– 0008 (accessed October 19, 2013).

Calhoun, Charles W. *Benjamin Harrison*. New York: Henry Holt, 2005.

"Cancer Facts and Figures for 2013." American Cancer Society. http://www.cancer.org/acs/groups/content/@epidemiologysurveilance/documents/document/acspc-036845.pdf (accessed January 7, 2014).

"Care of JFK by Dr. Max Jacobson, aka Dr. Feelgood." Suburban Emergency Management Project, Biot Report #678, January 7, 2010. http://www.semp.us/s/biot_reader.php?BiotID=678 (accessed August 17, 2011).

Caroli, Betty Boyd. *First Ladies.* New York: Oxford University Press, 1987.

_____. *First Ladies: From Martha Washington to Laura Bush.* New York: Oxford University Press, 2003.

Carrell, Jennifer. *The Speckled Monster: A Historical Tale of Battling Smallpox.* New York: Plume/Penguin, 2004.

Carter, Rosalynn. *First Lady from Plains.* Fayetteville: University of Arkansas Press, 1994.

Castro, Tony. *Mickey Mantle: America's Prodigal Son.* Washington, D.C.: Potomac, 2002.

Centers for Disease Control and Prevention. "Leading Causes of Death in Females United States." http://www.cdc.gov/women/lcod/2010/index.htm (accessed December 22, 2013).

Challinor, Joan Ridder. "Louisa Catherine Johnson Adams: The Price of Ambition." Ph.D. diss., American University, Washington, D.C., April 20, 1982.

Cheney, William Fitch. "Reminiscences of Three Eminent San Francisco Physicians." *California State Journal of Medicine* 8 (August 21, 1923): 325–7.

Chesley, Leon C. "The Origin of the Word 'Eclampsia.'" *Obstetrics and Gynecology* 39, no. 5 (May 1972): 802–4.

Chitwood, Oliver Perry. *John Tyler: Champion of the Old South.* New York: Russell and Russell, 1964.

Choate, Jean. *Eliza Johnson in Perspective.* New York: Nova History, 2006.

"Chronological History of ACS Recommendations for the Early Detection of Cancer." http://www.cancer.org/healthy/findcancerearly/cancerscreeningguidelines.html (accessed July 19, 2013).

Clark, Allen C. *Life and Letters of Dolly Madison.* Washington: W.F. Roberts, 1914.

Clark, James C. *The Murder of James A. Garfield: The President's Last Days and the Trial and Execution of His Assassin.* Jefferson, NC: McFarland, 1993.

Claxton, Jimmie Lou Sparkman. *Eighty-Eight Years with Sarah Polk.* New York: Vantage, 1972.

Clements, Kendrick A. *Woodrow Wilson: World Statesman.* Boston: Twayne, 1987.

"Cleveland, Frances." Biography. National First Ladies' Library. http://www.firstladies.org/biographies/firstladies.aspx?biography=23 (accessed December 16, 2013).

Clinton, Catherine. *Mrs. Lincoln: A Life.* New York: HarperCollins, 2009.

Clinton, Hillary. *Living History.* New York: Scribner, 2003.

"Colchester, Charles J." http://www.mrlincolnswhitehouse.org/content_inside.asp?ID=179&sub.htm. (accessed 12 February 2012).

Colditz, Graham A., Ruth Bonita, et al. "Cigarette Smoking and Risk of Stroke in Middle-Aged Women." *New England Journal of Medicine* 318 (April 14, 1988): 937–941.

Coleman, Elizabeth Tyler. *Priscilla Cooper Tyler and the American Scene, 1816–1889.* Birmingham: University of Alabama Press, 1955.

Collins, Gail. *William Henry Harrison.* New York: Henry Holt, 2012.

"Comparing Rheumatoid Arthritis and Osteoarthritis." http://www.webmd.com/rheumatoid-arthritis/tc/comparing-rheumatoid-arthritis-and-osteoarthritis-topic-overview (accessed October 24, 2013).

Consequences of United States Population Changes Report. Select Committee on Population, U.S. House of Representatives, 1979, p. 3

"Consumption." http://ask.yahoo.com/20020417.html (accessed 26 January 2012).

Coolidge, Grace. *Grace Coolidge: An Autobiography.* Edited by Lawrence Wilander and Robert Ferrell. Worland, WY: High Plains, 1992.

Cooper, John Milton, Jr. *Woodrow Wilson: A Biography.* New York: Random House, 2009.

Crapol, Edward. *John Tyler: The Accidental President.* Chapel Hill: University of North Carolina Press, 2006.

Cresson, W.P. *James Monroe.* Chapel Hill: University of North Carolina Press, 1946.

Crook, W.H. *Memories of the White House: The Home Life of Our Presidents from Lincoln to Roosevelt; Being Personal Recollections of Colonel W.H. Crook.* Boston: Little, Brown, 1911.

Crosby, Molly Caldwell. *The American Plague: The Untold Story of Yellow Fever, the Epidemic That Shaped Our History.* New York: Berkley, 2006.

Cunningham, Noble E., Jr. *The Presidency of James Monroe.* Lawrence: University Press of Kansas, 1996.

"Cushing, Clinton." Obituary. *Journal of the American Medical Association* 42, no. 21 (May 21, 1904): 1369.

Daniel, Thomas M. *Captain of Death: The Story of Tuberculosis.* Rochester, NY: University of Rochester Press, 1997.

David, Lester, and Irene David. *Ike and Mamie.* New York: G.P. Putnam's Sons, 1981.

Davidson, Jonathan R.T., and Kathryn M. Connor. "The Impairment of Presidents Pierce and

Coolidge after Traumatic Bereavement." *Comprehensive Psychiatry* 49 (2008): 413–419.

Davidson, Jonathan R.T., Kathryn M. Connor and Marvin Swartz. "Mental Illness in U.S. Presidents Between 1776 and 1974: A Review of Biographical Sources." *Journal of Nervous and Mental Disease* 194 (January 2006): 47–51.

Davis, C.A., and P. O'Brien. "Stroke and Pregnancy." *Journal Neurology, Neurosurgery and Psychiatry* 79 (2008): 240–245.

Davis, Edward Parker. *The Man and the Hour.* Privately published, 1919.

De Bow, J.D.B. *Mortality Statistics of the Seventh Census of the United States, 1850.* Washington, D.C.: A.O.P. Nicholson, 1855.

Decatur, Stephen, and Tobias Lear. *Private Affairs of George Washington, from the Records and Accounts of Tobias Lear, Esquire, His Secretary.* New York: Da Capo, 1969.

"Deep Vein Thrombosis (DVT)." Mayo Clinic. http://www.mayoclinic.com/health/deep-vein-thrombois/DS01005 (accessed August 26, 2013).

"Deep Vein Thrombosis Overview." Society of Interventional Radiology. http://www.sirweb.org/patients/deep-vein-thrombosis/ (accessed August 26, 2013).

Degregorio, William. *The Complete Book of U.S. Presidents.* New York: Wings Books, 1993.

Deppisch, Ludwig M. "Homeopathic Medicine and Presidential Health." *PHAROS* 60, no. 4 (Fall 1997): 5–10.

_____. "President Cleveland's Secret Operation." *PHAROS* 58, no. 3 (Summer 1995): 11–16.

_____. *The White House Physician: A History from Washington to George W. Bush.* Jefferson, NC: McFarland, 2007.

DeToledo, John C., Bruno B. Toledo and Meredith Lowe. "The Epilepsy of First Lady Ida Saxton McKinley." *Southern Medical Journal* 93, no. 3 (March 2000), 267–271.

Dhawan, Vivek, et al. "Long-term Effects of Repeated Pregnancies (Multiparity) on Blood Pressure Regulation." *Cardiovascular Research* 64 (2004): 179–186.

Donald, David Herbert. *Lincoln.* New York: Simon & Schuster, 1995.

Dorland's Illustrated Medical Dictionary. 23rd ed. Philadelphia: W.B. Saunders, 1957.

Dormandy, Thomas. *The White Death: A History of Tuberculosis.* London: Hambledon, 1999.

Dubos, Rene, and Jean Dubos. *The White Plague: Tuberculosis, Man, and Society.* New Brunswick, NJ: Rutgers University Press, 1987.

Dubovoy, Sina. *Ellen A. Wilson: The Woman Who Made a President.* New York: Nova History, 2003.

Dubriwny, Tasha N. "Constructing Breast Cancer in the News: Betty Ford and the Evolution of the Breast Cancer Patient." *Journal of Communication Inquiry* 33, no. 2 (April 2009): 104–125.

Duffy, John. "The Impact of Malaria on the South." In *Disease and Distinctiveness in the American South,* edited by Todd Savitt and James Harvey Young. Knoxville: University of Tennessee Press, 1988.

Dunlap, Annette. *Frank: The Story of Frances Folsom Cleveland, America's Youngest First Lady.* Albany: State University of New York Press, 2009.

Duran-Reynals, M.L. *The Fever Bark Tree: The Pageant of Quinine.* Garden City, NY: Doubleday, 1946.

Ebrahim, Shah, and Rowan Harwood. *Stroke: Epidemiology, Evidence and Clinical Practice.* Oxford: Oxford University Press, 1999.

Edelson, Ed. "Stroke Risk in Women Smokers Goes Up by Each Cigarette." http://health.usnews.com/health-news/family-health/heart/article/2008/08/14/stroke-risk-in-women-smokers (accessed 8 September 2012).

Edith Bolling Wilson Birthplace and Museum. "The Genealogy of Edith Bolling Wilson." http://edithbollingwilson.org/the-genealogy-of-edith-bolling-wilson/ (accessed March 4, 2013).

Egido, Jose Antonio, Olga Castillo, et al. "Is Psycho-Physical Stress a Risk Factor for Stroke? A Case-Control Study." *Journal of Neurology Neurosurgery Psychiatry* 10 (September 2012): 1136.

Eisenhower, John S.D., ed. *Letters to Mamie.* Garden City, NY: Doubleday, 1978.

_____. *Zachary Taylor.* New York: Henry Holt, 2008.

Eisenhower, Julie Nixon. *Pat Nixon: The Untold Story.* New York: Simon & Schuster, 1986.

_____. *Special People.* New York: Simon & Schuster, 1977.

Eisenhower, Mamie. Interview by Dr. John Wickman for the Eisenhower Library, August 15, 1972: OH #12, 92–3.

_____. Medical Record. Pueblo Hospital, 1931.

_____. Medical Record. Walter Reed Army Medical Center, January 4, 1946, George P. Robb, M.D.

_____. Medical Records, Walter Reed Army Medical Center, 1951–1957, Thomas Mattingly, M.D.

"Eisenhower, Mamie." Biography. National First Ladies' Library. http://www.firstladies.org/biographies/firstladies.aspx?biography=35 (accessed March 15, 2013).

Eisenhower, Susan. *Mrs. Ike.* New York: Farrar, Straus and Giroux, 1996.

Ellis, Joseph J. *First Family: Abigail and John Adams.* New York: Alfred A. Knopf, 2010.

Ellison, David L. *Healing Tuberculosis in the Woods: Medicine and Science at the End of the*

Nineteenth Century. Westport, CT: Greenwood, 1994.

Emerson, Jason. *The Madness of Mary Lincoln.* Carbondale: Southern Illinois University Press, 2007.

Entezami, Pouya, et al. "Historical Perspective on the Etiology of Rheumatoid Arthritis." *Hand Clinics* no 1 (February 27, 2011): 1–10.

"Epilepsy Across the Spectrum: Promoting Health and Understanding." Consensus Report, Institute of Medicine, March 30, 2012.

"Erysipelas." Pubmed Health, National Library of Medicine. http://www.ncbi.nlm.nih.gov/public medhealth/PMH0001643/ (accessed January 19, 2012).

Evans, W.A. *Mrs. Abraham Lincoln: A Study of Her Personality and Her Influence on Lincoln.* Carbondale: Southern Illinois University Press, 2010.

Ferling, John. *John Adams.* New York: Henry Holt, 1992.

Ferrell, Robert H. *Grace Coolidge: The People's Lady in Silent Cal's White House.* Lawrence, KS: Vantage, 2008.

_____. *Ill-Advised: Presidential Health and Public Trust.* Columbia: University of Missouri Press, 1992.

_____. *The Strange Deaths of President Harding.* Columbia: University of Missouri Press, 1996.

_____, ed. *The Eisenhower Diaries.* New York: W.W. Norton, 1981.

Fett, Sharla M. *Working Cures: Healing, Health, and Power on Southern Slave Plantations.* Chapel Hill: University of North Carolina Press, 2002.

Fields, Joseph E., ed. *"Worthy Partner": The Papers of Martha Washington.* Westport, CT: Greenwood, 1994.

Fields, William S., and Noreen A. Lemak. *A History of Stroke: Its Recognition and Treatment.* New York: Oxford University Press, 1989.

"Fillmore, Abigail." Biography. National First Ladies' Library. http://www.firstladies.org/biographies/firstladies.aspx?biography=14 (accessed October 29, 2013).

Finney, J.M.T. *A Surgeon's Life: The Autobiography of J.M.T. Finney.* New York: G.P. Putnam's Sons, 1940.

"Finney, John Miller Turpin." Obituary. *Annals of Surgery* 119, no. 4 (April 1944), 616–621.

Fix, Julie K. "Elizabeth Monroe." In *American First Ladies: Their Lives and Their Legacy,* 2d ed., edited by Lewis L. Gould. New York: Routledge, 2001.

Flexner, James Thomas. *Washington: The Indispensable Man.* New York: Signet New American Library, 1984.

Ford, Betty, with Chris Chase. *Betty: A Glad Awakening.* New York: Jove, 1988.

_____. *The Times of My Life.* New York: Ballantine, 1978.

"Ford, Betty." http:///www.fofweb.com/History/HistRefMain.asp?Pin=firstladies34 (accessed July 26, 2013).

"The Fox Sisters: Spiritualism's Unlikely Founders." http://www.historynet.com/the-fox-sisters-spiritualisms-unlikely-founders.htm (accessed 12 February 2012).

Francis, Samuel W. "Biographical Sketch of General R.C. Wood." *Medical and Surgical Reporter* 20 (April 10, 1869): 275–6.

Freeman, Douglas Southall. *Washington.* New York: Simon & Schuster, 1992.

Freud, Sigmund, and William C. Bullitt. *Thomas Woodrow Wilson: A Psychological Study.* Boston: Houghton Mifflin, 1966.

Friedlander, Walter J. "The Rise and Fall of Bromide Therapy in Epilepsy." *Arch Neurol* 57 (December 2000): 1782–5.

Gara, Larry. *The Presidency of Franklin Pierce.* Lawrence: University Press of Kansas, 1991.

"Gardner." In *Directory of Deceased American Physicians, 1804–1929,* vol. 1. Edited by Arthur Wayne Hafner, et al. Chicago: American Medical Association, 1993.

Geer, Emily Apt. *First Lady: The Life of Lucy Webb Hayes.* Kent, OH: Kent State University Press, 1984.

"Gibbons, Henry, Jr." Obituary. *Journal of the American Medical Association* 57, no. 16 (October 14, 1911): 1300.

Gibson, Paul. "Hypertension and Pregnancy." http://emedicine.medscape.com/article/261435-overview (accessed 21 December 2011).

Gilbert, Robert E. *The Tormented President: Calvin Coolidge, Death, and Clinical Depression.* Westport, CT: Praeger, 2003.

Gould, Lewis L. *American First Ladies: Their Lives and Legacy,* 2d ed. New York: Routledge, 2001.

_____. *Helen Taft: Our Musical First Lady.* Lawrence: University Press of Kansas, 2010.

_____. *Lady Bird Johnson: Our Environmentalist First Lady.* Lawrence: University Press of Kansas, 1999.

_____, ed. *My Dearest Nellie: The Letters of William Howard Taft to Helen Herron Taft, 1909–1912.* Lawrence: University Press of Kansas, 2011.

Grant, Julia Dent. *The Personal Memoirs of Julia Dent Grant.* Carbondale: Southern Illinois University Press, 1975.

"Grant, Julia." Biography: National First Ladies' Library. http://www.firstladies.org/biographies/firstladies.aspx?biography=19 (accessed 19 February 2013).

"Grant, Ulysses S." Missouri Civil War Sesquicentennial. http://mocivilwar150.com/history/figure/300 (accessed December 3, 2011).

"Graves' Disease." "Diffuse Thyrotoxic Goiter." PubMed Health. http://www.nlm.nih.gov/pub medhealth/PMH0001398/ (accessed 5 June 2011).

Graves' Disease Foundation. Onsite Support Bulletin Board, post by Dianne Smith November 15, 1996. http://ngdf.org/phpBB/ngdf/view topic.php?f+4&t+372 (accessed June 7, 2011).

Graves' Disease Foundation: Onsite Support Bulletin Board, posts by Shannon Gwen June 8, 1997. http:/ngdf.org/phpBB/ngdf/viewtopic. php?f=4&t=3185 (accessed June 7, 2011).

"Graves, Robert James, 1796–1853: Milestones in European Thyroidology." European Thyroid Association. http://www.eurothyroid.com/about/met/graves.php (accessed 9 June 2011).

Grayson, Cary. *Woodrow Wilson: An Intimate Memoir*. 2d ed. Washington: Potomac, 1960.

Greene, John Robert. *Betty Ford: Candor and Courage in the White House*. Lawrence: University Press of Kansas, 2004.

Groopman, Jerome. "A Child in Time." *New Yorker*, October 24, 2011.

Gurewitsch, David. The Eleanor Roosevelt Papers Project. http://www.gwu.edu/-erpapers/teach inger/glossary/gurewitsch-david.cfm (accessed June 20, 2013).

Gutin, Myra G. *Barbara Bush: Presidential Matriarch*. Lawrence: University Press of Kansas, 2008.

Hahnemannian Monthly. Homeopathic Medical Society of the State of Pennsylvania, May 1901.

Hall, Marshall. *The Threatenings of Apoplexy and Paralysis, etc.* The Cronian Lectures, delivered at the Royal College of Physicians, March 1851.

Hamilton, Holman. *Zachary Taylor: Soldier in the White House*. Indianapolis: Bobbs-Merrill, 1951.

_____. *Zachary Taylor: Soldier of the Republic*. Indianapolis: Bobbs-Merrill, 1941.

"Hardin, Bernard Lauriston." Obituary. *Journal of the American Medical Association* 107, no. 2 (July 11, 1936): 145.

"Harrison, Anna." Biography. National First Ladies' Library. http://www.firstladies.org/bio graphies/firstladies.aspx?biography=9 (accessed October 27, 2013).

Hart, Craig. *A Genealogy of the Wives of American Presidents and Their First Two Generations of Descent*. Jefferson, NC: McFarland, 2004.

Harvey, A. McGehee. "Medical Students on the March: Brown, MacCallum and Opie." *Johns Hopkins Medical Journal* 134 (June 1974): 330–4.

_____, Gert H. Brieger, Susan L. Abrams and Victor A. McKusick. *A Model of Its Kind: A Centennial History of Medicine at Johns Hopkins*, vol. 1. Baltimore: Johns Hopkins University Press, 1989.

"Hayes, Lucy." Biography. National First Ladies' Library. http://www.firstladies.org/biographies/

firstladies.aspx?biography=20 (accessed 19 February 2013).

Heckscher, August. *Woodrow Wilson: A Biography*. New York: Macmillan, 1991.

Heinrichs, Ann. *Louisa Catherine Johnson Adams*. New York: Children's, 1998.

Heller, Milton F., Jr. *The Presidents' Doctor: An Insider's View of Three First Families*. New York: Vantage, 2000.

Herron, Nancy L. *Ida Saxton McKinley: Indomitable Spirit or Autocrat of the Sickbed* in *Inventing a Voice: The Rhetoric of American First Ladies of the Twentieth Century*. Edited by Molly Meijer Wertheimer. Lanham, MD: Rowman and Littlefield, 2004.

Heymann, C. David. *Bobby and Jackie: A Love Story*. New York: Atria, 2009.

_____. *A Woman Named Jackie*. New York: Carol, 1994.

Hill, Clint. *Mrs. Kennedy and Me*. New York: Gallery, 2012.

Hinsdale, Burke A., and Isaac Newton Demmon. *History of the University of Michigan*. Ann Arbor: University of Michigan Press, 1906.

"Hirschfelder, Joseph Oakland." In *Directory of Deceased American Physicians, 1804–1929*, vol. 1. Edited by Arthur Wayne Hafner, et al. Chicago: American Medical Association, 1993.

Hirschhorn, Norbert, and Robert G. Feldman. "Mary Lincoln's Final Illness: A Medical and Historical Reappraisal." *Journal of the History of Medicine* 54 (October 1999): 511–542.

"The History and Stigma of Epilepsy." Introduction. *Epilepsia* 44 (Suppl. 6, 2003): 12–14.

History of the Medical Society of the District of Columbia. Washington, D.C: Medical Society of the District of Columbia, 1909.

Holloway, Laura C. *The Ladies of the White House; or, In the Home of the Presidents: Being a Complete History of the Social and Domestic Lives of the Presidents from Washington to the Present Time, 1789–1881*. Philadelphia: Bradley, 1881.

Holt, Marilyn Irvin. *Mamie Doud Eisenhower: The General's First Lady*. Lawrence: University Press of Kansas, 2007.

Holton, Woody. *Abigail Adams*. New York: Free, 2009.

Homeopathic Recorder. International Hahnemannian Association, 1892, pp. 271–2.

Honyman, Robert. Virginia Center for Digital Research at University of Virginia. http://www2. vcdh.virginia.edu/xslt/servlet/XSLTServlet? xml=/xml_docs/Dolley/Glossary.xml&xsl=/ xml_docs/Dolley/glossary.xsl&area= glossaryr#H (accessed October 2011).

Hoogenboom, Ari. *Rutherford B. Hayes: Warrior and President*. Lawrence: University Press of Kansas, 1995.

"Hoover, Lou." Biography. National First Ladies'

Library. http://www.firstladies.org/biographies/ firstladies.aspx?biography=32 (accessed May 8, 2013).

Horsley, Scott. "Civil Liberties Groups Call For Obama to Enact NSA Changes." NPR, http:// www.npr.org/2013/12/19/25559764/civil-liberties-groups-call (accessed January 1, 2014).

Humphreys, Margaret. *Malaria, Poverty, Race and Public Health in the United States.* Baltimore: Johns Hopkins University Press, 2001.

"Hunt, Harriot Kezla, 1805–1875." http://www. jiffynotes.com/a_study_guides/book_notes_ add/amer_000 (accessed January 16, 2012).

Hysteria. http://en.wikipedia.org/wiki/Female_ hysteria (accessed November 5, 2013).

"Irish in New York City." http://www.irishinnyc. freeservers.com/custom.html (accessed November 20, 2011).

Jacoby, Ann, and Joan K. Austin. "Social Stigma for Adults and Children with Epilepsy." *Epilepsia* 48 (Suppl. S9, December 2007): 6–9.

"Jane Pierce." *American President: A Reference Resource.* http://millercenter.org/president/ pierce/essays/firstlady (accessed January 2, 2012).

Jay, Venita. "A Portrait in History: Prosper Menière." *Archives of Pathology* (February 2000), 124, 192.

Jerrard-Dunne, Paula, Geoffrey Cloud, Ahmad Hassan and Hugh S. Markus: "Evaluating the Genetic Component of Ischemic Stroke Subtypes: A Family History Study." *Stroke* 34 (2003): 1364–1369.

"Johnson, Eliza." Biography. National First Ladies' Library. http://www.firstladies.org/biographies/ firstladies.aspx?biography=18 (accessed 27 March 2012).

"Johnson, Eliza." NNDB. http://www.nndb.com/ people/091/000127707/ (accessed January 26, 2010).

Joyner, James. "Laura Bush Skin Cancer Flap." Outside the Beltway, December 19, 2006. http:// www.outsidethebeltway.com/laura_bush_ skin_cancer_flap/ (accessed June 19, 2011).

"Kahlo, George Dwight." Obituary. *Journal of the American Medical Association* 66, no. 9 (February 26, 1916): 671.

Kaplan, Louis. *The Strange Case of William Mumler, Spirit Photographer.* Minneapolis: University of Minnesota Press, 2008.

Keckley, Elizabeth. *Behind the Scenes; or, Thirty Years as a Slave, and Four Years in the White House.* Los Angeles: Indo-European, 2011.

Keko, Don. "Louisa Adams: The Reclusive First Lady." http://www.examiner.com/article/louisa-adams-the-reclusive-first-lady (accessed January 3, 2012).

Kelly, Howard A. *A Cyclopedia of American Medical Biography Comprising the Lives of Eminent Deceased Physicians and Surgeons from 1610 to 1910.* New York: W.B. Saunders, 1920.

_____, and Walter L. Burrage. *American Medical Biographies.* Baltimore: Norman, Remington, 1920.

"Kennedy, Jackie." "Female Celebrity Smoking List." http://smokingsides.com/asfs?K/Kennedy. html (accessed April 26, 2013).

Kennedy, Jacqueline. *Historic Conversations with Arthur Schlesinger, Jr., 1964.* New York: Hyperion, 2011.

"Kennedy, Jacqueline." Biography, National First Ladies' Library. http://www.firstladies.org/ biographies/firstladies.aspx?biography=36 (accessed April 15, 2013).

Kent, Deborah. *Jane Means Appleton Pierce.* New York: Children's, 1998.

Ketcham, Ralph. *James Madison.* Charlottesville: University of Virginia Press, 1990.

Kirschmann, Anne Taylor. *A Vital Force: Women in American Homeopathy.* New Brunswick, NJ: Rutgers University Press, 2004.

Kittner, Steven J., et al. "Pregnancy and the Risk of Stroke." *New England Journal of Medicine* 335 (September 12, 1996): 768–774.

Knab, Douglas. *ABMS Compendium of Certified Medical Specialists*, vol. 3. Evanston, IL: American Board of Medical Specialties, 1986–7.

Knoles, George H. *The Presidential Campaign and Election of 1892.* Stanford: Stanford University Press, 1942.

Koblentz, Stuart J. *Marion.* Charleston, SC: Arcadia, 2004.

Kumar, Seema, Sarah Nadeem, et al. "A Stimulatory TSH Receptor Antibody Enhances Adipogenesis via Phosphoinositide 3-Kinase Activation in Orbital Preadipocytes from Patients with Graves' Ophthalmopathy." *Journal of Molecular Endocrinology* 46, no. 3 (June 2011): 156–163.

Lane, Dorothy S., Anthony P. Polednak and Mary Ann Burg. "The Impact of Media Coverage of Nancy Reagan's Experience on Breast Cancer Screening." *American Journal of Public Health* 79, no. 11 (November 1989): 1551–2.

"Lane, Harriet." Biography. National First Ladies' Library. http://www.firstladies.org/biographies/ firstladies.aspx?biography=16 (accessed February 3, 2014).

Lasby, Clarence G. *Eisenhower's Heart Attack.* Lawrence: University Press of Kansas, 1997.

Lash, Joseph P. *Eleanor and Franklin.* New York: W.W. Norton, 1971.

_____. *Eleanor: The Years Alone.* New York: W.W. Norton, 1972.

"Laudanum." http://www.reference.com/browse/ laudanum (accessed March 8, 2012).

"Laudanum." Wikipedia, http://en.wikipedia.org/ wiki/Laudanum (accessed March 8, 2012).

"Laudanum. What Is Laudanum?" http://www.

laudanumonline.com.drupal/content/what-laudanum (accessed March 8, 2012).

Leahy, Christopher. "Torn Between Family and Politics: John Tyler's Struggle for Balance." *Virginia Magazine of History and Biography* 114, no. 3 (2006): 322–355.

Leamer, Laurence. *The Kennedy Women.* New York: Villard, 1994.

Leaming, Barbara. *Mrs. Kennedy: The Missing History of the Kennedy Years.* New York: Free, 2001.

Learning Center, American Diagnostic Corporation. "History of the Sphygmomanometer." http://adctoday.com/learning-center/about-sphygmomanometers/history-sphygmomanometer (accessed January 7, 2014).

"Leech." Wikipedia, http:en.wikipedia.org/wiki/Leech (accessed 27 February 2012).

Leech, Margaret. *In the Days of McKinley.* New York: Harper, 1959.

Lerner, B.H. "Revisiting the Death of Eleanor Roosevelt: Was the Diagnosis of Tuberculosis Missed?" *International Journal of Tuberculosis and Lung Disease* 5, no. 12 (December 2001): 1080–5.

Lerner, Barron. "Charting the Death of Eleanor Roosevelt." http://www.fathom.com/feature/35672/index.html (accessed March 20, 2012).

Lerner, Barron H. "What Can We Learn from Eleanor Roosevelt's Death?" http://www.huffingtonpost.com/barron-h-lerner/eleanor-roosevelt-end.html (accessed June 18, 2013).

Lertzman, Richard A., and William J. Birnes. *Dr. Feelgood.* New York: Skyhorse, 2013.

Levin, Phyllis Lee. *Abigail Adams.* New York: St. Martin's, 1987.

"Life Expectancy by Age, 1850–2004." http://www.info please.com/ipa/A0005140.html (accessed June 18, 2009).

"Locock, Sir Charles." Obituary. *British Medical Journal* (July 31, 1875): 151.

"Louisa Adams: The Chocoholic Resurfaces." My Year with the First Ladies, http://firstladyblog.typepad.com/my-year-with-the-first-la/2011/04/first-ladies-history-louisa-adams-the-chocoholic-resurfaces.html (accessed January 3, 2012).

Lungren, John C., and John C. Lungren, Jr. *Healing Richard Nixon.* Lexington: University of Kentucky Press, 2003.

Lustig, L.R., and A. Lalwani. "The History of Menière's Disease." *Otolaryngologic Clinics of North America* 30, no. 6 (December 1997): 917–45.

Lyons, Albert S., and R. Joseph Petrucelli, II. *Medicine: An Illustrated History.* New York: Harry C. Abrams, 1987.

"Madison, Dolley." Biography. National First Ladies' Library. http://www.firstladies.org/bio graphies/firstladies.aspx?biography=4 (accessed February 9, 2010).

Magro, G., et al. "Clinico-Pathological Features of Breast Myxoma: Report of a Case with Histogenetic Considerations." *Virchows Arch* 456, no. 5 (May 2010): 581–6.

Mahan, Russell L. *Lucy Webb Hayes: A First Lady by Example.* New York: Nova Science, 2011.

"Malaria." Johns Hopkins School of Public Health, http://www.jhsph.edu/_archive/2009.07.10_malaria/Malaria_Background.html#US (accessed 2010).

"Malaria." World Health Organization, October 2011. http://www.who.int/mediacentre/factsheets/fs094/en/index.html (accessed November 19, 2011).

"Malaria Mortality Rates Remain Unacceptably High, Senior UN Official Says." UN News Centre, http://www.un.org/apps/news/story.asp?NewsID=34465&Cr=malaria (accessed November 19, 2011).

Mariano, Connie. *The White House Doctor: My Patients Were Presidents; A Memoir.* New York: St. Martin's, 2010.

Martin, James N., Jr., Brad D. Thigpen, et al. "Stroke and Severe Preeclampsia and Eclampsia: A Paradigm Shift Focusing on Systolic Blood Pressure." *Obstetrics and Gynecology* 105, no. 2 (February 2005): 246–253.

Martin, Joel, and William J. Birnes. *The Haunting of the Presidents: A Paranormal History of the US Presidency.* Old Saybrook, CT: Konecky and Konecky, 2003.

Mattern, David B., and Holly C. Shulman, eds. *The Selected Letters of Dolley Payne Madison.* Charlottesville: University of Virginia Press, 2003.

"Mattingly, Thomas William." Brigadier General, United States Army. http://www.arlington cemetery.net/tmatting.htm (accessed June 14, 2010).

May, Gary. *John Tyler.* New York: Times/Henry Holt, 2008.

Maynard, Nettie Colburn. *Séances in Washington: Abraham Lincoln and Spiritualism During the Civil War.* Toronto: Ancient Wisdom, 2011.

"Mayo, Charles H." Obituary. *British Medical Journal* (June 3, 1959): 159–160.

McAdoo, Eleanor Wilson. *The Priceless Gift: The Love Letters of Woodrow Wilson and Ellen Axson Wilson.* Westport, CT: Greenwood, 1962.
_____. *The Woodrow Wilsons.* New York: Macmillan, 1937.

McCallops, James S. *Edith Bolling Gault Wilson: The Unintended President.* New York: Nova History, 2003.

McCullough, David. *John Adams.* New York: Simon & Schuster, 2001.

McFeely, William S. *Grant: A Biography.* New York: W.W. Norton, 1982.

McIntire, Ross T. *White House Physician.* New York: G.P. Putnam's Sons, 1946.

McIntosh, Shona J., and Rose Anne Kenny. "Carotid Sinus Syndrome in the Elderly." *Journal of the Royal Society of Medicine* 187 (December 1994): 798–800.

"McKinley, Ida." Biography. National First Ladies' Library, http:www.firstladies.org/biographies/firstladies.aspx?biography=25 (accessed June 25, 2010).

McMillen, Sally G. *Motherhood in the Old South: Pregnancy, Childbirth and Infant Rearing.* Baton Rouge: Louisiana State University Press, 1990.

McWhinnie, Douglas L., and David N.H. Hamilton. "The Rise and Fall of Surgery for the 'Floating' Kidney." *British Medical Journal* 288 (March 17, 1984): 845–7.

Medical and Surgical Register of the United States and Canada. Detroit: R.L. Polk, 1917.

"Medical Ethics." "Confidentiality and Duty to Report." University of Illinois at Chicago College of Medicine, Ethics in Clerkships. http://www.uic.edu/depts/mcam/ethics/confidentiality.htm (accessed January 3, 2014).

Medical Mirror 3 (1892), 471–2; 514.

"Menière's Disease." http://www.entnet.org/HealthInfomration/menieresDisease.cfm (accessed March 19, 2013).

Menière's Society. "Managing Menière's Disease." http://www.menieres.org.uk/managing_md_the_task.html (accessed March 19, 2013).

Millard, Candice. *Destiny of the Republic: A Tale of Madness, Medicine and the Murder of a President.* New York: Doubleday, 2011.

Miller, Kristie. *Ellen and Edith: Woodrow Wilson's First Ladies.* Lawrence: University Press of Kansas, 2010.

Miller, Virginia. "Dr. Thomas Miller and His Times." *Records of the Columbia Historical Society* 3 (1900), 303–323.

"Mind Games: A Look at Phrenology in the 1830s." Skeptic Report, http:/www.skepticreport.com/sr/?p=558 (accessed December 15, 2011).

Minor, Michael, and Larry F. Vrzalik. "A Study in Tragedy: Jane Means Pierce, First Lady." *Manuscripts* 40, no. 3 (Summer 1988), 177–89.

Mitchell, Stewart, ed. *New Letters of Abigail Adams, 1788–1901.* Boston: Houghton Mifflin, 1947.

Monroe, Dan. *The Republican Vision of John Tyler.* College Station: Texas A&M University Press, 2003.

"Monroe, Elizabeth." Biography. National First Ladies' Library, http://www.firstladies.org/biographies/firstladies.aspx?biography=5 (accessed November 3, 2012, October 23, 2013).

"Monroe, Elizabeth." Facts on File History Database Center, http://www.fofweb.com/History/MainPrintPage.asp?iPin=firstladies (accessed November 3, 2012).

Monroe, James. *The Autobiography of James Monroe,* edited by Stuart Gerry Brown. Syracuse, NY: Syracuse University Press, 1959.

_____. *The Papers of James Monroe, 1776–1794.* Edited by Daniel Preston. Westport, CT: Greenwood, 2003.

Moore, Anne Chieko. *Caroline Lavinia Scott Harrison.* New York: Nova History, 2005.

Moore, James N., Jr. "Stroke and Severe Preeclampsia and Eclampsia: A Paradigm Shift Focusing on Systolic Blood Pressure." *Obstetrics and Gynecology* 106, no. 2 (February 2005): 246–254.

Morgan, George. *The Life of James Monroe.* Boston: Small, Maynard, 1921.

Morris, Edmund. *Colonel Roosevelt.* New York: Random House, 2010.

Morris, Sylvia Jukes. *Edith Kermit Roosevelt: Portrait of a First Lady.* New York: Coward, McCann and Geoghegan, 1980.

Mowbray, Jay Henry, ed. "Joseph Norton Bishop." In *Representative Men of New York,* vol. 1. New York: New York Press, 1898.

Murphy, David. *A Texas Bluebonnet: Lady Bird Johnson.* New York: Nova Science, 2011.

Murphy, Jim. *An American Plague: The True and Terrifying Story of the Yellow Fever Epidemic of 1793.* New York: Clarion, 2003.

Mushet, William Boyd. *So-Called Nervous Apoplexy, on Congestion of the Brain and Serous Effusion.* London: John Churchill, 1866.

Myers, J. Arthur. *Tuberculosis: A Half Century of Study and Conquest.* St. Louis: Warren H. Green, 1970.

Nabel, Elizabeth G., and Eugene Braunwald. "A Tale of Coronary Artery Disease and Myocardial Infarction." *New England Journal of Medicine* 366 (January 5, 2012): 54–63.

Nagel, Paul C. *The Adams Women: Abigail and Louisa Adams, Their Sisters and Daughters.* New York: Oxford University Press, 1987.

_____. *Descent from Glory: Four Generations of the John Adams Family.* New York: Oxford University Press, 1983.

_____. *John Quincy Adams: A Public Life, a Private Life.* Cambridge, MA: Harvard University Press, 1997.

Nancy Reagan Breast Center. Simi Valley Hospital, http://www.simivalleyhospital.com/services/cancer/Nancy_Reagan.php (accessed July 14, 2013).

National Health Care Conference. www.irishhealth.com/article.html?id=14108 (accessed February 11, 2009).

Nattinger, Ann Butler, et al. "Effect of Nancy Reagan's Mastectomy on Choice of Surgery for Breast Cancer by U.S. Women." *Journal of the*

American Medical Association 279, no. 10 (1998): 762–766.

Neely, Mark E., Jr., and R. Gerald McMurtry. *The Insanity File.* Carbondale: Southern Illinois University Press, 1986.

Nelson, Anson, and Fanny Nelson. *Memorials of Sarah Childress Polk.* Spartanburg, SC: Reprint, 1980.

Nevins, Allan. *Grover Cleveland: A Study in Courage.* New York: Dodd, Mead, 1948.

Nichols, Roy Franklin. *Franklin Pierce: Young Hickory of the Granite Hills.* Norwalk, CT: Easton, 1931.

"N.Y. Judge: NSA Spying 'Imperils Civil Liberties of Every Citizen' but 'Legal,'" *New American,* December 27, 2013.

"Obamacare and Confidentiality," Patheos.com, September 18, 2013.

O'Brien, Michael. *Mrs. Adams in Winter.* New York: Farrar, Straus and Giroux, 2010.

Packard, Jerrold. *The Lincolns in the White House: Four Years That Shattered a Family.* New York: St. Martin's Griffin, 2005.

Packard, Randall M. *The Making of a Tropical Disease: A Short History of Malaria.* Baltimore: Johns Hopkins University Press, 2007.

"Patient Privacy Goes Out the Window and into the Obamacare Data Hub." American Thinker, November 9, 2013.

Paulson, George. "James Fairchild Baldwin, MD, 1850–1930: An Extraordinary Surgeon." Medical Heritage Center at Ohio State University. *House Call* 9, no. 1 (Fall 1905), 1–2.

Peskin, Allan. *Garfield.* Kent, OH: Kent State University Press, 1978.

Peterson, Barbara Bennett. *Sarah Childress Polk: First Lady of Tennessee and Washington.* New York: Nova History, 2002.

Peterson, Helen Stone. "First Lady at 22." *Virginia Cavalcade* 11 (1961), 14–19.

Peterson, Norma Lois. *The Presidencies of William Henry Harrison and John Tyler.* Lawrence: University Press of Kansas, 1989.

"Phrenology, the History of." http:/www.phrenology.org/intro.html (accessed December 15, 2011).

"Pierce, Jane." Biography. National First Ladies' Library, http://www.firstladies.org/biographies/firstladies.aspx?biography=15 (accessed February 14, 2011).

"Pope, Gustavus William." In *History of Homeopathy Biographies,* by Sylvain Cazalet. http://www.homeoint.org/history/bio/p/popegw.htm (accessed 13 February 2011).

"Portmann, E. Odo." In *Directory of Deceased American Physicians, 1804–1929,* vol. 2. Edited by Arthur Wayne Hafner, et al. Chicago: American Medical Association, 1993, p. 1244.

"Postpartum Depression." MayoClinic.com, http://www.mayoclinic.com/health/postpartum-depression/DS00546 (accessed April 25, 2013).

"Potassium Bromide." Wikipedia, http://en.wikipedia.org/wiki/Potassium_bromide (accessed July 1, 2010).

Pray, Steven W. "Ménière's Disease." Medscape, http://www.medscape.com/viewarticle/509085_2?pa=SYenn1R3OKikkgP%2FeFKQuu%2BC525D2cB2h2t4%2BvRiMnghdgfPvHvy8Pq7ORlu7IzpyDBGK1Oqidp4D2%2FHGprWCA%3D%3D (accessed January 7, 2014).

"Presidential Notes: Louisa Catherine Adams." http://www.essortment.com/presidential-notes-louisa-catherine-adams (accessed January 3, 2012).

Proceedings of the 60th Annual Meeting of the Massachusetts Homeopathic Medical Society. Boston, April 10–11, 1900.

"Puerperal Fever." Wikipedia, http://en.wikipedia.org/wiki/Puerperal_fever#Famous_Victims (accessed January 23, 2012).

Quaife, Milo Milton. *The Diary of James K. Polk During His Presidency.* Chicago: A.C. McClurg, 1910.

Randolph, J. *Life and Character of Philip Syng Physick.* Philadelphia: T.K. and P.G. Collins, 1839.

Rayback, Robert J. *Millard Fillmore: Biography of a President.* Newtown, CT: American Political Biography, 1998.

"Reagan, Nancy." Biography. National First Ladies' Library and Museum, http://www.firstladies.org/biographies/firstladies.aspx?biography=41 (accessed July 17, 2013).

Reagan, Nancy, with William Novak. *My Turn: The Memoirs of Nancy Reagan.* New York: Random House, 1989.

Reagan, Ronald. *The Reagan Diaries.* Edited by Douglas Brinkley. New York: HarperCollins, 2007.

Reeves, Thomas. *A Question of Character: A Life of John F. Kennedy.* New York: Free/Macmillan, 1991.

Remini, Robert. *John Quincy Adams.* New York: Henry Holt, 2002.

Riley, Valerie J., and John Spurlock. "Vesicovaginal Fistula." http://emedicine.medscape.com/article/267943-overview (accessed July 28, 2009).

Rixey, Presley Marion. "Guarding the Health of Our Presidents." *Better Health* (June 1925).

Roach, Mary. *Stiff: The Curious Lives of Human Cadavers.* New York: W.W. Norton, 2004.

Robar, Stephen F. *Frances Clara Folsom Cleveland.* New York: Nova History, 2002.

Robbins, Peggy. "President Tyler's First Ladies." *American History Illustrated* 18 (January 1984), 9.

Roberts, John B., II. *Rating the First Ladies.* New York: Citadel, 2003.

Robson, K.J. "Advances in Mammographic Imaging." *British Journal of Radiology* (2010): 83, 273–275

Rocco, Fiammetta. *The Miraculous Fever Tree.* Great Britain: HarperCollins, 2003.

Roos, Charles A. "Physicians to the Presidents, and Their Patients: A Bibliography." *Bulletin of the Medical Library Association* 49 (1961).

"Roosevelt, Alice Hathaway Lee." Theodore Roosevelt Center at Dickinson State University, http://www.theodorerooseveltcenter.org/Learn-About-TR/Themes (accessed December 18, 2013).

"Roosevelt, Edith Carow." Biography. National First Ladies' Library, http://www.firstladies.org/biographies/firstladies.aspx?biography=26 (accessed December 18, 2013).

Rosenkrantz, Barbara Gutman, ed. *From Consumption to Tuberculosis.* New York: Garland, 1994.

Ross, Ishbel. *The General's Wife: The Life of Mrs. Ulysses S. Grant.* New York: Dodd, Mead, 1959.

_____. *Grace Coolidge and Her Era.* Plymouth, VT: Calvin Coolidge Memorial Foundation, 1988.

Rothman, Sheila. *Living in the Shadow of Death: Tuberculosis and the Social Experience of Illness in American History.* New York: Basic, 1994.

Rothstein, William G. *American Physicians in the 19th Century: From Sects to Science.* Baltimore: Johns Hopkins University Press, 1985.

Rowland, Lewis P., ed. *Merritt's Textbook of Neurology*, 9th ed. Baltimore: Williams and Wilkins, 1995.

Ruffin, Sterling. *American Physicians and Surgeons in the United States and Canada.* Minneapolis: Midwest, 1931.

"Ruffin, Sterling." Obituary. *Medical Annals of the District of Columbia* 18 (1949).

"Ruffin, Sterling." Obituary. *Transactions of the American Clinical Climatological Association* 61 (1949): xlv-xlvi.

Russell, Francis. *The Shadow of Blooming Grove: Warren G. Harding in His Times.* New York: McGraw-Hill, 1968.

Russell, Jan Jarboe. *Lady Bird: A Biography of Mrs. Johnson.* New York: Scribner, 1999

Russell, Thomas R. "Remembering Oliver H. Beahrs." *Oncology Times* 28, no. 7 (April 10, 2006): 33–34.

Rutenberg, Jim. "The First Lady's Skin Cancer." The Caucus, http://thecaucus.blogs.nytimes.com/2006/12/19/the-first-ladys-skin-cancer (accessed August 31, 2013).

Rutkow, Ira M. "Philip Syng Physick." *Archives of Surgery* 136, no. 8 (August 2001), 968.

Sai-Ching, Jim Yeung. "Graves' Disease." Medscape. http://emedicine.medscape.com/article/120619-overview#a0199 (accessed January 7, 2014).

Sale, Sara L. *Bess Wallace Truman: Harry's White House "Boss."* Lawrence: University Press of Kansas, 2010.

Sandburg, Carl. *Abraham Lincoln: The Prairie Years and the War Years.* New York: Harcourt Brace Jovanovich, 1954.

Saunders, Francis Wright. *Ellen Axson Wilson: First Lady Between Two Worlds.* Chapel Hill: University of North Carolina Press, 1985.

Savitt, Todd L. *Fevers, Agues, and Cures: Medical Life in Old Virginia, an Exhibition.* Richmond: Virginia Historical Society, 1990.

_____, and James Harvey Young, eds. *Disease and Distinctiveness in the American South.* Knoxville: University of Tennessee Press, 1988.

"Sawyer, Carl." Obituary. *Journal of the American Medical Association* 196, no. 3 (June 27, 1966): 154.

"Sawyer, Carl." *Polk's Medical Registry and Directory*, 1917.

Scarry, Robert J. *Millard Fillmore.* Jefferson, NC: McFarland, 2001.

Schneider, Dorothy, and Carl Schneider. *First Ladies: A Biographical Dictionary.* New York: Facts on File, 2001.

Scott, Paula Spencer. "Nancy Reagan's Fall Wasn't Her First." http://www.caring.com/blogs/fyi-daily/nancy-reagans-fall-wasnt-her-first (accessed July 14, 2013).

Seager, Robert, II. *And Tyler Too: A Biography of John and Julia Gardiner Tyler.* New York: McGraw-Hill, 1963.

Severance, Frank H., ed. *Millard Fillmore Papers*, vol. 2. Buffalo: Buffalo Historical Society, 1907.

Severn, Bill. *Frontier President: The Life of James K. Polk.* New York: Ives Washburn, 1965.

Sewall, Thomas. *Examination of Phrenology.* Washington City: Honans, 1837.

Shaw, John. *Lucretia.* New York: Nova History, 2004.

Shepherd, Jack. *Cannibals of the Heart: A Personal Biography of Louisa Catherine and John Quincy Adams.* New York: McGraw-Hill, 1980.

Shultz, Suzanne. *Body Snatching: The Robbing of Graves for the Education of Physicians in Early Nineteenth Century America.* Jefferson, NC: McFarland, 1992.

Sievers, Harry J. *Benjamin Harrison: Hoosier President.* Newtown, CT: American Political Biography, 1996.

Sievers, Harry J., S.J. *Benjamin Harrison: Hoosier Statesman.* New York: University, 1959.

_____. *Benjamin Harrison: Hoosier Warrior.* Chicago: Henry Regnery, 1952.

Smith, Elbert B. *The Presidencies of Zachary Taylor and Millard Fillmore.* Lawrence: University Press of Kansas, 1988.

Smith, F.B. *The Retreat of Tuberculosis, 1850–1950.* London: Croom Helm, 1988.

Smith, Gene. *When the Cheering Stopped: The Last Years of Woodrow Wilson.* New York: William Morrow, 1964.

Smith, Jean Edward. *Grant.* New York: Simon & Schuster, 2001.

Smith, Sally Bedell. *Grace and Power: The Private World of the Kennedy White House.* New York: Random House, 2004.

"Smoking Tied to Miscarriage Risk." http://www.abs-cbnnews.com/lifestyle/01/01/11/smoking-tied-miscarriage (accessed April 22, 2013).

Smyth, Peter, PA. "Graves, Robert James, 1796–1853." Milestones in European Thyroidology. European Thyroid Association. http://www.eurothyroid.com/about/met/graves.php (accessed 9 June 2011).

Snyder, Howard. Incomplete manuscript on Dwight D. Eisenhower, 1946, p. 14.

Socolofsky, Homer E., and Allan B. Spetter. *The Presidency of Benjamin Harrison.* Lawrence: University Press of Kansas, 1987.

Sodeman A.C., J. Moller, et al. "Stress as a Trigger of Attacks in Menière's Disease." *Laryngoscope* 114, no. 10 (October 2004): 1843–8.

Sotos, John G. *The Physical Lincoln Sourcebook: An Annotated Medical History of Abraham Lincoln and His Family.* Mount Vernon, VA: Mount Vernon Book Systems, 2008.

Southern Journal of Homeopathy. Letter to the editor, May 11, 1896, p. 112.

"Stress Management Therapy for Menière's Disease." http:///www.clinical trails.gov/ct2/show/NCT01099046 (accessed March 19, 2013).

"Surgical Management of Strabismus," (chapter 1). History of Strabismus Surgery. http://www.cybersight.org/bins/volume_oage.asp?cid=1-2161–2252 (accessed February 20, 2013).

"Taft, Florence: Puerperal Eclampsia." *Proceedings of the Annual Session of the International Hahnemannian Association* (1895): 279–288.

"Taft, Helen." Biography: National First Ladies Museum. http://www.firstladies.org/biographies/firstladies.aspx?biography=27 (accessed November 20, 2013).

Taft, Helen Herron. *Recollections of Full Years.* New York: Dodd, Mead, 1914.

Taylor, George B. "The Inaugural Essay on Apoplexia of Apoplexy, Submitted to the Faculty of the University of Pennsylvania for the Degree of Doctor of Medicine." 1824.

Taylor, Lloyd C., Jr. "A Wife for Mr. Pierce." *New England Quarterly* 28, no. 3 (September 1955), 339–348.

"Taylor, Margaret." Biography. The First Ladies' National Library and Museum. http://www.firstladies.org/biographies/firstladies.aspx?biography+13 (accessed November 12, 2012).

Taylor, Robert. *Saranac: America's Magic Mountain.* Boston: Houghton Mifflin, 1986.

Teo, S.H., K.K. Teh, L. Azura and Yo Ng. "The Great Mimic Again? A Case of Tuberculosis Knee." *Malaysian Orthopedic Journal* 5, no. 3 (2011): 32.

"Thyroid Newsmakers: Barbara Bush." http://www.coulditbemythyroid.com/Book-Exprts/nsmaker-BBush.html (accessed April 18, 2011).

"Toxemia: Preeclampsia and Hypertension in Pregnancy." http://www.pregnancycrawler.com/toxemia.html (accessed June 8, 2012).

Transactions of the 44th Session of the American Institute of Homeopathy. Atlantic City, NJ, 1891.

Transactions of the 45th Session of the American Institute of Homeopathy. Washington, D.C., June 13–17, 1892.

Trefousse, Hans L. *Andrew Johnson: A Biography.* New York: W.W. Norton, 1989.

Trudeau, Edward Livingston. *An Autobiography.* New York: Lea and Febiger, 1915.

"Truman, Bess." Biography. National First Ladies' Library and Museum. http://www.firstladies.org/biographies/firstladies.aspx?biography=34 (accessed May 28, 2013).

Truman, Margaret. *Bess W. Truman.* New York: Macmillan, 1986.

_____. *First Ladies.* New York: Random House, 1995.

"Tuberculosis in the White House." *Medical Record* 42 (October 29, 1892).

"Tyler, Julia." Biography. National First Ladies' Library. http://www.firstladies.org/biographies/firstladies.aspx?biography=11 (accessed December 19, 2013).

"Tyler, Julia Gardner." American President: A Reference Resource. http://millercenter.org/president/tyler/essays/firstlady/julia (accessed April 2, 2013).

Tyler, Lyon G. *The Letters and Times of the Tylers*, vol. 1. Richmond, VA: Whittet & Shepperson, 1884.

_____. *The Letters and Times of the Tylers*, vol. 2. Richmond, VA: Whittet & Shepperson, 1885.

Unger, Harlow G. *The Last Founding Father: James Monroe and a Nation's Call to Greatness.* Philadelphia: Da Capo, 2009.

"Van Valzah." In *Directory of Deceased American Physicians, 1804–1929*, vol. 2, edited by Arthur Wayne Hafner, et al. Chicago: American Medical Association, 1993.

van Wyhe, John. *The History of Phrenology on the Web.* http://www.historyof phrenology.org.uk/overview.htm (accessed December 15, 2011).

Vasavada, Sandip P., and Raymond Rackley. "Vesicovaginal and Ureterovaginal Fistula." http://emedicine.medscape.com/article/452934-overview (accessed July 28, 2009).

Venzke, Jane Walter, and Craig Paul Venzke. "The

President's Wife, Jane Means Appleton Pierce: A Woman of Her Time." http://www.nhhistory. org/s/Revealing_Relationships_Presidents_ wife.pdf (accessed February 27, 2011).

Vikse, Bjorn Egil, Lorentz M. Irgens, et al.: "Preeclampsia and the Risk of End-Stage Renal Disease." *New England Journal of Medicine* 359 (2008): 800–9.

Waggoner, Ashley. "Sixth First Lady Louisa Adams: Accidental Social Activist." Suite101. com. http://ashley-waggoner.suite101.com/ sixth-first-lady-louisa-adams-a80524 (accessed January 3, 2012).

Walker, Jane C. *John Tyler: A President of Many Firsts.* Blacksburg, VA: McDonald and Woodward, 2001.

Wall, L. Lewis. "Thomas Addis Emmet, the Vesicovaginal Fistula, and the Origins of Reconstructive Gynecologic Surgery." *International Urogynecology Journal* 13 (2002): 145–155.

"Washington, Martha." Biography. National First Ladies' Museum. http://www.firstladies.org/ biographies/firstladies.aspx?biography=11.

Watson, Robert P. *First Ladies of the United States: A Biographical Dictionary.* Boulder, CO: Lynne Rienner, 2001.

_____. *The Presidents' Wives: Reassessing the Office of the First Lady.* Boulder, CO: Lynne Rienner, 2000.

Watson, Robert P., and Anthony J. Eksterowicz, eds. *The Presidential Companion: Readings on the First Ladies.* Columbia: University of South Carolina Press, 2003.

Weber, Peter C., and Warren Y. Adkins, Jr. "The Differential Diagnosis of Menière's Disease." *Otolaryngologic Clinics of North America* 30, no. 6 (December 1997): 977–986.

Weinstein, Edwin A. *Woodrow Wilson: A Medical and Psychological Biography.* Princeton, NJ: Princeton University Press, 1981.

Wharton, Anne Hollingsworth. *Martha Washington.* New York: Scribner's, 1899.

"What Is Menière's Disease? What Causes Menière's Disease?" Medical News Today. http://www.medicalnewstoday.com/articles/ 163888.php (accessed March 19, 2013).

Wijetunga, Mevan N., and Irwin J. Schatz. "Carotid Sinus Hypersensitivity." http:// emedicine.medscape.com/article/153312- overview (accessed 11 May 2010).

Wikander, Lawrence E., and Robert H. Ferrell, eds. *Grace Coolidge: An Autobiography.* Worland, WY: High Plains, 1992.

Wilson, Brenda J., M. Stuart Watson, et al. "Hypertensive Diseases of Pregnancy and Risk of Hypertension and Stroke in Later Life: Results from Cohort Study." *BMJ* 326 (2003): 845.

Wilson, Edith Bolling. *My Memoir.* Indianapolis: Bobbs-Merrill, 1938, 1939.

Withey, Lynne. *Dearest Friend: A Life of Abigail Adams.* New York: Simon & Schuster, 2002.

Wolf, Philip A., Ralph B. D'Agostino, et al. "Cigarette Smoking as a Risk Factor for Stroke." *Journal of the American Medical Association* 259, no. 7 (1988): 1025–1029.

Wood, Robert C. Robert C. Wood's Medical Officer's Files, National Archives and Records Administration.

Woodward, Bob, and Carl Bernstein. *The Final Days.* New York: Simon & Schuster, 1976.

Wootton, James E. *Elizabeth Kortright Monroe* (pamphlet). Charlottesville, VA: Ash Lawn-Highland, 1987.

"Yellow Fever Epidemic of 1793." Wikipedia. http://en.wikipedia.org/wiki/Yellow_Fever_ Epidemic_of_1793 (accessed October 9, 2011).

Young, Hugh. *Hugh Young: A Surgeon's Autobiography.* New York: Harcourt, Brace, 1940.

Young, Nancy Beck. *Lou Henry Hoover: Activist First Lady.* Lawrence: University Press of Kansas, 2004.

Zall, Paul. *Dolley Madison.* Huntington, NY: Nova History, 2001.

Newspaper Articles and Television

Altman, Lawrence. "Every Time Bush Says 'Ah,' Second Guessers of His Doctor Cry 'Aha.'" *New York Times*, 18 February 1992.

Amherst (NH) Farmer's Cabinet, April 9, 1841, vol. 39 no. 33, page 2.

"Amphetamines Used by a Physician to Lift Moods of Famous Patients," *New York Times*, December 4, 1972.

Anderson, Jack. "Kennedy's Most Pressing Date." *Los Angeles Times*, August 6, 1963, p. 6.

"Appointments by the President." *Baltimore Sun*, May 13, 1844.

"Appointments by the President," *The Madisonian*, May 4, 1841.

Associated Press. "List of Presidential Rankings," February 16, 2009.

"The Attempt at Assassination," *Washington National Intelligencer*, February 9, 1835.

"Barbara Bush Being Treated for Graves' Disease, a Thyroid Disorder," *Los Angeles Times*, March 30, 1989.

"Barbara Bush Hospitalized for Pneumonia in Texas," *New York Times*, December 31, 2013.

"Barbara Bush, Prescribing Mammograms," *Washington Post*, September 21, 1989

"Barbara Bush Says She Fought Depression in '76," *Washington Post*, May 20, 1990.

"Barbara Bush Says Thyroid Condition Caused Weight Loss," *New York Times*, March 30, 1989.

"Barbara Bush to Aid Group in Boston Speech

Planned for Thyroid Fund." *Boston Globe*, July 21, 1992.

"Bess Truman Home, Happy," *Los Angeles Times*, June 22, 1981.

"Bess Truman in Hospital," *Los Angeles Times*, November 22, 1978.

"Bess Truman Leaves Hospital," *New York Times*, December 18, 1978.

"Betty Ford, Former First Lady, Dies at 93," *New York Times*, July 8, 2011.

"Brief Illness Sidelines Mrs. Carter in Caracas," *Washington Post*, June 12, 1977.

Bryk, William. "Dr. Feelgood Past and Present." *New York Sun*, September 20, 2005. http://www.nysun.com/out-and-about/dr-feelgood/20251/ (accessed September 16, 2011).

"Bush's Physicians Say Thyroid Gland Disrupted Heart," *New York Times*, May 8, 1991.

"Calvin Coolidge Jr., Dies of Blood Poisoning." *Atlanta Constitution*, July 8, 1924.

"Calvin Coolidge Jr. Is Seriously Ill," *New York Times*, July 5, 1924.

"Capital Society Events," *Washington Post*, February 15, February 22, March 4, March 14, 1928.

"Care-Giving's First Lady," *Washington Post*, November 7, 1994.

"Columbian College in the District of Columbia." *American Mercury*, December 31, 1821.

"Condition of Coolidge Boy Is Unchanged, but Serious," *Washington Post*, July 5, 1924.

"Coolidges Depart for a Sunday Cruise," *New York Times*, July 20, 1924.

"Court Rules That First Lady Is 'De Facto' Federal Official," *New York Times*, June 23, 1993.

"Death Notices." *Baltimore Sun*, April 11, 1845.

"Death of White House Chatelaine Brings Gloom to Nation's Capital," *Washington Post*, August 7, 1914.

"Doctor Thomas Sewall." *Baltimore Sun*, March 24, 1845.

"Dr. Thomas Sewall," *New Hampshire Patriot and State Gazette*, April 17, 1845.

"Dr. W.W. Johnston's Funeral Tomorrow," *Washington Times*, March 23, 1902.

"Doctors Remove Benign Lump from Breast of Rosalynn Carter," *Toledo Blade*, April 29, 1977.

"Doctors Step Up Therapy Program for Mrs. Nixon," *Los Angeles Times*, July 14, 1976.

"The Doctor's World: A White House Puzzle: Immunity Ailments," *New York Times*, May 27, 1991.

Dwyer, Devin. "Barbara Bush May Be Released from Hospital." *ABC News*, March 30, 2010.

Dwyer, Devin, Ann Compton and Gina Sunseri. "Former First Lady Barbara Bush Had 'Mild Relapse' of Graves' Disease." *ABC News*, March 31, 2010.

"Ex-1st Lady OK After Hip Surgery," *Chicago Tribune*, May 8, 1981.

Face the Nation. CBS, December 24, 2006.

"Fear for Hillary Clinton as She Is Rushed to Hospital with Blood Clot Just Three Weeks After Suffering Concussion," *Daily Mail* (UK), December 31, 2012.

"First Lady Begins Radiation Treatment," *Washington Post*, January 4, 1990.

"First Lady Cancels Trip to Australia," *Los Angeles Times*, August 27, 2007.

"First Lady Heckled at Holy Sites in Jerusalem," *Los Angeles Times*, March 23, 2005.

"First Lady Laura Bush Had a Skin Cancer Tumor Removed from Her Right Shin," MSNBC, December 19, 2006.

"First Lady Laura Bush to Undergo Surgery for Pinched Nerves in Neck," *Fox News*, September 7, 2007.

"First Lady Makes Short Kabul Visit," *Los Angeles Times*, March 31, 2005.

"First Lady Marks First Year Since Cancer Surgery," *Los Angeles Times*, October 18, 1988.

"First Lady Quits Hospital Today," *New York Times*, August 13, 1963.

"First Lady Ready for Folksy Ways," *New York Times*, March 31, 1952.

"First Lady Sees Play in Guadalupe." *Arizona Republic*, June 17, 2006.

"First Lady Starts Radiation Therapy for Eyes," *New York Times*, January 4, 1990.

"First Lady Welcomed Home by Crowd, Jazz Combo," *Los Angeles Times*, October 23, 1987.

"First Lady Will Undergo Surgery," *Los Angeles Times*, September 8, 2007.

"First Lady's Health Is Whose Business?," *Chicago Tribune*, November 1, 1987.

"Form of Cortisone Prescribed for First Lady's Eye Ailment," *New York Times*, August 23, 1989.

"Frail Nancy Reagan Soldiers On," *National Enquirer*, March 4, 2013.

"Funeral for Coolidge's Son at 4 p.m. Today." *Chicago Daily Tribune*, July 9, 1924.

"General Delaney Dies; Physician to Taft," *Wilkes-Barre Record*, November 13, 1936.

Goldberg, Jonah. "The Irony of Michelle Obama's Water Campaign." *Los Angeles Times*, October 1, 2013.

"Good News—Twice for Harry Truman," United Press International, May 19, 1959.

"Grover's Baby." *Atlanta Constitution*, October 4, 1891.

"Harding's Widow Is Seriously Ill," *New York Times*, November 3, 1924.

"Herbert Hoover Jr. to Convalesce at Asheville," *The Lewiston Star*, October 16, 1930.

"Hillary Clinton Making 'Excellent Progress,' Doctors Say," *USA Today*, January 1, 2013.

"Hillary Clinton Recovering at Home Following Concussion Caused by Fall," *Guardian* (UK), December 15, 2012.

"If It Only Were a Boy!" *Chicago Daily Tribune*, October 4, 1891.

"Important Surgical Operation." *Baltimore Sun*, November 6, 1839.

"In Breast Cancer, Treatment Dilemma Persists," *Washington Post*, October 20, 1987.

The Indianapolis News, October 24, 25, 1892.

"Jack Jones: Pat Nixon's Doctors Optimistic," *Los Angeles Times*, July 9, 1976.

"Jacqueline and Baby 'Doing Fine,'" *Washington Post*, November 26, 1960.

"Jon Nordheimer: Doctors Say Mrs. Nixon Is Showing Improvement," *New York Times*, July 10, 1976.

"Kennedy Alters Schedule to Stay Close to New Son," *New York Times*, November 26, 1960.

"Kennedy Baby Dies at Boston Hospital; President at Hand," *New York Times*, August 9, 1963.

"Kennedy Reaches Ill Wife's Side," *Washington Post*, August 29, 1956.

"Kennedy Son Yawns, Gurgles at Baptism," *Los Angeles Times*, December 9, 1960.

"Kennedys Have Daughter," *Washington Post*, November 28, 1957.

"Lady Bird Johnson, 94, Dies; Eased a Path to Power," *New York Times*, July 12, 2007.

"Laura Bush Has Surgery for Pinched Nerve," *New York Times*, September 8, 2007.

"Laura Bush Says She First Thought Skin Cancer Was an Insect Bite," *USA Today*, December 24, 2006.

"Laura Bush: Skin Cancer 'No Big Deal,'" *Washington Post*, December 19, 2006.

"The Manic Lawrence," *Washington Globe*, February 4, 1835.

"Mastectomy Is Not the Only Choice," letter to the editor, *Chicago Tribune*, October 31, 1987.

"Mastectomy Seen as Extreme for Small Tumor," *New York Times*, October 18, 1987.

"Memorandum of the Particulars of a Conversation with R. Lawrence," *Connecticut Courant*, February 7, 1835.

"More Surgery Options Tied to Changing Medical Views," *Los Angeles Times*, October 17, 1987.

"More Women Seek X-Rays of Breasts," *New York Times*, November 1, 1987.

"Most Breast Lesions Not Malignant, Experts Say," *Chicago Tribune*, October 17, 1987.

"Mrs. Carter 'Just Fine' Following Minor Surgery," *Ellensburg Daily Record*, August 15, 1977.

"Mrs. Cleveland a Mother," *Washington Post*, October 4, 1891.

"Mrs. Eisenhower and a Rumor," *New York Times*, November 3, 1973.

"Mrs. Eisenhower Sick; May Miss Wedding," *New York Times*, December 20, 1968

"Mrs. Ford Faces a Breast Biopsy," *New York Times*, September 28, 1974.

"Mrs. Ford Is Reported Cancer-Free," *New York Times*, November 7, 1976.

"Mrs. Ford Ready to Leave Hospital," *New York Times*, October 11, 1974.

"Mrs. Ford Resumes Her Role as Hostess," *New York Times*, October 24, 1974.

"Mrs. Harding Back in Washington," *New York Times*, January 3, 1924.

"Mrs. Harding Dies After Long Fight," *New York Times*, November 22, 1924.

"Mrs. Harding Ill, but Not Seriously; Not a Breakdown, and She Will Be Out Soon," *New York Times*, September 7, 1922.

"Mrs. Harding Past Crisis of Illness," *New York Times*, September 12, 1922.

"Mrs. Harding Still in Critical State; Shows Slight Gain," *New York Times*, September 9, 1922.

"Mrs. Harding Worse; Recovery Not Sure; Specialists Called," *New York Times*, September 8, 1922.

"Mrs. Harrison's Illness," *Frank Leslie's Weekly*, September 29, 1892, p. 227.

"Mrs. Hoover Dies of Heart Attack," *New York Times*, January 8, 1944.

"Mrs. Kennedy Bears Son," *Chicago Daily Tribune*, November 25, 1960.

"Mrs. Kennedy Rests at Home," *Washington Post*, August 16, 1963.

"Mrs. Kennedy Told to Curb Her Activities," *Chicago Tribune*, August 14, 1963.

"Mrs. McKinley Dies in Canton Cottage," *New York Times*, May 27, 1907.

"Mrs. McKinley's Condition Is Reportedly Grave," *New York Times*, June 5, 1901.

"Mrs. McKinley's Life and Character," *Los Angeles Times*, June 14, 1901.

"Mrs. T. Roosevelt Dies at Oyster Bay," *New York Times*, October 1, 1948.

"Mrs. Taft Can't Meet Guests," *New York Times*, May 22, 1909.

"Mrs. Taft Ill Here, President with Her," *New York Times*, May 15, 1911.

"Mrs. Taft Still Ill; Not at Garden Party," *New York Times*, May 29, 1909.

"Mrs. Taft Still Improves" *New York Times*, May 20, 1909.

"Mrs. Taft Will Rest," *New York Times*, May 20, 1911.

"Mrs. Taft's Illness Due to Social Causes," *New York Times*, May 19, 1909.

"Mrs. Truman Has Operation; Tumor Removed from Left Breast," *Chicago Daily Tribune*, May 19, 1959.

"Mrs. Truman Home in 'Excellent' Condition," *Chicago Daily Tribune*, June 4, 1959.

"Mrs. Truman Retires with Nation's Esteem," *Los Angeles Times*, January 18, 1953.

"Mrs. Truman's Cheerfulness Reason Plain," *Los Angeles Times*, March 30, 1952.

"Mrs. W.H. Taft Dies; President's Widow," *New York Times*, May 22, 1943.

"Mrs. Wilson Dies in the White House," *Los Angeles Times*, August 7, 1914.

"Mrs. Wilson Dies in White House," *New York Times*, August 7, 1914.

"Mrs. Wilson Needs Rest," *New York Times*, June 21, 1913.

"Mrs. Wilson Won't Even Discuss Remarriage," *New York Times*, October 2, 1925.

"Nancy Reagan Defends Her Decision to Have Mastectomy," *New York Times*, March 5, 1988.

"Nancy Reagan Has Tumor Removed from Her Face," *New York Times*, August 30, 1990.

"Nancy Reagan Hospitalized with Broken Pelvis," *People*, October 15, 2008.

"Nancy Reagan Urges Breast Checkups," *Chicago Tribune*, October 21, 1987.

"The Nation: Bush Resumes Hyperspeed; Is He Up to It?," *New York Times*, June 2, 1991.

"The Nation: The Most Fear of Tumors," *Time*, October 7, 1974.

"New Attitudes Ushered In by Betty Ford," *New York Times*, October 17, 1987.

New Hampshire Gazette, March 10, 1834.

New York Daily Times, March 23, 1853.

New York Times, July 16, 1879.

New York Times, October 2, 1925.

New York Tribune, October 25, 1892.

"Newborn Kennedy Son Ill," *Chicago Tribune*, August 8, 1963.

"No Hope for Mrs. McKinley," *New York Times*, May 24, 1907.

"No Hope for Mrs. McKinley," *New York Times*, May 25, 1907.

"No Hope for Mrs. McKinley," *New York Times*, May 26, 1907

"Obama's NSA Plan to Pre-Empt Privacy Board," *USA Today*, January 9, 2014.

"Obituary," *Washington Intelligencer*, September 12–13, 1842.

"Obituary: John W. Walsh, 87, Kennedy Obstetrician," *New York Times*, November 25, 2000.

"Obituary of Dr. Franklin A. Gardner," *New York Times*, February 13, 1903.

"Obituary of Letitia Tyler." *Baltimore Sun*, September 14, 1842, page 4.

"Obituary of Letitia Tyler," *Washington Globe*, September 13, 1842.

"Off for Canton Home," *Washington Post*, July 6, 1901.

"Official Announcements: Bulletins from the Bedside." Associated Press to *Los Angeles Times*, May 17, 1901.

"Operate on Calvin, Jr.; Doctors Battle for Boy's Life," *Los Angeles Times*, July 6, 1924.

"Operation on President's Son Called Success: Father and Mother Spent Night at Hospital." *Atlanta Constitution*, July 6, 1924.

"Pat Leaves Hospital, Says She 'Feels Fine,'" *Los Angeles Times*, July 23, 1976.

"Pat Nixon, Former First Lady, Dies at 81," *New York Times*, June 23, 1993.

"Pat Nixon Returns Home After Stroke," *Los Angeles Times*, August 23, 1983.

"Pat Nixon Suffers Stroke, Spends 5 Days in Hospital," *Los Angeles Times*, August 22, 1983.

"Pat Reading 'That' on the Day of Stroke," *Chicago Tribune*, August 9, 1976.

"Perform Operation on Mrs. Harding," *New York Times*, November 8, 1924.

"President Is Well After Operation to Ease Prostate," *New York Times*, January 6, 1987.

"President's Son Is Seriously Ill; Foot Is Poisoned," *Atlanta Constitution*, July 5, 1924.

"Prognosis Good Even If Lesion Is Cancerous," *Washington Post*, October 17, 1987.

Radcliffe, Donnie. "Appreciation: Pat Nixon: Cloth Coat, Ironclad Devotion," *Washington Post*, June 23, 1993.

"Radiation Therapy Is Weighed for Mrs. Bush," *New York Times*, December 1, 1989.

"Robert B. Semple Jr.: A Stoic Pat Nixon Is Recalled by Aide," *New York Times*, August 14, 1976.

"Rosalynn Carter Has Benign Lump Taken from Breast," *New York Times*, April 28, 1977.

"Rosalynn Carter Reported 'Fine' After Surgery," *Washington Post*, August 16, 1977.

Safire, William. "Political Spouse," *New York Times*, June 24, 1993.

"2d Son Born to Kennedys; Has Lung Illness," *New York Times*, August 8, 1963.

"Senate Committee Names 3 Leading Physicians to Examine Fall for Them and Make a Report," *New York Times*, January 31, 1924.

"Services Today for President's Son," *New York Times*, July 9, 1924.

"Stable: Barbara Bush Learned After Two Hours of Tests," *Orlando Sentinel*, November 29, 1989.

"Standing by for Mrs. Nixon," editorial, *Chicago Tribune*, July 10, 1976.

"Stroke Hospitalizes Mrs. Truman," *Los Angeles Times*, September 28, 1981.

"Successful Neck Surgery for First Lady Laura Bush," *Fox News*, September 8, 2007.

"Teddy Roosevelt's Widow Dies at 87." *Chicago Daily Tribune*, October 1, 1948.

"Temperance Lecture on a Large Scale," *New Hampshire Sentinel*, December 29, 1841.

Tennessee Williams letter to the editor, *New York Times*, December 6, 1972.

"Therapy Expert Aids Mrs. Nixon," *Los Angeles Times*, July 15, 1976.

Trafford, Abigail. "Me, Bush and Graves' Disease: Many Thyroid Patients Face an Emotional Roller Coaster," *Washington Post*, May 26, 1991.

"Truman's Widow Bess Dead at 97," *Chicago Tribune*, October 19, 1982.

"2009 Historians Presidential Leadership Survey," C-SPAN, 2012.

"Van Valzah Renounces Allopathy," *New York Times*, November 29, 1882.

"What Laura Bush Can Teach You About Skin Cancer," *ABC News*, December 19, 2006.

"White House Defends Laura Bush's Decision Not to Disclose Skin Cancer Removal," *Fox News,* December 19, 2006.

"White House Stayed Quiet on Laura Bush Cancer Surgery," *Independent* (UK), December 20, 2006.

"Wife of Sen. Kennedy Loses Unborn Baby," *Chicago Daily Tribune*, August 24, 1956.

"World Briefing," *New York Times*, October 1, 2003.

Letters, Notes and Diaries

Axson, Ellen. Savannah, Georgia, to Ellen Axson Wilson, Bryn Mawr, Pennsylvania, April 1, 1887.

Axson, Stockton. Brooklyn, New York, to Ellen Axson Wilson, Princeton, New Jersey, November 7, 1897.

Brown, Louisa Hoyt. Gainesville, Georgia, to Ellen Axson Wilson, Bryn Mawr, Pennsylvania, November 20, 1885.

_____. Gainesville, Georgia, to Woodrow Wilson, Bryn Mawr, Pennsylvania, April 16, 17, 1886; March 16, 1887.

Churchville, Lida Holland. Washington, D.C., to the author, September 5, 2009.

Daugherty, Harry. To Florence Harding, February 16, 1923.

Davis, Edward P. Philadelphia, to Dr. Cary T. Grayson, Washington, D.C., July 22, 1913; February 12, 1914; February 24, 1914.

_____. Philadelphia, to Dr. Cary T. Grayson, the White House, April 7, 1914; May 16, 1914.

Dimmick, Mary Lord. Diary entries, May 20, 1892. Benjamin Harrison Home.

_____. Indianapolis, to Mrs. Putzi, September 23, 1891. Benjamin Harrison Home.

_____. Loon Lake, New York, to May Saunders Harrison, Cape May, New Jersey, July 28, 1892.

Eisenhower, Dwight D. Versailles, France, to Mamie Eisenhower, Washington, D.C., September 23, 1944.

Erwin, Beth. To Ellen Axson Wilson, Bryn Mawr, Pennsylvania, December 27, 1885.

Fillmore, Millard. Buffalo, New York, to Julia, his sister, April 12, 1953. Buffalo and Erie County Historical Society.

_____. Note: "Funeral Expenses of Mrs. F at Washington," April 17, 1853. Special Collections, Penfield Library, SUNY Oswego.

_____. Washington, D.C., to Franklin Pierce, Washington, D.C., March 28, 1853. Special Collections, Penfield Library, State University of New York at Oswego.

Gardner, Franklin A. Letters to Benjamin Harrison, September 5, 1898; January 15, 22, 1899. Library of Congress Benjamin Harrison collection.

Gardner, Mrs. Franklin. Notes to Benjamin Harrison, March 18, 1892; April 1, 1892.

Grayson, Cary. Letter to Colonel Edward House, August 20, 1914. House Papers.

Hardin, B.L. To Florence Harding, December 11, 1922.

_____. To Florence Harding, undated.

Harding, Florence. To Evalyn McLean, February 5, 1923.

Harrison, Benjamin. Indianapolis, to Dr. F.E. Doughty, New York, November 10, 1897; June 3, 1898.

_____. Indianapolis, to Dr. E.L. Trudeau, Saranac Lake, New York, March 22, 1899. Library of Congress Benjamin Harrison Collection.

_____. To Russell Harrison, October 11, 1892. Library of Congress, Benjamin Harrison Collection.

_____. United States Senate, to Dr. Thomas A. Emmet, New York, June 13, 1883.

_____. United States Senate, to his cousin Maggie, February 12, 1883.

Howe, George. To Ellen Axson Wilson, Gainesville, Georgia, May 2, 1886.

Hoyt, Mary E. Rome, Georgia, to Ellen A. Wilson, Bryn Mawr, Pennsylvania, October 9, 1885; November 7, 1885, December 13, 1885, February 23, 1887; March 13, 1887.

_____. Rome, Georgia, to Woodrow Wilson, Bryn Mawr, Pennsylvania, November 10, 1885; August 30, 1887.

Monroe, James. Albemarle County, Virginia, to Charles Everett, Albemarle County, Virginia, January 13, 1810.

_____. Albemarle County, Virginia, to Charles Everett, Albemarle County, Virginia, July 1, 1820. *Tyler's Historical Quarterly* 5: 18. New York: Kraus Reprint, 1967.

_____. Albemarle County, Virginia, to Charles Everett, Albemarle County, Virginia, July 9, 1820.

_____. Albemarle County, Virginia, to Elizabeth Trist, Albemarle County, Virginia, March 6, 1810.

_____. Oak Hill, Virginia, to James Madison, Montpelier, Virginia, March 20, 1829.

_____. Oak Hill, Virginia, to Samuel Gouverneur, New York, New York, February 24, 1826.

_____. Oak Hill, Virginia, to Samuel Gouverneur, New York, New York, December 29, 1826. James Monroe Papers, Manuscripts and Archives Division, New York Public Library.

_____. Oak Hill, Virginia, to Samuel Gouverneur, New York, New York, September 23, 1830. James Monroe Papers, Manuscripts and Archives Division, New York Public Library.

_____. Washington, D.C., to Charles Everett, July 6, 1824.

_____. Washington, D.C., to Charles Everett, Albemarle County, Virginia, November 13, 1823. *Tyler's Historical Quarterly* 5: 21. New York: Kraus Reprint, 1967.

_____. Washington, D.C., to Charles Everett, September 1, 1824. *Tyler's Historical Quarterly* 5: 23. New York: Kraus Reprint, 1967.

_____. Washington, D.C., to Dr. Charles Everett, Richmond, Virginia, December 2, 1822. *Tyler's Historical Quarterly* 5: 18. New York: Kraus Reprint, 1967.

Pierce, Jane. To her deceased son Bennie, January 23, 1853. New Hampshire Historical Society Manuscript, Franklin Pierce Papers, accession no. 1929–001.

Scott, John. To Henry Scott, May 3, 1858. Benjamin Harrison Home.

Taft, William. To Helen Herron Taft, October 31, 1909. Physicians in William Howard Taft's Life. http:///www.apneos.com/physicians.html (accessed September 8, 2012).

_____. To Robert Taft, May 18, 1909. Physicians in William Howard Taft's Life. http:///www.apneos.com/physicians.html (accessed September 8, 2012).

Taylor, (Colonel) James, M.D. To General Howard Snyder, M.D., October 27, 1950.

Tyler, Letitia. To Mary Tyler Jones, March 25, 1836. Library of Congress, John Tyler Collection.

Wilson, Woodrow. To Mary Allen Hulbert, June 21, 1914.

_____. To Alfred P. Wilson, July 23, 1914.

_____. To E.P. Davis, July 26, 1914.

_____. To J.R. Wilson, August 6, 1914.

Young, Hugh. Baltimore, to Joel Boone, Washington, D.C., April 18, 1928. Library of Congress, Joel Boone Papers.

Interviews by the Author

Anthony, Carl. E-mail July 28, 2013.

Calhoun, Charles W. E-mail, March 27, 2012.

Capps, Jennifer. E-mail, March 30, 2012.

Cole, Tiffany. James Madison's Montpelier, e-mail November 8, 2011.

Davidson, Jonathan. E-mail, April 18, 2012.

Eisenhower, Julie Nixon. E-mail, May 31, 2010.

Ellis, Joseph. Telephone, December 3, 2011.

Husu, Emanuel. E-mail, September 22, 2013.

Lein, Howard. E-mail, November 18, 2009.

Levenson, Alan. E-mails, April 15, 2011; April 18, 2012; August 10, 2011.

Mariano, Connie. E-mail, July 1, 2013.

Miller, Kristie. E-mail, March 7, 2013.

Miller, Nancy R. University of Pennsylvania Archives and Records Center. E-mail February 4, 2005.

Patterson, Nancy Hord. Telephone, June 13, 2011.

Schermer, Craig. E-mail, September 6, 2008.

Smith, Hugh. Personal, April 19, 2013.

Tubb, Richard. Personal, August 13, 2011.

Tyler, Harrison. Telephone, July 3, 2009.

Index